THE OPIATE NARCOTICS
Neurochemical Mechanisms in
Analgesia and Dependence

THE OPIATE NARCOTICS
Neurochemical Mechanisms in Analgesia and Dependence

The International Narcotic Research Club Conference
May 21-24, 1975
Airlie House, Virginia

Executive Committee, INRC

Avram Goldstein (Secretary)
*Department of Pharmacology, Stanford University and
Addiction Research Foundation
Palo Alto, California, U.S.A.*

Sydney Archer
*Department of Chemistry
Renssalaer Polytechnic Institute
Troy, New York, U.S.A.*

H. O. J. Collier
*Research Department
Miles Laboratories, Ltd.
Slough S. L. 24LY, England*

A. Herz
*Max-Planck-Institut für Psychiatrie
Deutsche Forschungsanstalt für Psychiatrie
Munich, Germany*

H. W. Kosterlitz
*Unit for Research on Addictive Drugs
Marischal College
Aberdeen, Scotland*

H. Takagi
*Department of Pharmacology
Kyoto University
Kyoto, Japan*

Julian E. Villarreal
*Department of Behavioral Pharmacology
Laboratorios Miles de Mexico
Mexico, 22, D.F.*

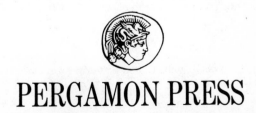

PERGAMON PRESS

New York / Toronto / Oxford / Sydney / Braunschweig

PERGAMON PRESS INC.
Maxwell House, Fairview Park, Elmsford, N.Y. 10523

PERGAMON OF CANADA LTD.
207 Queen's Quay West, Toronto 117, Ontario

PERGAMON PRESS LTD.
Headington Hill Hall, Oxford

PERGAMON PRESS (AUST.) PTY. LTD.
Rushcutters Bay, Sydney, N.S.W.

PERGAMON GmbH
D - 3300 Braunschweig, Burgplatz 1

Library of Congress Cataloging in Publication Data

International Narcotic Research Club.
The opiate narcotics.

1. Opiate habit — Congresses.
2. Opium — Physiological effect — Congresses.
I. Goldstein, Avram. II. Title.
RC568.06I57 1975 615'.782 75-15864
ISBN 0-08-019869-4
Simultaneous Publication with *Life Sciences*
Vol. 16, No. 12 and Vol. 17, No. 1

Printed in the United States of America
by Shandling Lithographing Co., Inc./602 W. Rillito St., Tucson, Arizona 85705

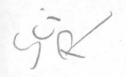

Preface

The systematic accumulation of knowledge in a particular field of science is sometimes punctuated by periods of very rapid, almost explosive progress. Research on the opiate narcotics appears to be in such a phase right now. To truly understand the action of any drug, one has to comprehend the several steps in a connected chain of events: the interaction of the drug with its specific receptor, the immediate biochemical consequence of that interaction, the resultant alteration of physiologic function, and finally how that produces what we recognize as the pharmacologic effect of the drug in an experimental animal or in man. Rapid strides are now being made in understanding all these steps in the actions of the opiate narcotics.

The **International Narcotic Research Club** is a very informal association of investigators who have been meeting approximately annually for exchange of current research information in this field. At our previous conferences in San Francisco (1972), Chapel Hill (1973), and Cocoyoc, Mexico (1974) it has been the policy not to publish anything, in order to preserve the atmosphere of informality and to encourage free speculation. The recent rapid advances alluded to in the previous paragraph, however, led us to believe that publication of the proceedings of the 1975 conference would be useful. In order to achieve very rapid publication — the only kind that is worthwhile in a fast-moving field of research — we asked all authors to bring camera-ready manuscripts to the conference. Accordingly, although the proceedings are in a sense pre-edited by the invitations extended to the various speakers, the publication itself has not been edited except with respect to minor matters of format. Authors bear sole responsibility for their contributions to this volume.

On behalf of the International Narcotic Research Club I express appreciation to all the participants, to Dr. B. B. Brodie, and to Susan Brandes of *Life Sciences,* to Mr. Robert Miranda of Pergamon Press; to the National Institute on Drug Abuse for generous travel grants used especially to facilitate the attendance of young scientists; and to Barbara Judson, who was responsible for coordinating all aspects of the conference and the publication.

Avram Goldstein

Palo Alto, California
May 1975

Contents

III. Cyclic Nucleotides and Mechanism of Opiate Action

IV. Effects of Opiates on Neurotransmitters and Neuromodulators

V. Effects of Opiates on Single Neurons

VI. Hypotheses on Neurochemical Mechanisms of Opiate Action in Analgesia

VII. Conference Summation

PURIFICATION AND PROPERTIES OF ENKEPHALIN - THE POSSIBLE ENDOGENOUS LIGAND FOR THE MORPHINE RECEPTOR[1]

John Hughes, Terry Smith, Barry Morgan[2] and Linda Fothergill[3]

Unit for Research on Addictive Drugs, University of Aberdeen,
Marischal College, Aberdeen, AB9 1AS, Scotland

(Received in final form May 24, 1975)

The purification and properties of a
peptide of low molecular weight (800-1200)
which has been extracted from the pig brain
is described.   This substance acts as an
agonist at opiate receptor sites.   It is
suggested that the peptide may have a wide
neurophysiological role in the brain and
possibly in other tissues.

There is mounting evidence that the brain contains an endogenous constituent which acts as an agonist at morphine receptor sites (1,2,3).
This substance, which we have termed enkephalin, loses its biological activity
on incubation with carboxypeptidase-A and leucine aminopeptidase, and appears
to be a low molecular weight peptide (1000).   We believe that enkephalin may
bear a similar relationship to morphine as acetylcholine does to muscarine or
nicotine.   The purification and study of the pure compound has now been
achieved.

[1]This study was supported by grants from the United States National Institute
on Drug Abuse (DA 00662) and from the U.K. Medical Research Council to H. W.
Kosterlitz.

[2]Present address: Pharmaceutical Division, Reckitt and Colman, Dansom Lane,
Hull.

[3]Department of Biochemistry, University of Aberdeen.

[4]We are most grateful for supplies of pig brains from MacIntosh & Co. and
Lawsons of Aberdeen, and from Burroughs Wellcome Laboratories, Kent.

Isolation of Enkephalin

Biological assays were carried out on the mouse vas deferens as previous-
described (3,4). A specific action at the morphine receptor was assumed if
the depression of the neurally evoked contractions was antagonised by naloxone
or by diallylnormorphinium iodide. The specificity of this test has been
discussed by Hughes (3). The quantitative estimation of enkephalin in a
sample was obtained by bracket assay with normorphine and the biological
activity expressed as μg-equivalents of normorphine.

The purification procedure is outlined in Table 1. Pig brains[4] were
extracted with 5 ml/g acetone as previously described (3); this yielded 0.3-
0.5 μg equivalents per kg of whole brain. Stages 1-3 yielded material
suitable for high efficiency liquid chromatography. Complete correspondence
between the biological activity and UV absorption at 280 nm was not obtained
until the final Sephadex G-15 step (Fig. 1). Gel chromatography was
particularly useful since adsorptive mechanisms as well as gel penetration
appear to operate during this separation as evidenced by the high partition
coefficient (K_d = 1.3). The overall recovery from all the steps averaged
50-55%, the ion exchange steps averaged 85% recovery and the gel filtration
95%. Siliconised glassware was exclusively used in the latter isolation
stages. The final freeze dried extract was a white amorphous powder.

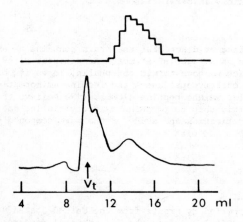

FIG. 1

Sephadex G-15 chromatography of enkephalin. The column
(100 x 0.4 cm) was developed with 1M acetic acid (0.2 ml/
min). Upper trace: biological activity on mouse vas
deferens. Lower trace: UV absorption at 280 nm. Vt =
salt peak corresponding to total liquid column volume.
Enkephalin eluted between 12-16 ml effluent volume.

TABLE 1

ISOLATION OF ENKEPHALIN

1. Acetone extraction, extraction of dried extract with MeOH to dissolve enkephalin and precipitate protein and salt. Transfer to aqueous phase and extract lipids with ether/ethyl acetate at pH 3.

2. Batch absorption on Dowex-50-H[+] at pH 3, wash with 0.1M NH₄ acetate pH 5.5 and elute with 0.2M NH₄ OH.

3. Batch absorption on Amberlite CG400-Formate at pH 8, wash with 0.1M NH₄ formate pH 6.8, elute with 0.1M formic acid.

4. Freeze dried sample absorbed on 20 x 1 cm Aminex-A5-NH₄[+] column at pH 3. Elution with 0.3M NH₄ formate pH 7.4 at 1 ml/min. Enkephalin emerges over fractions 80-95 ml.

5. Freeze dried sample dissolved in 1M acetic acid. Gel chromatography on 100 x 1 cm Sephadex G-15 column with 1M acetic acid. Activity recovered in fractions 75-90 ml corresponding to a K_d of 1.3.

6. Freeze dried sample dissolved in 0.07M NH₄ formate, injected onto 100 x 0.4 cm AE-SAX Pellionex[1] pellicular anion exchange column. Isocratic elution (1 ml/min) with 0.07M NH₄ formate in 25% MeOH. Enkephalin mainly elutes in fraction 10-18 ml but with considerable tailing.

7. Freeze dried sample rechromatographed on 100 x 0.4 cm Sephadex G-15 column with 1M acetic acid.

[1]Reeve Angel Chromatography Products.

Chemical Properties and Electrophoresis

Spot tests were made with 10-12 μg-equivalents on Whatman No. 1 paper. A pink spot was obtained with cadmium ninhydrin reagent and a positive chlorine reaction was seen with the Royden-Smith test for NH-groups. Ehrlich's reagent gave a blue-grey colour which differed from the normal purple for tryptophan. Spectrophotofluorometric analysis in aqueous solution showed one emission peak at 360 nm at an excitation wavelength of 275 nm (uncorrected spectra).

High voltage paper electrophoresis at 2.5-3 Kv was carried out at pH 2, 3.5 and 6.5, only one positive ninhydrin or chlorine spot was seen in each case. Parallel runs without staining showed that the biological activity corresponded to the ninhydrin/chlorine spot and could not be detected elsewhere on the paper. Enkephalin ran just behind aspartic acid at pH 2 and with valine at pH 6.5. Assuming a charge of 1 the electrophoretic mobility at pH 2 indicates a Mol. Wt. of around 800 according to the method of Offord (5). This conclusion however would be negated if substituted or unusual amino acids are present in the peptide.

Amino acid analysis after 6M HCl hydrolysis revealed the presence of glycine, methionine, phenylalanine and tyrosine with no basic amino acids. A tentative estimation of molar ratios indicates 3 gly, 1 phe, 1 met, 1 tyr with the probability of tryptophan or a derivative in unknown amounts. This gives a minimum Mol. Wt. of 924 which is in agreement with the electrophoretic

and gel filtration measurements.   The high content of aromatic amino acids
would also explain the strong absorption effects displayed by enkephalin.

Pharmacology

Neurally evoked contractions of the mouse vas deferens and guinea-pig
myenteric plexus are inhibited by enkephalin.   Rabbit and guinea-pig vasa
deferentia do not possess morphine receptors and these tissues are unaffected
by enkephalin.   The potency of enkephalin in the guinea-pig myenteric plexus
relative to normorphine was only 10-15% of that in the mouse vas deferens and
this has been attributed to enzymatic destruction (3).   Enkephalin showed no
antagonist action towards normorphine, mixtures of the two compounds gave
additive effects consistent with their effects when given singly.

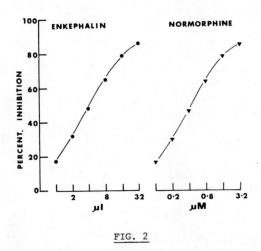

FIG. 2

Dose response curves for enkephalin and normorphine in the
mouse vas deferens.   Points are the means of 5 parallel
experiments, the standard error of each point was between
4-8%.

Dose response curves for normorphine and enkephalin are parallel in the
mouse vas deferens (Fig. 2) consistent with a common site of action.   The
actions of both normorphine and enkephalin were abolished by the narcotic
antagonists naloxone, naltrexone, N-diallylnormorphinium iodide and (±)
MR 1305[1].   Detailed studies were made on the interaction between naloxone and
enkephalin.   In parallel experiments full dose response curves to enkephalin
and normorphine were obtained in duplicate in the absence and in the presence
of naloxone.   The pA_2 values were derived from linear regression analysis of
the plot of (log dose ratio -1) v naloxone concentration.   In five
experiments the pA_2 for naloxone v normorphine was 8.60 ± 0.06 (slope =
0.98 ± 0.03, r = 0.995), whilst with enkephalin the pA_2 was 7.89 ± 0.06
(slope = 0.78 ± 0.02, r = 0.993).   The difference in the pA_2 values was
highly significant (p < 0.001).   There was a parallel shift in the enkephalin
dose response curves with naloxone and no depression of the maximum response
up to dose ratios of 30, higher dose ratios could not be obtained because of
the limited amounts available.   Quantitative studies on other antagonists are
not yet completed but similar results to naloxone are apparent in that
significantly more antagonist is required against enkephalin than normorphine;

4

this effect is particularly noticeable with weak antagonists such as N-diallylnormorphinium iodide. The implications of these results is discussed more fully by Kosterlitz and Hughes elsewhere in this volume.

It has been shown that the laevo (-) isomers MR 1452[1] and GPA 1843[2] are 20-50 times more potent narcotic antagonists than their corresponding dextro (+) isomers MR 1453 and GPA 1847 (6). Complete antagonism of enkephalin was seen with GPA 1843 at 0.2 μM, whereas GPA 1847 had no effect at 2 μM and only completely antagonised enkephalin at 18-54 μM (Fig. 3). Similarly the (-) isomer MR 1452 was at least twenty times more active against enkephalin than the (+) isomer MR 1453. These results indicate a stereospecific interaction between these antagonists and enkephalin.

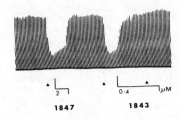

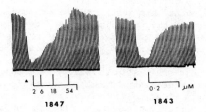

FIG. 3

Stereoselective antagonism of enkephalin in the mouse vas deferens. The triangles mark injections of enkephalin. In the first experiment (upper panel) a rapid reversal was obtained with the (-)-isomer GPA 1843 (0.4 μM) whereas the (+)-isomer had little effect at 2.0 μM. Note that a further injection of enkephalin was without effect in the continued presence of GPA 1843.

In the second experiment (lower panel) the (+)-isomer only completely reversed the effect of enkephalin at 54 μM. The (-)-isomer effected complete reversal at 0.2 μM.

Enkephalin has been found in the brains of pig, cow, guinea-pig, rabbit, rat and mouse. The brain distribution is uneven (3) with the greatest amounts occurring in areas known to be rich in morphine receptor binding sites (7). No activity was detected in rabbit or guinea-pig lung, liver or kidney, nor in the rat ileum. However, appreciable amounts were detected in the guinea-pig ileum (0.8 μg-equivalent per g).

---

[1] α-(3-furylmethyl)-5,9-dimethyl-2'-hydroxy-6,7-benzomorphan.
[2] 2-allyl-5-phenyl-9-methyl-2'-hydroxybenzomorphan.

Discussion

Enkephalin appears to be a unique peptide with specific activity at morphine sensitive neuroeffector junctions. The peptide has a Mol. Wt. in the 800-1200 range and contains a high proportion of glycine and aromatic amino acids and is unlike any other peptide so far described in the brain. Both a primary amino N-group and carboxy C-group appear to be present. The amino acid sequence determination is still in progress. At present we cannot be certain that there is just one single peptide with opiate receptor affinity and comparative studies will be particularly interesting in this respect.

The evidence for a specific action at opiate receptor sites is substantial. The peptide is selectively active on those tissues known to possess opiate receptor sites and its action is prevented by a wide range of narcotic antagonists. Stereospecificity of narcotic antagonist action is evident from the differential activity of (+) and (-) isomers against enkephalin. Other workers (1,2) have shown that a substance similar to ours binds stereo-specifically to opiate receptors and we have also shown a similar stereo-specific binding of enkephalin to opiate receptors in the guinea-pig brain (Hughes, Kosterlitz and Smokcum, unpublished results). It is possible that the kinetics of the interaction of enkephalin with the opiate receptor may not be identical to that of morphine and its congeners, but further studies with purified and synthetic material are needed to confirm this.

Enkephalin is rapidly destroyed by tissue extracts and by carboxypepti-dase-A. Attempts to prevent this destruction in the guinea-pig ileum have been unsuccessful so far and this has limited our investigations in this tissue. The development of an effective means of preventing this inactiva-tion should greatly advance our knowledge of the role of enkephalin.

It seems unlikely that enkephalin is solely concerned with the modulation of pain perception. Its wide distribution in the brain and presence in the guinea-pig ileum suggest a wider neurochemical role. We do not know yet whether enkephalin is invariably present in tissues containing opiate recep-tors although we have so far failed to detect it in the rat heart which does possess opiate receptors. It will be important to investigate other sites such as the mouse vas deferens and cat nictitating membrane. However, the problem of detecting very small quantities of the peptide have yet to be overcome.

References

1. L. TERENIUS and A. WAHLSTRÖM, Acta pharmac. tox. 35, Suppl. 1, 55 (1974)
2. J. HUGHES, Neurosciences Res. Prog. Bull. 13 (1), 55-58 (1975)
3. J. HUGHES, Brain Research 88, 295-308 (1975)
4. J. HUGHES, H. W. KOSTERLITZ and F. M. LESLIE, Br. J. Pharmac. 53, 371-381 (1975)
5. R. E. OFFORD, Nature 211, 591-593 (1966)
6. H. W. KOSTERLITZ and A. A. WATERFIELD, Ann. Rev. Pharmac. 15, 29-47 (1975)
7. M. J. KUHAR, C. B. PERT and S. H. SNYDER, Nature 245, 447-450 (1973)

MORPHINE-LIKE LIGAND FOR OPIATE RECEPTORS IN HUMAN CSF

Lars Terenius and Agneta Wahlström

Department of Medical Pharmacology, University of Uppsala, Uppsala, Sweden.

(Received in final form May 24, 1975)

Human CSF was fractionated chromatographically and tested for affinity to opiate receptors in synaptic plasma membrane preparations from rat brain. A unique fraction of an apparent molecular weight of 1000 to 1200 dalton, probably identical with that previously found by us in brain extracts, showed affinity. Since the active factor behaved similar to morphinomimetic analgesics in its interaction with the receptors and not like the narcotic antagonist naltrexone, it is termed MLF (morphine-like factor). The level of MLF varied between different individuals and was apparently lower in patients with trigeminal neuralgia than in other patients.

The opiate receptors are functionally specific, i.e., only narcotic analgesics and corresponding antagonists have a considerable affinity for the receptors, while a large number of neurotransmitters and other neuroactive agents lack affinity. We have earlier suggested that it is unlikely that an opiate receptor which mediates a physiologically important effect, should exist unless there is an endogenous ligand for this receptor. Results so far obtained (1,2) also point to the presence of at least one such principle in extracts of rat, rabbit and calf brain. Since this factor interacts with opiate receptors more like a morphinomimetic agent than like the antagonists naloxone or naltrexone, it is called MLF (morphine-like factor) for short.

We have earlier briefly reported that a similar factor is present also in human CSF (1). A detailed presentation of these findings is given below.

Material and Methods

Dihydromorphine (DHM), labelled with tritium by catalytic hydrogenation of morphine, at a specific activity of 59 or 76 Ci/mmole was obtained from New England Nuclear Corp., Boston, Mass., and from the Radiochemical Centre, Amersham, England, respectively. Naltrexone-15,16-^{3}H of 16 Ci/mmole was supplied through the courtesy of Dr. R.W. Willette, NIDA, Rockville, Md.

Nonlabelled drugs were from usual sources. Buffers were made out of reagent grade chemicals and bidistilled water.

Most tests on receptor affinity were run in a near-physiological buffer of the following composition: NaCl 124 mM, KCl 5 mM, KH_2PO_4 1.2 mM, $CaCl_2$ 0.75 mM, N-2-hydroxyethylpiperazine-N'-2-ethanesulfonic acid "HEPES" 26 mM. It was adjusted to pH 7.4 at 25°C. In a few cases, incubations were run in 50 mM Tris, pH 7.4 at 25°C, eventually supplemented with 100 mM NaCl.

Receptor preparations from synaptic plasma membranes of rat brains were obtained as described earlier (3). The receptor preparations were obtained on a large scale basis and aliquotes were stored at -70°C for up to 6 months with maintenance of receptor content.

The patients were being treated surgically at the Neurosurgical Clinic of the University Hospital, Uppsala. No patient except one, had any known previous history of opiate medication. The exception, patient K.T. was given 5 mg pethidine, i.m., in a single dose as premedication for operation.

The CSF (10-30 ml) was drawn from the lumbar region or from the ventricle (patient H.P.), stored on ice and ultrafiltered through an Amicon P10 filter (nominal cut-off 10,000 dalton) within 1-2 hours and it was then kept frozen at -20°C until subjected to chromatography. In a few cases, CSF aliquots were heated for 20 min at 70°C prior to ultrafiltration.

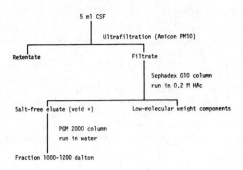

FIG. 1.

Fractionation scheme.

The chemical processing of the ultrafiltrate is shown in Fig. 1. The ultrafiltrate was run through a Sephadex G10 (Pharmacia, Uppsala, Sweden) column of 46 x 2.0 cm, eluted in 0.2 M HAc. The flow rate was 1 ml/min and the eluate ahead of the inorganic salts was collected. This eluate was lyophilized and redissolved in 1 ml of water. It was chromatographed on a PGM 2000 column of the following characteristics: dimensions 90 x 1.0 cm; sample load 1 ml; elution by water at 29 ml/h, 2.9 ml per fraction. This column was previously calibrated with peptides of known molecular weight. The receptor active fraction, at 1000-1200 dalton apparent molecular weight, was collected and lyophilized.

The fractions were tested for receptor affinity in a previously described procedure (3). The fractions were made up in HEPES-buffer and tested against labelled DHM of 0.8×10^{-9} M with synaptic plasma membrane (SPM) fraction of rat brain. Incubation at 25°C for 40 min was followed by centrifugation in the cold for 10 min. The SPM pellet was obtained by cutting the tips of the tubes which were digested by Soluene (Packard, LaGrange, Ill.). To the digests, 5 ml of scintillation cocktail was added and the tritium content was measured. Each experimental run included samples with no added fraction (controls) and those with 10^{-6} M nonlabelled DHM (carrier). The carrier values represent nonspecific (unsaturable) binding and were substracted from all experimental values. Receptor blocking activity was then expressed in percent of the corrected control value.

Definition: 1 relative unit in the receptor blocking assay will reduce the specific binding in 0.4 ml buffer under the above conditions by 50%. The amount of MLF is calculated from a log concentration-inhibition curve (2).

Testing of receptor blocking activity against tritium-labelled naltrexone followed the general procedure outlined above, except that the carrier samples

8

contained a lower concentration, 10^{-7}M, of nonlabelled material (=naltrexone).

The presence of inorganic salts was monitored by measuring Na$^+$ with an Eppendorf flame photometer. Assays for primary amines with fluorescamine (Fluram, Roche) were carried out at pH 8.1 (4). A standard curve with leucine was always run in parallel.

Results

The ultrafiltrate of CSF was desalted by passage through a Sephadex G10 column in 0.2 M acetic acid. The eluate ahead of the inorganic salts was collected. The salt concentration in the collected eluate was below detection levels. It was checked that MLF of brain extracts (2) was eluted in the same fraction. The collected eluate was freeze-dried and subjected to molecular sieving on the calibrated PGM 2000 column. The eluate from the column was continuously monitored for UV absorbance at 254 nm, for fluorescamine positive reaction (i.e., presence of primary amine groups) and for receptor affinity. The biologically active material occurred in a fraction of a calibrated m.w. 1000-1200 dalton. The peak of maximum receptor blocking affinity seemed to coincide with a UV peak. Considerable amounts of fluorescamine-reactive material was also present (Fig. 2). In a few cases, enough CSF was available to allow further fractiona-

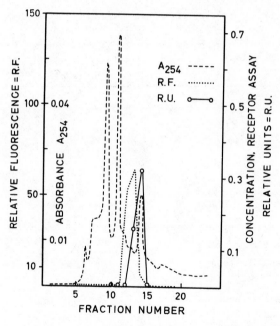

FIG. 2

Elution profile of prefractionated CSF sample on a PGM column in terms of UV absorption, fluorescence after reaction with fluorescamine, which reacts with primary amine groups, and receptor blocking activity. The units for receptor blockade are defined in Methods. The sample load was 1 ml originating from 15 ml of CSF.

tion of the active fraction on microcrystalline cellulose thin layers. Following electrophoresis in one dimension and chromatography in a second dimension, at least 5 ninhydrin- and fluorescamine-positive spots were observed.

In one single case, patient K.T. (Table 1), an additional peak of receptor blocking activity was found at higher calibrated m.w. (about 1400). It was also noted that heating of the CSF prior to ultrafiltration, reduced the high molecular UV absorbing components in the PGM eluate but did not change the amount of receptor blocking activity in the "active" fraction. Heating also gave UV absorbing components of a lower apparent molecular weight (which did not affect the receptor). A few tests were also run to check whether in non-heated CSF any receptor-blocking activity was concentrated over the ultrafilter (nominal cut-off 10,000 dalton). No such activity was detected at concentration factors of 10-20.

Table 1 shows the results of tests with CSF from various patients. The material tested was that in the interval 1000-1200 dalton (apparent molecular weight). This interval is wide enough to include all fractions showing any receptor blocking activity. It is apparent that receptor blocking activity was present in all samples except one, and that the concentration varied by 5 times at the most.

TABLE 1

Receptor blocking activity of MLF in CSF samples from
various patients. Trig. is trigeminal neuralgia.

Patient	Diagnosis	Receptor blocking activity (units/ml)[1]
R.W.	Trig.	-
H. Håk.	Trig.	0.08
A-L.E.	Trig.	0.09
A.P.	Trig.	0.10
A.K.	Trig.	0.11
P.E.	Trig.	0.11
H.N.	Trig.	0.14
K.T.	Trig. + neurologic disease	0.17[2]
H.P.	Intention tremor	0.20
P.S.	Cerebellar tumor	0.23
J.A.	Trig.	0.24
M.M.	Cerebral aneurysm	0.30
H.H.	Cerebral tumor	0.51

[1] Units are defined in Methods

[2] One more peak of receptor activity at higher apparent m.w.; not included here

The active fraction from CSF was also tested against a labelled morphine antagonist, naltrexone, in Na^+-rich and Na^+-free incubation media, respectively. The presence of high Na^+ concentration is known to reduce the competitive affinity of narcotic agonists while antagonists maintain their affinity (5,6). It was found (Fig.3) that MLF from brain extracts showed a 5-fold reduction in competitive affinity upon addition of Na+, a similar decrease was observed with fractions from CSF. This Na-effect should be compared with a 50-fold reduction for dihydromorphine and a 1.2-fold gain for naltrexone under the same testing conditions.

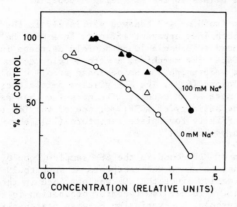

FIG. 3

Effect of MLF on the binding of tritium-labelled naltrexone to synaptic plasma membrane fraction of rat brain. Tests were run in a Tris-buffer in the absence (open symbols) and the presence (closed symbols) of 100 mM Na+. MLF from brain extracts was obtained as described previously (2). Triangles represent samples from CSF.

Discussion

The CSF is thought to communicate with the extracellular fluid of the brain (7). Molecules as large as albumin can pass freely. A water-soluble substance produced in the brain can therefore be expected to reach the CSF. The extent of this process will be dependent on the site of synthesis, the net synthesis and on fluid dynamics. Since opiate receptors involved in analgesia are situated in the periaqueductal gray matter (8) the levels of MLF in the CSF might possibly be closely related to those in receptor areas. It is even possible that such a factor is produced in the thalamic-hypothalamic area and reaches the receptors via CSF. These considerations suggest that analysis of MLF levels in CSF samples may be useful in defining its role under various physiologic and pathologic conditions, particularly in relation to severe pain.

Because of the limited volumes of CSF that can be drawn from a patient, the purification procedure had to be restricted to a few steps. However, the CSF is chemically very much less composite than total brain extracts. We have chosen to use an ultrafiltration step to remove proteins and similarly-sized molecules and desalting step on Sephadex gel to remove inorganic salts and low-molecular weight components. The remaining material, in the molecular weight interval 500-10,000 dalton was fractionated on a PGM 2000 column. This column gives a very good resolution of peptides from 2000 dalton and downwards (2). Since it is run in water, solutes are easily recovered.

In general, the results are satisfactory in the sense that evidence was obtained for the presence of MLF in exactly the same chromatographic fractions where we had previously detected activity in brain extracts. This was corroborated by the finding that MLF isolated from brain extracts (2) chromatographed as

MLF from CSF. Further chemical characterization of the active fraction from CSF indicates that it is considerably less complex than the corresponding fraction from brain extracts. The specific activity in terms of fluorescamine-reactive groups was also slightly higher in the CSF fraction despite the fact that a less elaborate procedure was followed for its purification. All presently available chemical evidence points to the MLF being a peptide.

MLF isolated from brain or CSF behaved similarily in the assay with labelled naltrexone since both lost apparent affinity in a high Na^+ medium. The addition of high Na^+ is known to cause a 10 to 50-fold decrease in affinity with "pure" analgesic agonists like morphine, a 2 to 3-fold decrease in affinity with partial agonists like nalorphine and no decrease at all with "pure" antagonists like naltrexone or naloxone (6,9). The MLF gives a 5-fold decrease (Fig.3) and is therefore behaving more as an agonist like morphine than as an antagonist. It is interesting that the affinity of $ACTH_{1-28}$, one of the few peptides known to possess considerable affinity for opiate receptors (10), shows a 10-fold reduction upon the addition of high Na^+.

The concentrations of MLF found in the CSF samples, would, if identical to those in receptor areas, saturate the receptors at most to 10-15%. This can of course be an underestimation since the CSF was obtained in the lumbar region. It is also possible that a rather low receptor occupation is sufficient to overcome an activation threshold. The variation between patients is likely to be real, because every chromatogram was run on the same specified column under identical conditions with continuous monitoring of UV-absorption, and measurements of ionic content and primary amine groups. The case material is too small to allow definite conclusions but it is suggestive, that patients with trigeminal neuralgia seem to have lower levels than patients with other diagnoses. A causal relationship may therefore exist. It is clear, however, that further progress in this field will require more extensive studies both on the chemical and clinical sides.

Acknowledgement

We wish to thank our collegues of the Neurosurgical Department of the University Hospital for CSF samples, and Mrs. I. Eriksson and Mrs.L.Bennich-Björkman for technical assistance. Labelled naltrexone was kindly donated by Dr. R.W. Willette, NIDA, Rockville, Md., nonlabelled naltrexone by Dr. M.J. Ferster, Endo Labs, Brussels, Belgium. The work was supported by the Swedish Medical Research Council (B75-25X-3766-04).

References

1. L. TERENIUS, and A. WAHLSTRÖM, Acta pharmac. tox. 35 Suppl. I 55 (1974).

2. L. TERENIUS, and A. Wahlström, Acta physiol. scand. 94 74-81 (1975).

3. L. TERENIUS, Acta pharmac. tox. 34 88-91 (1974).

4. S. UNDENFRIEND, S. STEIN, P. BÖHLEN, W. DAIRMAN, W. LEIMGRUBER, and M. WEIGELE, Science 178 871-872 (1972).

5. E.J. SIMON, J.H. HILLER, and I. EDELMAN, Proc.natn. Acad. Sci. 70, 1947-1949 (1973).

6. C.B. PERT, G. PASTERNAK, and S.H. SNYDER, Science 182 1359-1361 (1973).

7. E.A. BERING Jr., Fed. Proc. PT.1. 33 2061-2063 (1974).

8. A. HERZ, and H.-J. TESCHEMACHER, Adv. Drug Res. 6 79-119 (1971).

9. C.B. PERT, and S.H. SNYDER, Mol. Pharmacol. 10 868-879 (1974).

10. L. TERENIUS, J. Pharm. Pharmac. (1975) in press.

AN ENDOGENOUS MORPHINE-LIKE FACTOR IN MAMMALIAN BRAIN

Gavril W. Pasternak, Robert Goodman and Solomon H. Snyder

Departments of Pharmacology and Experimental Therapeutics and Psychiatry and the Behavioral Sciences, Johns Hopkins University School of Medicine, Baltimore Maryland 21205

(Received in final form May 24, 1975)

An endogenous morphine-like substance (MLF) found in rat and calf brains has a regional distribution correlating with that of opiate receptors, with the highest levels in the caudate and negligible amounts in the cerebellum. In binding assays MLF behaves like an opiate agonist. Sodium ion and enzyme and reagent treatment of membranes decrease its potency and manganese ion enhances it. MLF is localized in synaptosomal fractions, stored in an osmotically labile compartment, and can be degraded by carboxypeptidase A and leucine amino peptidase, implying a peptide structure. Its molecular weight is about 1000 as determined by gel chromatography.

The highly selective interactions of the opiate receptor (1-3) and its association with pain pathways (4, LaMott, Pert and Snyder, in preparation) suggest that some normally occurring substance, possibly a neurotransmitter of pain pathways, serves as an endogenous ligand for the opiate receptor. Hughes (5) has identified a morphine-like factor (MLF) in pig brain which mimics the ability of morphine to inhibit electrically induced contractions of the mouse vas deferens. The actions of the substance described by Hughes are antagonized by low concentrations of the opiate antagonist naloxone and its regional distribution in pig brain parallels the distribution of the opiate receptor in rat and monkey brains (6). Previously we observed that incubation of brain extracts released a substance which inhibits opiate receptor binding, possesses a regional distribution in rat brain resembling that of the opiate receptor, and is destroyed by carboxypeptidase A but not trypsin (7). Terenius also obtained preliminary evidence that brain extracts can inhibit opiate receptor binding (8). In the present study we describe the characteristics of a morphine-like factor in calf and rat brain whose properties are the same as those anticipated for the endogenous ligand of the opiate receptor.

METHODS

Brains were homogenized in 10 volumes of 0.32M sucrose with a Potter-Elvehjem homogenizer, centrifuged at 100,000 x g at 0°C for 1 hour. Pellet was resuspended in 2 volumes of 10mM Tris buffer (pH 7.7 at 25°C) and immersed in a boiling water bath for 15 minutes. The boiled tissue was then centrifuged at 100,000 x g for 1 hour at 0°C and the clear supernatant carefully pipetted off. This supernatant, which contains the morphine-like factor (MLF), was then either used or lyphilized and stored under liquid nitrogen.

[3]H-Opiate binding assays were performed as previously described (7). All values represent opiate-specific binding as were calculated from triplicate determinations which varied less than 10%.

Extracts of calf caudate nucleus inhibit opiate receptor binding in a concentration dependent fashion with 75μl of calf MLF inhibiting both ^{3}H-naloxone and ^{3}H-dihydromorphine 50%. In addition, inhibition of binding is seen with the following ^{3}H-opiates: levorphanol, levallorphan and diprenorphine. Thus it is likely that this inhibition is related to opiates in general. Rat MLF behaves identically to calf MLF in inhibition studies. Calf MLF is a competitive inhibitor of ^{3}H-naloxone binding, as determined by Lineweaver-Burke analysis.

All brain areas examined in both calf and rat show marked regional differences in the concentration of MLF (Table 1). (A unit of MLF is defined as that amount of MLF which, when added to 1 ml, yields 50% receptor occupancy. This value is determined according to Colquhoun (9), assuming classical binding interactions.) The regional distribution in both the rat and calf is remarkably similar and it correlates extremely well with the regional distribution of the opiate receptor (6) and with MLF distribution according to Hughes (5).

By studying the influence of ions upon opiate receptor binding it is possible to determine whether an agent has the properties of an opiate agonist or antagonist. Low concentrations of sodium but not of other monovalent cations such as potassium, selectively inhibit receptor binding of opiate agonists, and reduce the ability of opiate agonists to inhibit receptor binding of ^{3}H-naloxone (11,12). Similarly as little as 5mM NaCl markedly reduces the ability of MLF to inhibit ^{3}H-naloxone binding while as much as 100mM KCl has no influence on ^{3}H-naloxone binding (Figure 1). In contrast to the influence of sodium on the opiate receptor, low concentrations of manganese enhance the receptor binding of opiate agonists (10,13). The ability of caudate MLF to inhibit ^{3}H-naloxone binding is enhanced 43% by 1mM manganese. To exclude the possibility that MLF activity can be attributed to an endogenous divalent cation, we examined the influence of the chelating agent EDTA. At 5mM concentration, EDTA has no influence on the ability of MLF to inhibit naloxone binding (Figure 1). Identical results are obtained with rat MLF.

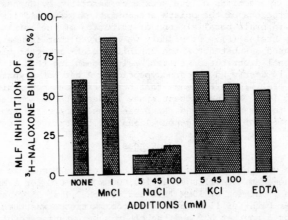

FIG. 1

Effect of ions and chelaters on MLF inhibition of ^{3}H-naloxone binding. Calf MLF was assayed with ^{3}H-naloxone (35,000cpm/ml) and the appropriate addition. MLF inhibition was determined by the binding remaining in samples with MLF and the addition to samples with only the addition. Thus, the inhibition is due to only MLF, not to the additions used. The experiment was repeated four times.

TABLE 1

Regional Localization of MLF in Rat and Calf Brain

MLF (Units)

Region	Calf	Rat
Caudate	5.4	4.8
Hypothalamus	2.8	
Spinal Cord	1.5	
Pons	1.2	
Cortex		0.8
Parietal Region	1.2	
Thalamus	0.6	
Medulla-Oblongata	0.6	1.4
Cerebellum	0.6	0
Corpus Callosum	0	

Brains were dissected and MLF prepared as described and amounts equivalent to 100 mg tissue wet weight were assayed in triplicate with ^{3}H-naloxone and 1mM $MnCl_2$ to determine inhibition. The experiment was repeated three times.

TABLE 2

MLF Inhibition of ^{3}H-Naloxone Binding in

Membranes Treated with Enzymes and Reagents

Treatment	MLF Inhibition
None	53%
Trypsin	20%
Chymotrypsin	30%
N-Ethylmaleimide	30%
Iodoacetamide	27%
p-Chloromercuribenzoate	34%

Rat brain membranes were prepared and treated with trypsin (0.5 μg/ml), chymotrypsin (50 μg/ml), N-ethylmaleimide (10 μM), iodoacetamide (5 mM), and p-chloromercuribenzoate (10 μM), for 20 min at 25°C and the reagents or enzymes washed out by centrifugation. Aliquots of the tissue were then assayed with ^{3}H-naloxone and 1mM $MnCl_2$ in the presence and absence of calf MLF (100μl). The experiment has been repeated three times.

Rat brain membranes treated with certain enzymes (14) and reagents (7, 15) show a dramatic decrease in agonist binding while antagonist binding is essentially unaffected. Accordingly, we examined the ability of MLF to inhibit ^{3}H-naloxone binding on treated membranes (Table 2). As with the ions, MLF behaves like an agonist on treated membranes, like results of Hughes (5).

If MLF is a modulator of synaptic activity in the brain, it might be anticipated to be localized to nerve terminals. Homogenizing the brain in 0.32 M sucrose with a loosely fitting Teflon pestle (Potter-Elvehjem) results in the formation of synaptosomes (16). When brain tissue is extensively distrupted by Polytron treatment, synaptosomes are not found and potential synaptosomal constituents are released into the supernatant fluid. Synaptosome containing pellets subjected to hypotonic lysis and sonification also release

TABLE 3

Subcellular Localization of Rat MLF

	MLF (Units)
Polytron Pellet	2.2
Potter-Elvehjem Pellet	6.8
Lysed Potter-Elvehjem Pellet	2.4
Supernatant from Lysed Potter-Elvehjem Pellet	3.2
P_1 (crude nuclear)	0.45
P_2 (crude mitochondrial)	2.7
P_3 (crude microsomal)	1.8
S_3 (supernatant)	0.87

Rat brains were either polytroned in 10 volumes 50mM Tris buffer or homogenized with a Potter-Elvehjem homogenizer (Teflon pestle and glass tube) in 10 vol. of 0.32M sucrose and centrifuged at 100,000 g for 60 min. MLF was then extracted from the pellets. A Potter-Elvehjem pellet was lysed by resuspension in 50mM Tris and sonification and then centrifuged 50,000 g x 30 min, The pellet was extracted for MLF and supernatant tested directly. A Potter-Elvehjem homogenate was subjected to differential centrifugation (16) and the pellets extracted for MLF. Fractions were assayed with ^{3}H-naloxone and 1mM $MnCl_2$. The experiment was repeated three times.

TABLE 4

Sensitivity of MLF to Enzymes

Treatment	Calf	Rat
None	49%	69%
Trypsin	50%	72%
Chymotrypsin	41%	44%
Leucine aminopeptidase	12%	38%
Carboxypeptidase A	25%	40%
Neuraminidase	49%	70%

Rat and calf MLF was prepared and reacted with trypsin (1 mg/ml), chymotrypsin (1 mg/ml), carboxypeptidase A (40 U/ml), Leucine aminopeptidase (448 U/ml), neuraminidase (50 µg/ml) or nothing at 37°C for 30 min. The enzymes were inactivated by boiling (Trypsin also had soybean trypsin inhibitor added - 4 mg/ml) and the mixtures tested in a binding assay with 1 mM $MnCl_2$ and ^{3}H-naloxone. The experiment was repeated three times.

their contents into the supernatant fluid. When the synaptosome-containing Potter-Elvehjem pellet is subjected to hypotonic lysis with sonification, about 60% of the recovered activity is released into the supernatant fluid and 40% remains in the residual pellet (Table 3). Pellets from homogenates subjected to Polytron treatment contain only a third as much MLF as the Potter-Elvehjem pellet, about the same amount as that in the residual Potter-Elvehjem pellet after lysis. Differential centrifugation (16) shows the highest levels in the P_2 fraction, consistent with a synaptosomal localization.

On Biogel P_2, the MLF shows a molecular weight of 1000 daltons, with $K_{AV}=0.23 (K_{AV}=(V_e-V_o)^2(V_t-V_o)^{-1})$. The material is stable to boiling for up to 15 minutes, but is degraded by a number of enzymes (Table 4), resembling results of Hughes (5).

REFERENCES

1. C.B. Pert and S.H. Snyder, Science 179:1011 (1973).

2. L. Terenius, Acta Pharmac. Tox. 33:377 (1973).

3. E.J. Simon, J.M. Hiller and I. Edelman, Proc. Nat. Acad. Sci. USA 70:1947 (1973).

4. A. Pert and T. Yaksh, Brain Res. 80:135 (19740.

5. J. Hughes, Brain Res. 88:295-308 (1975).

6. M.J. Kuhar, C.B. Pert and S.H. Snyder, Nature 245:447 (1973).

7. G.W. Pasternak, H.A. Wilson and S.H. Snyder, Mol. Pharmacol. in press (1975)

8. L. Terenius, Neurosciences Research Program, 13:39 (1975).

9. Colquhoun, D., Drug Receptors, p. 149, University Park Press, Baltimore (1973).

10. G.W. Pasternak and S.H. Snyder, Neurosciences Research Bulletin, 13:58 (1975).

11. C.B. Pert, G.W. Pasternak and S.H. Snyder, Science 182:1359 (1973).

12. C.B. Pert and S.H. Snyder, Mol. Pharmacol. 10:868 (1974).

13. G.W. Pasternak, A. Snowman and S.H. Snyder, Mol. Pharmacol. in press (1975).

14. G.W. Pasternak and S.H. Snyder, Mol. Pharmacol. in press (1975).

15. H.A.Wilson, G.W. Pasternak and S.H. Snyder, Nature 253:448-450 (1975).

16. E.G. Gray and V.P. Whittaker, J. of Anatomy 96:79 (1962).

ACKNOWLEDGEMENTS

These studies were supported by the Johns Hopkins Drug Abuse Research Center Grant DA-00266 from the United States Public Health Service. G.W.P. is the recipient of Drug Abuse Center Research Fellowship 1 F22-DA 01646-01. S.H.S. is the recipient of Research Scientist Development Award MH-33128.

A PEPTIDE-LIKE SUBSTANCE FROM PITUITARY THAT ACTS LIKE MORPHINE.

1. ISOLATION

H. Teschemacher*, K. E. Opheim, B. M. Cox and Avram Goldstein

Addiction Research Foundation and Stanford University (Department of Pharmacology), Palo Alto, California 94304, U.S.A.

(Received in final form May 24, 1975)

Summary

A method is described for extraction from bovine pituitary glands of a substance that shows several properties characteristic of opiates. The material inhibits the twitch tension of the electrically stimulated guinea pig longitudinal muscle-myenteric plexus preparation and of the electrically stimulated mouse vas deferens. This inhibition is reversed and blocked by the opiate antagonist naloxone. The extract also inhibits binding of the opiate agonist etorphine and the opiate antagonist naloxone to stereospecific binding sites in synaptic membranes of guinea pig brain. The inhibition of naloxone binding is decreased by Na^+ in the manner characteristic of opiate agonists. The physiologic role of the pituitary opioid remains to be investigated.

The highly specific interaction of opiates with opiate receptors in the brain (1-3) and the guinea pig ileum (4) suggested the existence of endogenous ligands for these receptors, as proposed by Goldstein in 1973 (5). The search for such endogenous opioids has been carried out by several groups in addition to our own. Terenius (6) reported the presence in brain of material that inhibits the binding of dihydromorphine to membrane-bound opiate receptors. Hughes (7) has recently reported on a substance in brain with pharmacologic properties like those of morphine, the distribution of which was like that of the opiate receptors. Our work with pituitary gland was prompted by the finding, recounted in the following paper (8), that crude preparations of adrenocorticotrophic hormone contain opioid activity. We describe here the isolation of a substance from bovine pituitary that has morphine-like action in two bioassay systems and also interacts with opiate receptors in synaptic membranes of guinea pig brain. The purification and characterization of the endogenous opioid(s) from pituitary are described in the following paper (8).

METHODS

Isolation Procedure. Initial attempts to extract pituitary glands with trichloroacetic acid, sodium chloride solutions, or acid-acetone yielded ambiguous results. Therefore, we turned to another procedure, which had proved successful in isolating pituitary peptide hormones (9,10). Bovine pituitary glands, obtained fresh at the slaughterhouse and frozen on dry ice, were homogenized in a Waring blendor with acetone (20 ml per g wet weight of tissue) at

---

*Present address: Max-Planck-Institut fur Psychiatrie, 8000 Munich 40, GERMANY.

Reprint requests to Addiction Research Foundation.

23°, and centrifuged. This and all subsequent centrifugation was carried out at 0°, 12,000 g for 10 min except as noted. To the dried and powdered sediment was added acetone (2.5 ml per g), and then glacial acetic acid (16 ml per g) was added slowly with stirring. The mixture was heated at 70° with stirring for 45 min under anhydrous conditions, and then centrifuged at 30°. The supernatant was saved, and the sediment was washed once with glacial acetic acid and acetone. To the combined supernatants were added 1/2 vol of acetone and 1/200 vol of 5M NaCl with vigorous stirring. After storage at 2° for 9-12 hr, the precipitate was centrifuged and discarded. An equal volume of ether was added to the supernatant, and 1 hr later the resulting precipitate was collected by centrifugation. This sediment was washed 3 times with acetone and twice with ether, then dried under vacuum. The dry powdered material was dissolved in water. The resulting yellow solution (pH 2.5) yielded a heavy precipitate on adjustment of the pH to 7.4. After centrifugation, the clear supernatant solution was used for the tests described under Results.

Guinea pig ileum preparation. Preparation, mounting, and electrical stimulation of the longitudinal muscle strip with attached myenteric plexus from the guinea pig ileum were performed as described by Kosterlitz et al (11), and by Schulz and Goldstein (12).

Mouse vas deferens. The method was essentially that described by Henderson et al (13). Male albino mice (35-40 g) were used. The vas deferens was placed immediately in a 35° Ringer solution bubbled with 95% O_2-5% CO_2, and mounted in the tissue bath within a few minutes. The equipment and the Ringer solution were the same as for the guinea pig ileum preparation. Electrical stimulation was with rectangular pulses, 1 msec duration, supramaximal voltage (50-100 V), 0.1 Hz.

Opiate receptor binding assay. Synaptic membranes from guinea pig brains were prepared in the customary manner (14-16). The binding of ^{3}H-etorphine and ^{3}H-naloxone (both 2.5 x 10^{-9} M) to opiate receptors in the membranes (1 g tissue wet weight/10 ml Tris HCl buffer, 0.1 M, pH 7.4) was measured by a filtration assay (17).

RESULTS

Fig. 1 shows the effect of the crude extract on the twitch tension of the guinea pig ileum preparation. There was a prompt inhibition, which was readily reversed by washing (panel A). The effect produced by extract from 1/40 of a pituitary gland was equivalent to that obtained with about 0.25 nmole of normorphine (50 nM in the 5-ml bath). Prolonged exposure to the extract produced a sustained inhibition, which, however, was promptly reversed by naloxone (panel B). In the preparation previously treated with naloxone, the inhibition was almost totally blocked (panel C).

Fig. 2 shows the effect of the crude extract on the mouse vas deferens. Here the inhibition was reversed only partially by naloxone, and correspondingly (not shown), pretreatment with naloxone caused only a partial blockade.

Fig. 3 shows the effect of extract on the stereospecific binding of the agonist etorphine and the antagonist naloxone to opiate receptors in synaptic membranes from guinea pig brain. The material extracted from 1/40 of a pituitary gland inhibited the stereospecific binding of etorphine by 89% and of naloxone by 65%. Increasing the sodium concentration opposed the effect of the extract on naloxone binding, indicating an inhibiting substance of agonistic character (2,18).

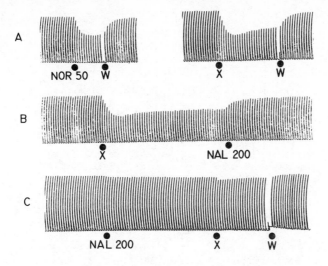

FIG. 1.

Effects of bovine pituitary extract on the responses of the isolated guinea pig ileum longitudinal muscle-myenteric plexus preparation to electrical stimulation. A longitudinal muscle strip from guinea pig ileum was suspended in Krebs solution at 37° and aerated with 95% O_2 + 5% CO_2. Tension changes induced by field electrical stimulation (0.1 Hz, 0.5 msec pulse duration, 80V) were recorded with a Grass FT. 03 transducer on a Grass polygraph. NOR = normorphine; NAL = naloxone; W = wash; X = extract from 1/40 of a pituitary gland. Figures refer to the bath concentration of drug (nM). Normorphine has been used as a standard because of its ready reversibility.

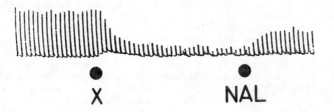

FIG. 2

Effect of bovine pituitary extract on the electrically stimulated mouse vas deferens. X = extract from 1/20 of a pituitary gland. NAL = naloxone, 1 μM final concentration in 5-ml bath.

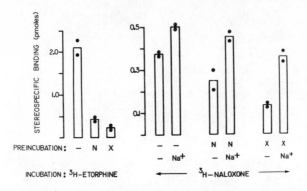

FIG. 3

Effect of bovine pituitary extract in the opiate receptor binding
assay. In each series, the nonspecific binding in the presence
of levorphanol (1 µM) was subtracted from the total binding to
obtain stereospecific binding, which is given as pmoles bound to
membranes obtained from 1 g wet weight of brain. Final volume
2 ml, containing synaptic membranes, radioactive ligand, and
the substance being tested for inhibitory effect. Preincubation:
15 min, 23°. Incubation: 15 min, 23°. N = normorphine (1 µM
in the etorphine set, 10 nM in the naloxone set). X = extract
from 1/40 of a pituitary gland. Na$^+$ = 100 mM NaCl. Duplicate
determinations are shown.

DISCUSSION

The effects of the pituitary extract on the guinea pig ileum preparation
and on the mouse vas deferens are typical of those seen with morphine and
other opiate narcotics. Although many substances nonspecifically inhibit the
electrically stimulated twitch in these tissues, reversal and blockade by
naloxone, as demonstrated here, has been observed only with opiates. The
interaction with stereospecific opiate receptor sites in synaptic membranes
from guinea pig brain, and the effects of Na$^+$ on this interaction constitute
confirmatory evidence that the pituitary substance behaves like a typical
opiate agonist. The same evidence argues against the alternative possibility,
that the substance releases an endogenous opioid in the tissues used for the
bioassay. As demonstrated in the following paper (8), the material is entire-
ly unlike any known natural or synthetic opioid in its physical and chemical
properties.

We can as yet only speculate on what the presence of an endogenous opioid
in the pituitary may signify. It could be synthesized in the hypothalamus and
act on the pituitary, like the hypothalamic releasing and release-inhibiting
peptide hormones. Indeed, since morphine stimulates or inhibits release of
several pituitary hormones (19) it could be concerned in the control of
pituitary functions. Alternatively, it could be produced or stored in the
pituitary and act at remote opiate sensitive tissues in the manner of a typical
pituitary hormone.

ACKNOWLEDGEMENTS

This work was supported by grants DA-972 and DA-1199 from the National Institute on Drug Abuse. We thank Madeline Rado and Rekha Padya for expert technical assistance.

REFERENCES

1. A. GOLDSTEIN, L.L. LOWNEY and B.K. PAL, Proc. Nat. Acad. Sci., U.S.A. 68, 1742-1747 (1971).

2. E.J. SIMON, J.M. HILLER and I. EDELMAN, Proc. Nat. Acad. Sci., U.S.A. 70, 1947-1949 (1973).

3. C.B. PERT and S.H. SNYDER, Science 179, 1011-1014 (1973).

4. H.W. KOSTERLITZ, J.A.H. LORD and A.J. WATT, In: "Agonist and Antagonist Actions of Narcotic Analgesic Drugs", Eds. H.W. Kosterlitz, H.O.J. Collier and J.E. Villarreal, pp. 45-61, Macmillan, London (1971).

5. A. GOLDSTEIN, Proc. Int. Symp. Alc. and Drug Res., Oct. 23-25, 1973. In: "Biological and Behavioural Approaches to Drug Dependence", Eds. H. Cappel and A.E. LeBlanc, Addiction Research Foundation, Toronto (1975).

6. L. TERENIUS and A. WAHLSTROM, Acta Pharmacol. Toxicol. 35 (Suppl.), 55 (1974).

7. J. HUGHES, Brain Res. 88, 295-309 (1975).

8. B.M. COX, K.E. OPHEIM, H. TESCHEMACHER and AVRAM GOLDSTEIN, Life Sci., 16 1777-1782 (1975).

9. R.W. PAYNE, M.S. RABEN and E.B. ASTWOOD, J. Biol. Chem. 187, 719-731 (1950).

10. O. KAMM, T.B. ALDRICH, I.W. GROTE, L.W. ROWE and E.P. BUGBEE, J. Amer. Chem. Soc. 50, 573-601 (1928).

11. H.W. KOSTERLITZ, R.J. LYDON and A.J. WATT, Brit. J. Pharmacol. 39, 398-413 (1970).

12. R. SCHULZ and A. GOLDSTEIN, J. Pharm. Exp. Ther. 183, 404-410 (1972).

13. G. HENDERSON, J. HUGHES and H.W. KOSTERLITZ, Brit. J. Pharmacol. 46, 764-766 (1972).

14. E.G. GRAY and V.P. WHITTAKER, J. Anat. (London) 96, 79-88 (1962).

15. V.P. WHITTAKER, I.A. MICHAELSON and R.J.A. KIRKLAND, Biochem, J. 80, 293-303 (1964).

16. L. TERENIUS, Acta Pharmacol. Toxicol. 33, 377-384 (1973).

17. C.B. PERT and S.H. SNYDER, Proc. Nat. Acad. Sci., U.S.A. 70, 2243-2247 (1973).

18. C.B. PERT, G. PASTERNAK and S.H. SNYDER, Science 182, 1359-1361 (1973).

19. R. GEORGE and P. LOMAX, In: "Chemical and Biological Aspects of Drug Dependence", Eds. S.J Mule and H. Brill, pp. 523-543, CRC Press, Cleveland (1972).

A PEPTIDE-LIKE SUBSTANCE FROM PITUITARY THAT ACTS LIKE MORPHINE

2. PURIFICATION AND PROPERTIES

B. M. Cox, K. E. Opheim, H. Teschemacher and Avram Goldstein

Addiction Research Foundation and Stanford University (Department of
Pharmacology), Palo Alto, California 94304, U.S.A.

(Received in final form May 24, 1975)

Summary

We have demonstrated the existence of a peptide-like opioid
in bovine and porcine pituitary, and determined some of its properties. It is an opioid agonist on the guinea pig myenteric
plexus-longitudinal muscle preparation, and on the mouse vas
deferens, and it binds to opiate receptors in homogenates of
guinea pig brain. Its physiologic role and its possible presence
in hypothalamic or other brain regions remain to be determined.

In the preceding paper Teschemacher et al (1) demonstrated the presence
in bovine pituitary of a substance that behaved like a typical opiate agonist
in two bioassays, and inhibited the binding of opiates to synaptic membranes
from guinea pig brain. The observations of Krivoy and his colleagues
that the development of tolerance to morphine was accelerated by a vasopressin
derivative (2), and that adrenocorticotrophic hormone (ACTH), tetracosactin, or
β-melanocyte stimulating hormone (β-MSH) antagonised morphine action on the
spinal cord (3,4) led us to test a crude porcine ACTH preparation (Sigma or
Calbiochem, Grade B) for opioid properties. The results were positive, both
in the guinea pig ileum longitudinal muscle-myenteric plexus preparation (5)
(Fig. 1) and in the opiate receptor binding assay (6,7). However, synthetic
human ACTH and α-MSH (kindly supplied by Dr. C. H. Li) and tetracosactin
(Synacthen , Ciba) were without opioid activity in our assay systems at concentrations up to 10^{-5}M. (i.e. a 10-fold increase above the ACTH concentration
in effective doses of the crude ACTH preparation). We have tested a number of
other synthetic samples of peptides that occur naturally in the pituitary or
hypothalamus, including lysine-vasopressin, oxytocin, luteinising hormone releasing hormone, substance P, Pro-Leu-Gly-NH_2 (MSH-RIH) and somatostatin. Only
the latter produced an inhibition of the guinea pig ileum and this effect was
not blocked by naloxone. We have therefore attempted to purify the active
opioid contaminant in the crude ACTH preparation, which is similar to the principle isolated from bovine pituitary (1).

Purification

Separated fractions of the crude material were assayed for opioid activity on the guinea pig ileum preparation. Activity was expressed in normorphine equivalent units, one unit producing an inhibitory effect equivalent to
that produced by one nanomole of normorphine in the 5-ml tissue bath.

An initial electrophoretic fractionation of the ACTH preparation showed
that the opioid material had a net positive charge in 0.2M NH_4OH (pH 10.5),
whilst the major part of the protein moved toward the anode. This suggested a
cation-exchange column fractionation. The crude ACTH was applied to a

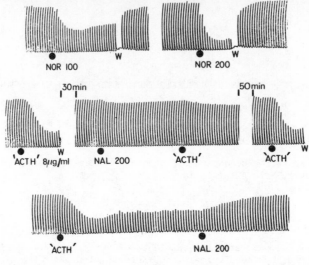

FIG. 1

Effects of a crude ACTH preparation on the responses of the isolated guinea pig ileum longitudinal muscle-myenteric plexus preparation to electrical stimulation. A longitudinal muscle strip from guinea pig ileum was suspended in Krebs solution at 37° and aerated with 95% O_2 + 5% CO_2. Tension changes induced by field electrical stimulation (0.1 Hz, 0.5 msec pulse duration, 80V) were recorded with a Grass FT. 03 transducer on a Grass polygraph. NOR = normorphine; NAL = naloxone; W = wash; "ACTH" = ACTH (Sigma, Grade B). Figures refer to the bath concentration of drug (nM). Normorphine has been used as a standard because of its ready reversibility.

---

carboxymethylcellulose column (BioRad Laboratories Cellex CM, 1.0 x 8.5 cm) in 0.1M NH_4OH, and the column was then eluted sequentially with 25 ml portions of 0.1M NH_4OH, distilled water, 0.1M formic acid, and 0.1N HCl. After lyophilization of each fraction and resolubilisation in distilled water, the opioid activity was found predominantly in the HCl eluate and we have designated it 'pituitary opioid peptide 1' (or POP-1) (Fig. 2). Virtually all of the opioid activity was recovered whilst the protein content was reduced by 95% as determined by the Lowry procedure (using bovine serum albumin as standard) (8). A similar fractionation of the material obtained by Teschemacher et al (1) from frozen bovine pituitary also yielded an active opioid in the HCl eluate.

Chemical properties

POP-1 was dialysable, but eluted in the void volume on a Sephadex G-15 column (minimum excluded molecular weight 1500). Comparison of the elution volume of the opioid activity with the elution volumes of peptides of known molecular weight on Sephadex G-25 gave an apparent molecular weight of 1750 (Fig. 3) in two separate determinations.

POP-1 was stable to heating in water at 100° for 30 min, and did not lose activity on standing for 30 min at 23° in 0.25N HCl, or 0.25N NaOH. TLC of crude ACTH and synthetic ACTH on silica gel (Eastman Chromagram, n-butanol: pyridine: acetic acid: water, 30:20:6:24, ninhydrin), showed that the opioid activity was coincident with ACTH (R_f:0.4). Paper electrophoretic fractionation of POP-1 indicated that the component with opioid activity moved as a

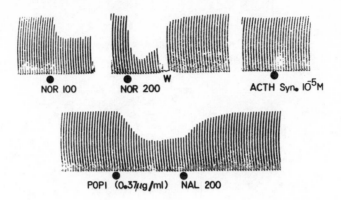

NOR 100   NOR 200   ACTH Syn. 10^{-5}M

POP1 (0.37μg/ml)   NAL 200

FIG. 2

Effects of the purified fraction POP-1 and synthetic ACTH on the guinea pig
ileum preparation. Method and nomenclature as in Fig. 1. POP-1 was prepared by CM-cellulose fractionation of the crude ACTH (see text). Concentration refers to reactivity in the Lowry protein determination with bovine
serum albumin as a standard. Synthetic ACTH (ACTH Syn) was kindly supplied
by Dr. C. H. Li.

---

single band toward the cathode in 0.2M NH_4OH (pH 10.5) (mobility 7 x 10^{-6}
cm^2/V·sec). A second fractionation in 0.1M formic acid (pH 2.5) after trans-
ferring this material to a new paper, revealed two components with opioid activity. Both migrated toward the cathode, the major one, with a mobility at pH
2.5 of 12 x 10^{-6} cm^2/V·sec, and a minor component representing about 10% of
the activity with a mobility of 96 x 10^{-6} cm^2/V·sec (Beckman Model R Paper
electrophoresis system, constant voltage 300V).

We have **sought further** information concerning the nature of POP-1 by
degradation studies. There was very rapid loss of opioid activity when
POP-1 or the crude ACTH was incubated with α-chymotrypsin or trypsin
(Fig. 4). The inactivation by trypsin was substantially inhibited by soybean
trypsin inhibitor. Even in the absence of added inhibitor a residual level
of activity appeared relatively resistant to inactivation by either enzyme.
The recovery of the ileum preparation following exposure to the material remaining after trypsin incubation was considerably more rapid than following
exposure to POP-1 (Fig. 5), and we tentatively attribute this residual activity to a product of the tryptic digestion of POP-1. A similar incomplete
trypsin digestion was observed with the bovine pituitary extract (1).

There was no loss of opioid activity when POP-1 was incubated with a
mixture of carboxypeptidases A and B (carboxypeptidase A, 33 μg/ml,
1.7u/ml; carboxypeptidase B, 33 μg/ml, 5.8 u/ml; 37°, 30 min). Under these
conditions hippuryl-phenylalanine, 5mM, was rapidly hydrolysed. Leucine
aminopeptidase (100μg/ml, 9.5 u/ml), ribonuclease (7 μg/ml, 0.525 u/ml),
phosphodiesterase (20 μg/ml, 0.008 u/ml), phospholipase A, (25μg/ml, 30 u/ml)
and phospholipase D (25 μg/ml, 0.5 u/ml) (incubations at 37° for 30 mins, all
enzymes from Sigma) also had no effect on opioid activity. Cyanogen bromide
treatment was without effect.

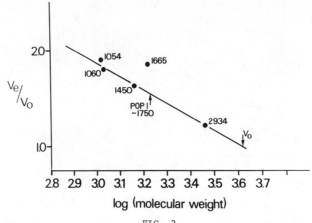

FIG. 3

Molecular weight determination of the opioid component of POP-1 on Sephadex G-25. A Sephadex G-25 column (1.5 x 50 cm) was set up in 0.1 M acetic acid with 0.15M NaCl (Total volume, V_T, approx. 75 ml). The flow rate was 0.3 ml/min and 3-ml fractions were collected. The void volume (V_o) was determined by blue dextran elution; the recorded elution volume of applied samples was chosen at the peak of eluted material as determined by UV absorbance or radioactivity. Each point indicates the average elution position from 2 separate determinations with each of the following peptides: lysine vasopressin (M.W. 1054), bradykinin (1060), bacitracin (1450), and tetracosactin (2934). Duplicate determinations of α-MSH (1665) show that this compound deviated from the behavior of the other peptides. The elution position of POP-1 was determined by assay on the guinea pig ileum preparation after lyophilization and solubilization in water.

Pharmacological properties

It is clear that the crude ACTH and POP-1 produced a naloxone reversible inhibition of the guinea pig ileum preparation. A similar effect was produced by the crude ACTH extract on the mouse vas deferens preparation (9). We estimate that the crude ACTH contained about 13 normorphine equivalent units/mg protein on the ileum preparation; estimations on two mouse vasa deferentia gave a value of 16 units/mg. POP-1 had an activity on the ileum preparation of 350 to 400 units/mg (based on the Lowry protein reactivity). As with normorphine or other typical opiate agonists, the responses of the ileum to injected acetylcholine were not affected by POP-1 whilst responses to serotonin were substantially depressed.

The crude ACTH and POP-1 both inhibited the stereospecific binding of ^{3}H-etorphine (2.5 nM) and ^{3}H-naloxone (2.5 nM) to synaptic membranes from guinea pig brain. The inhibitory effect on ^{3}H-naloxone binding was reduced in the presence of Na[+] (100 mM), suggesting that the material has predominantly agonist activity (7,10).

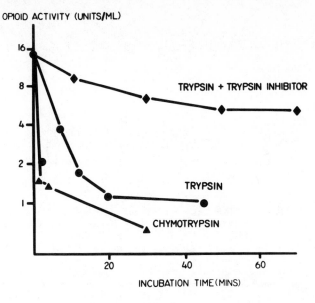

FIG. 4

Inactivation of the pituitary opioid peptide by trypsin and chymotrypsin. Samples of POP-1 at a concentration of 15 normorphine equivalent units/ml were incubated with a) α-chymotrypsin (Sigma, Type II from bovine pancreas, 60 u/mg, 10 μg/ml), or b) trypsin (Sigma, Type I from bovine pancreas, 9700 u/mg, 10 μg/ml), or c) trypsin 10 μg/ml, plus soybean trypsin inhibitor (Sigma, 20 μg/ml), in 0.1 M Tris-HCL buffer pH 7.4 at 37°. Samples were assayed for opioid activity on the guinea pig ileum preparation at appropriate times after the start of the incubation. The enzymes and inhibitor were without effect on the bioassay at these concentrations.

Discussion

These results show that there is present in extracts from porcine and bovine pituitary a material with typical opioid agonist properties. This material appears to be a trypsin and chymotrypsin sensitive peptide with a molecular weight of about 1750. Trypsin and chymotrypsin sensitivity imply the presence of basic and aromatic amino acid residues. The lack of effect of carboxypeptidases and leucine amino peptidase suggest that both amino and carboxyl terminals are masked, or that the peptide is cyclic. The insensitivity to cyanogen bromide suggests that there are no critically placed methionine residues. The electrophoretic behavior implies a predominance of basic amino acids. The general similarity in chemical and physical properties of the pituitary opioid to several of the known hypothalamic releasing and release inhibiting hormones is noteworthy. Its tissue of origin, enzyme sensitivity, molecular weight, ionic properties, and persistence of effect on the ileum preparation clearly differentiate it from the endogenous substance with opioid properties described by Hughes (11).

29

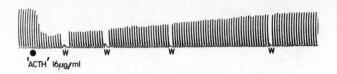

'ACTH' 16μg/ml

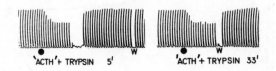

'ACTH'+ TRYPSIN 5'   'ACTH'+ TRYPSIN 33'

FIG. 5

Rapid reversibility of the opioid activity from pituitary following incubation with trypsin. A sample of the crude ACTH was incubated with trypsin
(100 μg/ml). The initial activity was very persistent, but after incubation with trypsin the residual activity on the ileum was rapidly reversed
by washing.

Acknowledgements

This work was supported by National Institute on Drug Abuse grants
DA-972 and DA-1149 and by the Drug Abuse Council. We thank Rekha Padhya,
Madeline Rado, and Stephen S. Wilmarth for technical assistance. We are
grateful to Dr. C. H. Li for the gift of synthetic ACTH and α-MSH, to CIBA
Pharmaceutical Company for a gift of Synacthen.

References

1. H. TESCHEMACHER, K.E. OPHEIM, B.M. COX and A. GOLDSTEIN, Life Sci. 16
    1771-1776 (1975).
2. W.A. KRIVOY, E. ZIMMERMANN and S. LANDE, Proc. Nat. Acad. Sci., U.S.A. 71,
    1852-1856 (1974).
3. W.A. KRIVOY, D. KROEGER, A. NEWMAN TAYLOR and E. ZIMMERMANN, Eur. J.
    Pharmacol. 27, 339-345 (1974).
4. E. ZIMMERMANN and W.A. KRIVOY, Prog. Brain Res. 39, 383-394 (1973).
5. H.W. KOSTERLITZ, R.J. LYDON and A.J. WATT, Brit. J. Pharmacol. 39, 398-413
    (1970).
6. C.B. PERT and S.H. SNYDER, Science 179, 1011-1014 (1973).
7. E.J. SIMON, J.M. HILLER and I. EDELMAN, Proc. Nat. Acad. Sci., U.S.A. 70,
    1947-1949 (1973).
8. O.H. LOWRY, N.J. ROSEBROUGH, A.L. FARR and R.J. RANDALL, J. Biol. Chem.
    193, 265-275 (1951).
9. G. HENDERSON, J. HUGHES and H.W. KOSTERLITZ, Brit. J. Pharmacol. 46,
    764-766 (1972).
10. C.B. PERT, G. PASTERNAK and S.H. SNYDER, Science 182, 1359-1361 (1973).
11. J. HUGHES, Brain Res. 88, 295-309 (1975).

OPIATE-SPECIFIC DISPLACEMENT OF STEROID HORMONES FROM MICROSOMES

Frank S. LaBella[1]

Department of Pharmacology and Therapeutics, Faculty of Medicine
University of Manitoba, Winnipeg, Manitoba, Canada R3E 0W3[2]
(Received in final form May 24, 1975)

Summary

Opiates displaced [^{3}H]-testosterone in relation to their pharmacological potencies from binding sites on rat liver microsomes. The
drugs competed less effectively with progesterone and least with corticosterone. Other drugs tested, including centrally acting ones, were
ineffective. These results support our hypothesis that opiate action
is mediated through steroid hormone receptors.

Opiates and steroid hormones are both derivatives of perhydrophenanthrene
and may produce euphoria, nausea, vomiting, analgesia, sedation, hypo- or hyper-
thermia, convulsions, respiratory depression, inhibition of the hypothalamus-
pituitary axis, and permanent effects on sexual development and behavior (1-3).
Both compounds are concentrated, metabolized, bound stereospecifically, and produce their effects in the hypothalamus and limbic system (4,5), and show similar withdrawal syndromes (1,6). Thus, opiates appear to mimic steroid hormones.
Due to unavailability of [^{3}H]-opiate of high specific activity, [^{3}H]-steroid
binding to brain tissue or fractions was examined but was unsatisfactory due to
excessive non-competitive binding. Liver microsomes, however, did exhibit displaceable binding of labelled steroid.

Methods

Liver microsomes were isolated by centrifugation from 3-month old male
Sprague-Dawley rats and suspended in 0.01 M TRIS-HCl buffer, pH 7.4. [^{3}H]-tes-
tosterone, corticosterone, or progesterone (ca.100 Ci/mmol, New England Nuclear)
2×10^{-9} M, microsomes (15 mg of liver equiv.), and competing drug were incubated in a total volume of 0.4 ml buffer for 60 min at 4 C. The microsomes were
sedimented by centrifugation for 15 min and the supernatant aspirated. The
pellet was dissolved in 0.3 ml of 2N KOH at 65 C and 0.2 ml added to an appropriate scintillation medium. In several experiments drugs were tested at 6
dilutions, and the concentrations causing 50% depletion of bound steroid (ED_{50})
calculated.

Results and Discussion

Of a large number of substances tested, including compounds with major actions on the CNS, only opiates and steroids were effective in diminishing the
binding of [^{3}H]-steroid (Table I). Of the three labelled steroids tested, testosterone was most effectively displaced from the liver microsomes by the opiates,

---

[1]Associate of the MRC. [2]Supported by the Medical Research Council and the Non-
Medical Use of Drugs Directorate, Health and Welfare Canada.

In the study cited, the narcotic antagonists were as efficacious as the agonists in displacing labelled opiate and in our study in displacing labelled steroid. Morphine was only 1/60th as potent as methadone and about as potent as codeine. This finding was confirmed with different preparations of the drug and suggests that morphine is metabolized _in vivo_ to a more active metabolite.

TABLE I

RELATIVE POTENCIES OF DRUGS DISPLACING [^{3}H]-TESTOSTERONE FROM LIVER MICROSOMES

Drug	ED$_{50}$(μM)	Drugs with no effect at 10^{-5}M (< 10% displacement)	
Testosterone	0.1	Dopamine	Phenobarbital
Methadone	0.5	Serotonin	Pentobarbital
Corticosterone	1.2	Noradrenaline	Diphenylhydantoin
Meperidine	1.5	Melatonin	LH-RH
Levallorphan	2.3	Glutamate	GH-IH
Levorphanol	5.3	Glycine	TRH
Propoxyphene	13	Caffeine	Insulin
Naloxone	15	Thyroxine	Atropine
Nalorphine	16		
Codeine	30		
Morphine	30		

It should be noted that methadone more effectively displaced [^{3}H]-testosterone than did another steroid, corticosterone. Progesterone, however, was almost as effective as testosterone; both lack the 11-OH group found in corticosterone, and this substitution may inhibit binding. When [^{3}H]-progesterone was used the opiates competed much less effectively, although their relative potencies were essentially the same as when they competed with labelled testosterone. With [^{3}H]-corticosterone, the opiates competed least effectively. Competition of opiates with [^{3}H]-estradiol has not been adequately examined in this system because of the apparent high degree of non-displaceable binding shown by this steroid.

The opiate-specific competition for steroid binding sites supports the proposal that these drugs mimic steroid hormones. Opiates may potentiate endogenous steroid in target cells by displacement from sequestering sites and/or by inhibition of metabolism. We are currently carrying out competitive binding studies with [^{3}H]-opiate and brain tissue. In other studies from our laboratory (7) the absence of morphine antinociception in gonadectomized, but not adrenalectomized, rats strongly suggests that opiate action is mediated through receptors for endogenous sex steroid.

References

1. L.S. GOODMAN and A. GILMAN (eds.), The Pharmacological Basis of Therapeutics, pp. 237, 1538, 1604, MacMillan, London (1970).
2. W.R. BUCKETT, Adv. Steroid Biochem. Pharmacol. 3, 39-65 (1972).
3. J.W. SLOAN, in: Narcotic Drugs, D.H. Clouet, ed., pp. 262-282 (1971).
4. M.J. KUHAR, C.B. PERT and S. SNYDER, Nature 245, 447-450 (1973).
5. B.S. McEWEN, R.E. ZIGMOND and J.L. GERLACH, in: The Structure and Function of Nervous Tissue, G.H. Bourne, ed., 5, pp. 205-291 (1972).
6. P.H. HENNEMAN, D.M.K. WANG and J.W. IRWIN, J. Am. Med. Ass. 158, 384-386 (1955).
7. C. PINSKY, S.J. KOVEN and F.S. LaBELLA, this issue.

EVIDENCE FOR ROLE OF ENDOGENOUS SEX STEROIDS IN MORPHINE ANTINOCICEPTION

Carl Pinsky, Sheldon J. Koven and Frank S. LaBella

Department of Pharmacology and Therapeutics, Faculty of Medicine,
University of Manitoba, Winnipeg, Manitoba R3E OW3[1]

(Received in final form May 24, 1975)

Summary

The effect of morphine on responses to sustained mild pain
was tested in male white rats with gonads and (or) adrenals removed. Morphine was ineffective in gonadectomized rats; adrenalectomy alone increased the effectiveness of morphine over that
in sham-operated controls. Morphine antinociception may involve
some actions of endogenous steroids.

Endogenous substances may be involved in an adaptive system which functions in mammals to relieve the subjective distress of chronically-maintained
pain or noxious stimuli (1-4). LaBella (preceding paper, this issue) has
suggested that morphine analgesia may involve endogenous steroids, therefore
we examined the responses to sustained mild pain in rats deprived of their
major sources of endogenous steroids; i.e. by removal of the gonads and (or)
adrenals.

Methods

Male Sprague-Dawley white rats, 140-160 g, were prepared in three groups
of nine each: (i) adrenalectomized, (bilaterally); (ii) "steroidectomized"
(bilateral adrenalectomy with gonadectomy); (iii) sham-operated. The experimental groups were maintained for 4-6 da on standard feed with 0.9% saline
to drink ad lib., the sham-operated group had feed and water ad lib. Rats
were placed on a hotplate at 44.5 + 0.1 C and observed for 15 min while the
number of times they licked their paws was recorded. The 15-min experimental
period was divided into 22 epochs of 1.0 min each; each epoch overlapped its
predecessor by 20.0 seconds (Fig. 2). Latency to the first instance of paw-
licking was measured. Either saline or morphine sulphate (BDH) 5.0 mg kg^{-1}
was injected i.p. 20 min prior to placing the rat on the hotplate.

Results

Morphine (M) significantly increased latency ($p < 0.02$) to first paw-lick
in the sham-operated rats (Sh; Fig. 1), as compared to their saline-treated
(S) controls. The narcotic had a greater effect in the adrenalectomized (Ad)
rats ($p < 0.005$) but had no effect on latency in steroidectomized (St) rats
(Fig. 1). Responses to sustained (15 min) mild hotplate pain are shown in
Fig. 2. Morphine (M) significantly reduced the area under the curve (measured
over epochs 7-17, where paw-licking was greatest and locomotor excitement least)
as compared with the saline control group in adrenalectomized rats ($p < 0.02$).
The corresponding reduction was not significant in the sham-operated group
(Fig. 2). The narcotic slightly _increased_ the corresponding area in the ster-
oidectomized group.

[1]Supported by the Medical Research Council and the Non-Medical Use of
Drugs (NMUD) Directorate of Health and Welfare Canada

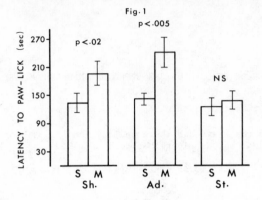

Fig. 1

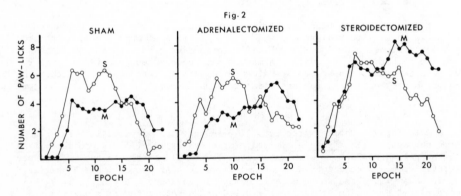

We have duplicated essentially these results with 21 rats from a different shipment. Also in that study we tested a group of gonadectomized rats (with unilateral adrenalectomy). The gonadectomized group did not respond to morphine either in latency or in measured curve area.

Fig. 2

Discussion

Our results indicate that, in male rats deprived of their gonads, morphine is ineffective in relieving the stress of mild pain. This suggests that mild pain may in some way mobilize an endogenous steroid of gonadal origin which acts to reduce nociception and that this substance, or its mobilizing mechanism, is potentiated by the morphine molecule. Moreover, adrenalectomy enhanced morphine antinociception. Hence the adrenals, in response to mild pain stress, may release a substance which antagonizes the effects of both the antinociceptive steroid and of morphine.

References

1. A. GOLDSTEIN, Life Sciences 14 615-623 (1974).
2. C.B. PERT and S.H. SNYDER, Science 179 1011-1014 (1973).
3. J. HUGHES, Brain Res. 88 295-308 (1975).
4. A. GOLDSTEIN, Invited Research Address, Can. Federation Biol. Soc. (1974).

STEREOSPECIFIC INCREASE BY NARCOTIC ANTAGONISTS OF
EVOKED ACETYLCHOLINE OUTPUT IN GUINEA-PIG ILEUM

Angela A. Waterfield and Hans W. Kosterlitz

Unit for Research on Addictive Drugs,
University of Aberdeen, Aberdeen, Scotland.

(Received in final form May 24, 1975)

In the myenteric plexus-longitudinal muscle preparation of the
guinea-pig ileum, naloxone (30-100 nM) increases the output of acetylcholine evoked by electrical field stimulation at 0.017 Hz and to a
lesser extent also at 10 Hz.   The stereospecific requirements for
this effect were studied with three pairs of optical isomers of
antagonists of the benzomorphan series.   The (-)-isomer of β-9-
methyl-5-phenyl-2-allyl-2'-hydroxy-6,7-benzomorphan (GPA 1843) which
had no agonist activity, had an effect similar to naloxone whereas the
(+)-isomer was inactive in this respect.   The (-)-isomer of
antagonists with even weak agonist activity gave variable results.
It is assumed that naloxone antagonises the action of enkephalin which
has been shown to be present in the guinea-pig ileum.   It is
recommended to establish the stereospecificity of an antagonist action
in order to exclude pharmacological effects not due to interaction
with opiate receptors.

Recently, it has been shown that the narcotic antagonist, naloxone, can
modify nociceptive reactions.   Thus, it reduces the antinociceptive effect of
electrical stimulation of the periaqueductal grey of the brain stem of rats
(1).   Naloxone also reduces the reaction time to nociceptive stimuli in rats
and mice (2).   These observations suggest the possibility that naloxone may
antagonize a neurotransmitter or neuromodulator which has an inhibitory effect
on the neuronal pathways responsible for the antinociceptive effects.

Since it cannot be excluded that a non-specific action of naloxone may
have contributed to the described effects, it was important to determine
whether the action of naloxone was stereospecific or not.   Very little is
known about the stereospecific requirements of pure antagonists although the
antagonist effect of compounds with dual agonist and antagonist actions is
highly stereospecific (3).   The main reason for this lack of information is
the small number of synthetic pure antagonists.

Under these circumstances, one of our in vitro models, the myenteric
plexus-longitudinal muscle preparation of the guinea-pig ileum was used to
study the effects of naloxone on the output of acetylcholine evoked by
electrical field stimulation.   When it was found that naloxone increased
the output, isomeric pairs of synthetic antagonists of the benzomorphan
series were examined for their relative agonist and antagonist properties.
The stereospecificity of the naloxone effect was then established with the
most suitable pair.

Methods

The methods used for the setting up of the myenteric plexus-longitudinal muscle preparation of the guinea-pig ileum, its stimulation by an electrical field (0.5 msec, supramaximal voltage), the collection of acetylcholine in the presence of physostigmine and its assay, have been described earlier (4).

Results

Properties of some Benzomorphan Antagonists with no or low Agonist Activity

Three pairs of benzomorphan antagonists were used. Two of them were N-furylmethyl analogues of the α-5,9-dialkyl-2'-hydroxy-6,7-benzomorphan series (Mr 1452/3 and Mr 2266/7) and the third was the N-allyl analogue of the β-9-methyl-5-phenyl-2'-hydroxy-6,7-benzomorphan series (GPA 1843/7). The structures are given in Fig. 1.

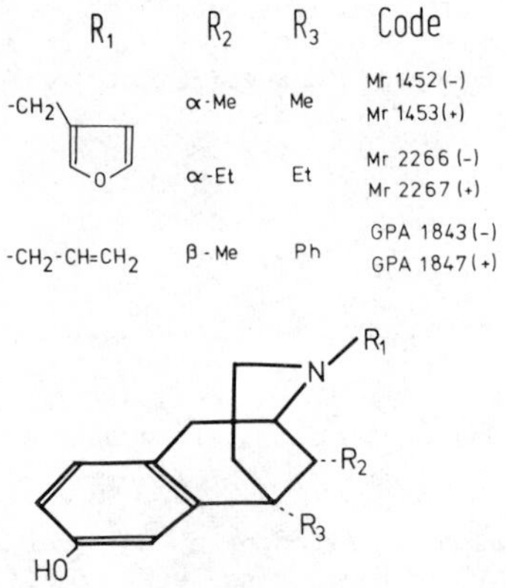

R_1	R_2	R_3	Code
-CH$_2$ (furyl)	α-Me	Me	Mr 1452 (-) / Mr 1453 (+)
	α-Et	Et	Mr 2266 (-) / Mr 2267 (+)
-CH$_2$-CH=CH$_2$	β-Me	Ph	GPA 1843 (-) / GPA 1847 (+)

FIG. 1

Structures of three pairs of benzomorphan antagonists.

TABLE 1

Assessment of antagonist potencies of stereoisomers of some benzomorphan antagonists with no or only low agonist ability

Compound	Number of observations	K_e (nM)	Relative potencies Agonist (Morphine = 1)	Relative potencies Antagonist (Naloxone = 1)
Mr 1452/3				
(-)	8	6.0 ± 0.32	low	0.20
(+)	9	132 ± 16	0	0.01
Mr 2266/7				
(-)	3	1.54 ± 0.09	low	0.79
(+)	5	41 ± 8.3	low	0.03
GPA 1843/7				
(-)	8	19.8 ± 3.9	0	0.062
(+)	7	1190 ± 415	low	0.001

The values of the equilibrium dissociation constants, K_e, are the means ± SEM. The compounds with low agonist activity had shallow dose-response curves with a maximum inhibition of the twitch of 30-40%. The Mr-compounds were supplied by C. H. Boehringer Sohn, Ingelheim (Dr. H. Merz) and the GPA-compound by Ciba-Geigy, Ardsley (Dr. F. H. Clarke).

The agonist and antagonist activities of these compounds were determined by assessment on the guinea-pig ileum (5). The antagonist potencies of the (+)-isomers were only 1.5 to 5% of the potencies of the corresponding (-)-isomers. Two of the (-)-isomers had weak agonist potency but the third (GPA 1843) was a pure antagonist (Table 1). Unfortunately, this compound had the lowest antagonist potency so that rather high concentrations were required to test for stereospecificity of the antagonist effects of naloxone; on the other hand, the difference between the potencies of the two stereoisomers was large.

Effect of Naloxone on evoked Acetylcholine Output from the Myenteric Plexus of the Guinea-Pig Ileum

In these experiments, the preparation of the longitudinal muscle with attached myenteric plexus was incubated in modified Krebs solution with 7.7 µM physostigmine sulphate for 1 hr to inactivate cholinesterase and obtain equilibrium between the various acetylcholine pools in the nerve terminals (M. Hutchinson and H. W. Kosterlitz, unpublished observations). The preparation was then stimulated repeatedly at 0.017 Hz (1/min) for 4 min and 10 Hz for 1 min until the outputs at the two frequencies remained constant. Naloxone hydrochloride was now added to the bath fluid to give a concentration of 100 nM and the preparation stimulated repeatedly at the two frequencies. The mean values of acetylcholine output before and after addition of naloxone are shown in Fig. 2. There was a mean increase of nearly 35% in the output due to stimulation at 0.017 Hz, the difference obtained by paired analysis being 277 ± 34 pmol g^{-1} pulse^{-1} (n = 22; P < 0.0005). At 10 Hz, the increase was 17%, with a difference of 1.55 ± 0.51 pmol g^{-1} pulse^{-1} (n = 7; P < 0.0125).

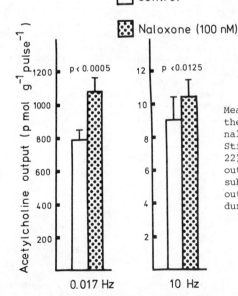

FIG. 2

Mean acetylcholine output in the absence and presence of naloxone (100 nM). Stimulation at 0.017 Hz (n = 22) or 10 Hz (n = 7). The output is given without subtraction of spontaneous output which is suppressed during stimulation (6).

When the effects of naloxone on the contractions of the preparation in the absence of physostigmine were studied, no potentiation was found. This result agrees with the findings of van Nueten and Lal (7) who, however, found an increase in the size of the contraction when the stimulation current was at just threshold strength.

Stereospecificity of the Increase in Acetylcholine Output caused by Narcotic Antagonists

In order to test for stereospecificity, the effects of the (-)-isomers were compared with those of the much less active (+)-isomers. It was important to choose a suitable concentration which gave unequivocal potentiation of the acetylcholine output with the (-)-isomers while the (+)-isomers were without effect.

Preliminary experiments showed that the most consistent results were obtained when the (-)-isomer of the compound was free of agonist potency. Since the N-(3-methylfuryl) compounds gave variable results they were found to be not very suitable although their antagonist potencies were closest to that of naloxone (Table 1). For instance, the (-)-isomer Mr 2266 (30-100 nM) increased the acetylcholine output caused by stimulation at 0.017 Hz in six out of ten experiments. The (+)-isomer had no significant effect on output. With the two isomers, Mr 1452 and Mr 1453, the results were not more definite.

The only compound of which the (-)-isomer had no agonist activity and of which the (+)-isomer was also available was β-9-methyl-5-phenyl-2-allyl-2'-hydroxy-6,7-benzomorphan (GPA 1843/7). Unfortunately the (-)-isomer had an antagonist potency of only 6% of that of naloxone (Table 1). It was therefore necessary to use a rather high concentration of this compound but neither the (-)-isomer nor the (+)-isomer had a non-specific depressant action at this concentration. As already stated the (-)-isomer was without agonist effect whereas the (+)-isomer caused a slight depression of the contraction of the longitudinal muscle of the guinea-pig ileum, an effect which was reversed by naloxone.

The design of the experiment consisted of continuous stimulation of the preparation at 0.017 Hz (1/min) with collection of the acetylcholine output for periods of 4 min every 10 min. When the output had become constant within the range of normal variation, the drug was added to give a concentration of 250 nM. After four to six collections of acetylcholine, the drug was washed out and further collections were made.

Typical experiments are shown in Fig. 3 in which the potentiation of acetylcholine by the (-)-isomer is shown whereas the (+)-isomer was ineffective.

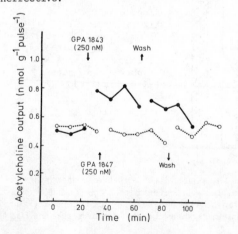

FIG. 3

Effects of optical isomers on the acetylcholine output due to stimulation at 0.017 Hz. (●), (-)-isomer, GPA 1843; (O), (+)-isomer, GPA 1847. Results obtained on separate preparations.

In six experiments with the (−)-isomer the mean increase in acetylcholine output was 121 ± 44 pmol g^{-1} pulse^{-1} (P < 0.025) whereas in four experiments with the (+)-isomer the difference was not significant (-42 ± 29 pmol g^{-1} pulse^{-1}). For a graphic presentation the first output of each experiment was taken to be 100 and the results before, during and after presence of the drug expressed as % of the first output (Fig. 4). Because of the large number of individual estimations, statistical evaluation had become more reliable; there was a highly significant increase in acetylcholine output due to the presence of the (−)-isomer (P < 0.001; 55 d.f.), whereas the effect of the (+)-isomer was now a decrease in output (P < 0.01; 36 d.f.). After washing out the drugs, there were no significant changes in output.

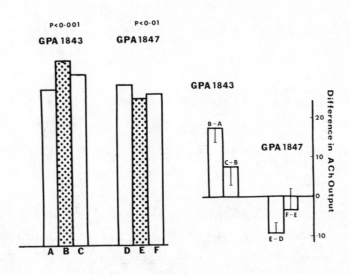

FIG. 4

The effects of the (−)-isomer, GPA 1843 and the (+)-isomer, GPA 1847 on the acetylcholine output due to stimulation at 0.017 Hz. A,D: before addition of drug; B,E: in presence of drug; C,F: after washing out of drug.

Discussion

The results presented in this paper show that the narcotic antagonist, naloxone, causes an increase in the output of acetylcholine from the myenteric plexus-longitudinal muscle preparation of the guinea-pig ileum when stimulated in vitro at 0.017 Hz (1/min) and to a lesser extent, at 10 Hz. The potentiation of acetylcholine output has been demonstrated to be stereo-specific since the (−)-isomer but not the (+)-isomer of β-9-methyl-5-phenyl-2-allyl-2'-hydroxy-6,7-benzomorphan has this effect.

These findings are indirect evidence of an endogenous ligand of the opiate receptor present in this preparation. Its functional importance appears to be the control of the output of acetylcholine from stimulated neurones of the myenteric plexus. Direct evidence for the presence of enkephalin in the guinea-pig ileum (0.8 μg equivalents of normorphine/g tissue) has been obtained recently (Hughes, Smith, Morgan and Fothergill, this volume).

It is of interest that naloxone does not increase the size of the contraction of the longitudinal muscle when the preparation is stimulated supra- or submaximally in the absence of physostigmine. This observation indicates that individual neurones appear to be fully activated even with submaximal stimulation, and that increase in the strength of stimulus leads to recruitment of further neurones.

In conclusion, it is important in _in_ _vitro_ or _in_ _vivo_ investigations to establish the stereospecificity of the action of a narcotic antagonist. This is particularly the case when the concentration of the antagonist is high or when circumstances are unusual, as for instance in the search for an endogenous ligand of the opiate receptor. Such a procedure will unmask pharmacological effects of antagonists which are not due to interaction with the opiate receptors.

Acknowledgements

Supported by grants from the U.S. National Institute on Drug Abuse (DA 00662) and the U.S. Committee on Problems of Drug Dependence, NRC-NAS.

References

1. H. AKIL, D. J. MAYER and J. C. LIEBESKIND, C.r. hebd. Séanc. Acad. Sci., Paris 274, 3603-3605 (1972)
2. J. J. JACOB, E. C. TREMBLAY and M.-C. COLOMBEL, Psychopharmacologia 37, 217-223 (1974)
3. H. W. KOSTERLITZ, H. O. J. COLLIER and J. E. VILLARREAL, Agonist and Antagonist Actions of Narcotic Analgesic Drugs. Macmillan, London (1972)
4. H. W. KOSTERLITZ, R. J. LYDON and A. J. WATT, Brit. J. Pharmacol. 39, 398-413 (1970)
5. H. W. KOSTERLITZ and A. J. WATT, Brit. J. Pharmacol. 33, 266-276 (1968)
6. H. W. KOSTERLITZ and A. A. WATERFIELD, Brit. J. Pharmacol. 40, 162-163P (1970)
7. J. M. VAN NUETEN and H. LAL, Archs int. Pharmacodyn 208, 378-382 (1974)

ANTAGONIST POTENCY AND RECEPTOR BINDING

Florin Ionescu*, Werner Klee†, and Robert Katz*

*Mid-Atlantic Research Institute,[1] 7315 Wisconsin Ave., Bethesda, MD 20014;
†National Institute of Mental Health, NIH, Bethesda, MD 20014.

(Received in final form May 24, 1975)

Receptor binding constants, using 3H-dihydromorphine and P_2
fraction of rat brain homogenate, have been determined for 28 narcotic antagonists. A good correlation (R = 0.92) has been obtained
between the binding constants and antagonist potency as determined
by Kosterlitz et al. using the guinea pig ileum preparation. It appears that the systems used in the correlation are useful in determining similarities or dissimilarities of guinea pig ileum and rat
brain receptors.

Binding constants (K_{RB}) for 28 antagonists were measured using 3H-dihydro-
morphine (3H-DHM) and the 10,000 g particulate fraction (P_2) of rat brain homogenate in, pH 8, sucrose-tris solution (1). The antagonist potencies (Ke) used

Table 1

No.	Compound	K_{RB} x 10^9	No.	Compound	K_{RB} x 10^9
1.	N-Me-allylnormor.	25.	15.	(−) BC 2887	2.
2.	Nalorphine	1.5	16.	Cyclazocine	0.8
3.	EN 2234A	2.	17.	Pentazocine	10.
4.	EN 1655A	1.	18.	(−) GPA 2163	12.
5.	EN 1620A	6.	19.	(+) GPA 1467	35.
6.	EN 1639A	0.2	20.	(−) GPA 1833	5.
7.	Naloxone	1.	21.	(−) GPA 3154	9.
8.	EFH-I-27-2	0.9	22.	(−) GPA 1894	23.
9.	EFH-I-47-1	20.	23.	(±) GPA 1364	50.
10.	Mr 1767-Ms	3.	24.	(−) GPA 1866	100.
11.	Levallorphan	0.62	25.	(±) Mr 1256-Ms	3.
12.	(−) BC 2605	0.5	26.	(−) Mr 1452-Ms	2.
13.	(−) BC 2888	0.2	27.	(±) Mr 1029-Ms	2.5
14.	(−) BC 2627	0.8	28.	Mr 1405-Cl	5.

in this study were all determined by Kosterlitz et al. (2,3), who used morphine
and the guinea pig ileum preparation in Krebs solution. A Hansch type multiple
regression analysis of the K_{RB} and the Ke values gave a relatively poor correlation (R = 0.70). From the plot (Figure 1), it is readily apparent that pentazocine provides the least fit in the regression line and, in fact, without
pentazocine, the correlation (0.92) is significantly improved.

[1]This research was supported by the National Institute on Drug Abuse
Grant DA-01037

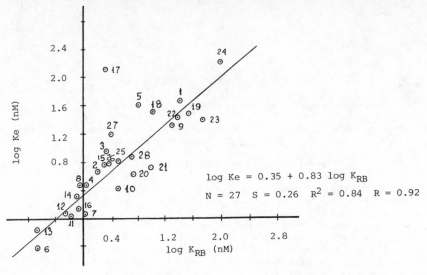

Figure 1

Correlation between antagonist potency (Ke) and receptor binding (K_{RB}).

Since Ke values presumably reflect binding to the guinea pig ileum receptor (GPIR), the above correlation suggests that the binding of 3H-DHM to rat brain receptor (RBR) and of morphine to GPIR is very similar. One might infer that GPIR and RBR are identical. However, recently a significant decrease in agonist binding, in the presence of Na^+, has been shown to occur (4,5). Taking this into account, it is reasonable to assume that 3H-DHM binding would be significantly different in the presence of sodium. Under such circumstances, the correlation obtained would indicate a proportionality in the two data sets in spite of the difference in the experimental conditions used for determination of Ke and K_{RB}. The present results, supplemented by K_{RB} values determined in the presence of NaCl should help us draw more definite conclusions about the identities of GPIR and RBR.

Acknowledgements

We wish to thank Drs. H.W. Kosterlitz and M. Hidalgo, and Mr. R. Streaty for their contribution.

REFERENCES

1. W.A. Klee and R. Streaty, *Nature 248* 61-63 (1974).
2. H. W. Kosterlitz and A.J. Watt, *Br. J. Pharmac. Chemother. 33* 266-276 (1968).
3. H. W. Kosterlitz, J.A.H. Lord, and A.J. Watt, in: *Agonist and Antagonist Actions of Narcotic Analgesic Drugs* (H.W. Kosterlitz, H.O.J. Collier, and J.E. Villareal, eds.), pp. 45-61. Baltimore, University Park Press (1973).
4. C.B. Pert, G. Pasternak, S.H. Snyder, *Science 182* 1359-1361 (1973).
5. C.B. Pert and S.H. Snyder, *Mol. Pharmacol. 10* 868-879 (1974).

OPIATE RECEPTORS AND THEIR INTERACTIONS WITH AGONISTS AND ANTAGONISTS

Eric J. Simon, Jacob M. Hiller, Irit Edelman,
Janice Groth and Kenneth D. Stahl

Department of Medicine, New York University Medical Center, New York, New
York 10016.[1]

(Received in final form May 24, 1975)

Independent evidence, derived from studies of the kinetics of
receptor inactivation by sulfhydryl reagents, is presented in support of a previously postulated allosteric model of the opiate receptor, in which sodium ions act as effectors. Scatchard analysis
provides evidence for cooperative binding, a characteristic of
allosteric systems. Both new and old evidence is cited which is
consistent with the hypothesis that agonists and antagonists bind
to the same receptor sites. These sites can exist in alternative
conformations that differ in their relative affinities for agonists
and antagonists.

Since the discovery of stereospecific binding sites for narcotic analgesics in animal brain (1,2,3) our laboratory has continued to devote much of
its research effort to the characterization and isolation of these sites.
Evidence from our laboratory and others is consistent with the hypothesis that
these binding sites represent pharmacological opiate receptors.
The present report deals with one aspect of our work in which we have
been studying the interaction of agonists and antagonists with receptor sites.
These studies have led us to postulate an allosteric model of the opiate
receptor, with sodium ions acting as allosteric effectors (4,5). We will present recent results which provide independent confirmation for this model.
Moreover, evidence will be presented which supports the contention that agonists and antagonists bind to the same site on the receptor.

Results

The Sodium Effect

Work in Snyder's laboratory (7) and our own (1) has led to the recogni-
tion that addition of sodium ions to the incubation medium results in an
increase in antagonist and a decrease in agonist binding. This is a highly
specific action of sodium, exhibited only somewhat by lithium and not at all
by the other alkali metal ions nor by other organic or inorganic cations.
Other cations, when added in sufficiently high concentrations, suppress the
binding of both agonists and antagonists. A study of the sodium effect in our
laboratory (4) has led us to conclude that the presence of Na^+ leads to an
increase in the affinity of antagonists and a decrease in the affinity of
agonists for the receptor. The total number of binding sites remains the
same. On the basis of these results we have postulated a model (4,5), according to which opiate receptors exist in (at least) two conformational states:

[1]Supported by grant DA-00017 from the National Institute on Drug Abuse.
Dr. Simon is a career scientist of the Health Research Council of the City of
New York.

a sodium-free state that binds a given agonist and a corresponding antagonist with about equal affinity and a sodium-dependent state which binds antagonists with considerably greater affinity than corresponding agonists.

Kinetics of Receptor Inactivation by Sulfhydryl Reagents and Protection by Opiates (6)

The inactivation of stereospecific etorphine binding by SH-reagents was reported by us earlier (1). We embarked on a detailed study of the kinetics of inactivation to learn more about the number of SH-groups involved and their functional significance. Most of these experiments were done with the alkylating agent N-ethylmaleimide (NEM), but similar results have been obtained with iodoacetamide and p-hydroxymercuribenzoate.

When membranes derived from a rat brain P_2 fraction were incubated with NEM for various periods there was a progressive decrease in the ability of membranes to bind labeled opiates stereospecifically. As shown in Fig. 1 the rate of inactivation follows pseudo-first order kinetics, consistent with the suggestion that alkylation of a single SH-group suffices to inactivate opiate binding. Identical results were obtained whether binding was assayed with the antagonist ^{3}H-naltrexone or the agonists ^{3}H-etorphine or ^{3}H-levorphanol.

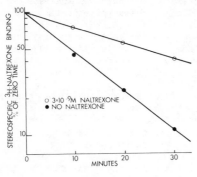

FIG. 1

Kinetics of receptor inactivation by NEM and protection by unlabeled naltrexone. A rat brain P_2 fraction was incubated with NEM (0.5 mM). Reaction was stopped by addition of tris-(2-carboxyethyl)-phosphine (2.5 mM) which rapidly destroys NEM. Stereospecific binding of ^{3}H-naltrexone was assayed as previously described (4). Results are expressed as percent of sample incubated zero time with NEM.

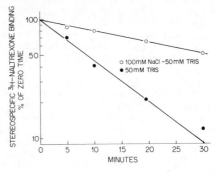

FIG. 2

Kinetics of receptor inactivation by NEM in the presence and absence of NaCl. Carried out as described in legend to Fig. 1.

It can also be seen from Fig. 1 that there is considerable protection against inactivation when incubation with NEM was carried out in the presence of unlabeled naltrexone. Similar protection has been observed with levorphanol. These experiments suggest that an SH-group essential for binding is located close to the opiate binding site of the receptor, though the possibility cannot be ruled out that the ligands induce a change in receptor conformation that make a distant SH-group less accessible to NEM.

Protection Against Inactivation by Sodium Ions

Fig. 2 shows the unexpected result we obtained when we carried out the incubation of P_2 membranes with NEM in the presence of 100 mM NaCl. The rate of inactivation of naltrexone binding (and of levorphanol and etorphine binding, not shown) was markedly slowed down in the presence of Na^+, from a half-time of 10 min. to one of 30 min. This is not due to an effect of NaCl on the alkylation reaction, since it was not observed when model SH compounds, such as glutathione, were reacted with NEM. We therefore postulated that the protective effect of Na^+ against SH-group inactivation is the result of a conformational change in the receptor molecule which renders SH-groups less accessible to NEM.

Our evidence suggests further that the alteration reflected in protection of SH-groups by Na^+ may be identical to that which results in enhanced antagonist and reduced agonist binding. Table 1 shows the effect of different alkali metal salts on the rate of inactivation by NEM. In addition to Na^+ only Li^+ has a slight protective effect, while K^+, Rb^+ and Cs^+ are totally inactive. When incubations were carried out in various concentrations of NaCl, protection was shown to increase from virtually none at 1 mM to maximal protection at 100 and 200 mM. The cation specificity as well as the concentration-response to Na^+ shown for the protection of SH-groups are identical to those previously reported for the changes in agonist and antagonist binding (4, 7).

TABLE 1

Effect of Cations on Receptor Inactivation by NEM

Time of Preincubation	Tris Only	KCl	RbCl	CsCl	LiCl	NaCl
(Min.)		^{3}H-naltrexone binding (% of zero time)				
5	73	72	75	-	81	85
10	45	51	51	50	65	78
20	22	24	27	24	42	65
30	12	11	17	12	32	48

All preincubations were carried out in the presence of 0.5 mM NEM in 50 mM Tris with appropriate salt added to final concentrations of 100 mM.

Properties of Opiate Receptors After Treatment With NEM

Pasternak and Snyder (8) reported recently that treatment with SH-reagents causes opiate receptors to "freeze" in the sodium-dependent form ("antagonist conformation" in the authors' language). Our evidence is not consistent with this suggestion. We have carried out binding studies after NEM treatment at concentrations of naltrexone and etorphine ranging from $10^{-10}M$ to $10^{-8}M$, in the presence and absence of NaCl. Such data for ^{3}H-naltrexone are shown in Fig. 3. It can be seen that the fraction of the binding remaining after NEM treatment is constant throughout the concentration range. Moreover, the dissociation constants of naltrexone are identical in control and NEM-treated membranes. Similar results for ^{3}H-etorphine are depicted in Fig. 4. In the absence of Na^+ the saturation curves in control and treated membranes again have similar half-saturation values (K_D's). In the presence of Na^+ the NEM-treated membranes exhibit a single K_D characteristic of the sodium-dependent conformation (2 nM), while controls show two K_D's (4), one due to the portion of receptors that remain in the sodium-free conformation ($K_D = 0.4$ nM). The latter appear to have been preferentially eliminated by NEM.

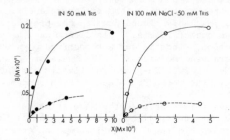

FIG. 3

Saturation curves for ^{3}H-naltrexone binding in NEM-treated membranes.
Binding was measured at ^{3}H-naltrexone concentrations between 10^{-10}M and
10^{-8}M. B = bound naltrexone and X = free naltrexone concentration
——— control, - - - - NEM-treated.

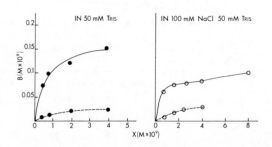

FIG. 4

Saturation curves for ^{3}H-etorphine binding in NEM-treated membranes.
Experiment identical to that in Fig. 3, except that binding of ^{3}H-etorphine
was measured.

We have also carried out a series of experiments which demonstrated that
conversion between the two conformational forms occurs very readily in receptors remaining active after NEM treatment. In fact, the sodium effect (enhancement of antagonist binding as well as reduction of agonist binding) was
consistently exaggerated after NEM treatment. We conclude from these results
that receptors whose SH-groups are alkylated are totally inactive in the
ligand concentration range studied, and that the residual active binding sites
have properties identical to receptors never exposed to NEM.

Cooperativity of Binding

A careful study of binding over a wide range of opiate concentrations
has yielded evidence for cooperativity of binding, a phenomenon normally
associated with allosteric (oligomeric) systems. Scatchard plots of the data
for ^{3}H-naltrexone binding in the presence and absence of NaCl are shown in

Fig. 5. The shapes of these curves are very similar to theoretical Scatchard plots for cooperative systems published by Changeux and Rubin (9). Scatchard plots for ^{3}H-etorphine binding are depicted in Fig. 6. The curve obtained in

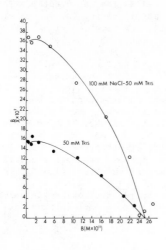

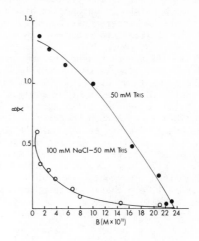

FIG. 5

Scatchard plots for saturation curves of ^{3}H-naltrexone binding in the presence and absence of NaCl. Binding was measured at ^{3}H-naltrexone concentrations ranging from 2 x 10[-11]M to 5 x 10[-8]M.

FIG. 6

Scatchard plots for saturation curves of ^{3}H-etorphine binding in the presence and absence of NaCl. Experiment identical to that in Fig. 5, except that binding of ^{3}H-etorphine was measured.

the absence of NaCl is similar to those for naltrexone, while the Scatchard plot for etorphine binding in 100 mM NaCl is biphasic, suggesting the presence of both conformations of the receptor, in agreement with out previous report (4). With the exception of the Scatchard plot for etorphine in NaCl, these curves bear little resemblance to those published by Pasternak and Snyder (8) for naloxone and dihydromorphine. The reason for the discrepancy is not known.

Discussion

The kinetics of receptor inactivation by sulfhydryl reagents in the presence and absence of NaCl lend independent support to the allosteric model of the opiate receptor. The shapes of the Scatchard plots of the saturation data provide evidence for cooperativity, a property considered essential for allosteric systems.

Our studies in NEM-treated membranes have provided evidence that receptors whose SH-groups have been alkylated are inactive throughout the range of drug concentrations studied. The residual active binding sites, rather than being "frozen" in one conformation, show ready and, in fact, more complete interconversion. This finding suggests a slight revision of our model: In the absence of Na[+] the receptor may exist in 2 forms (a dimeric and a monomeric form for purposes of discussion). The dimer is readily convertible to the Na[+]-dependent conformation, while the monomer is converted very slowly (dimerization may be the slow step). The residual Na[+]-free conformation that persists in 100 mM NaCl (4) may then be the monomer. Susceptibility to NEM inactivation seems to be even higher for the monomer than for the Na^+-free dimer, leaving, after NEM treatment, receptors greatly enriched in the dimeric form. This model could account for the absence of the Na^+-free conformation (monomer) in NaCl in NEM-treated membranes, as well as for the greater effect of Na^+ on agonist and antagonist binding. The latter finding is, in our view, also a possible interpretation of the differential inactivation of agonist binding by SH-reagents, observed by Wilson et al. (10), most markedly when binding took place in NaCl.

The evidence that agonists and antagonists bind to the same receptor site is as follows: Displacement experiments between agonists and antagonists exhibit competitive kinetics. The maximum number of binding sites is the same when estimated from agonist or antagonist binding. Sodium protects both agonist and antagonist sites against SH-group inactivation. Both agonists and antagonists can, in turn, protect against NEM inactivation of binding sites. In our hands, the effects of heat, chemical reagents and enzymes have been similar whether binding was measured with agonists or antagonists. Finally, as discussed earlier, the differential effects of protein reagents reported by Wilson et al. can be explained in ways other than the existence of separate binding sites for agonists and antagonists.

It is likely that more than one type of opiate receptor exists in animal and human brain. However, to date with our techniques we have obtained evidence for only one receptor which can exist in several states.

References

1. E.J. SIMON, J.M. HILLER and I. EDELMAN, Proc. Nat. Acad. Sci. U.S.A. 70, 1947-1949 (1973).

2. C.B. PERT and S.H. SNYDER, Science 179, 1011-1014 (1973).

3. L. TERENIUS, Acta Pharmacol. Toxicol. 32, 317-320 (1973).

4. E.J. SIMON, J.M. HILLER, J. GROTH and I. EDELMAN, J. Pharmacol. Exp. Therap. 192, 531-537 (1975).

5. E.J. SIMON, Neuroscience Res. Program Bull. 13, 43-50 (1975).

6. E.J. SIMON and J. GROTH, Proc. Nat. Acad. Sci. U.S.A. in press (1975).

7. C.B. PERT and S.H. SNYDER, Mol. Pharmacol 10, 868-879 (1974).

8. G.W. PASTERNAK and S.H. SNYDER, Nature 253, 563-565 (1975).

9. J.P. CHANGEUX and M.M. RUBIN, Biochemistry 7, 553-561 (1968).

10. H.A. WILSON, G.W. PASTERNAK and S.H. SNYDER, Nature 253, 448-450 (1975).

DIFFERENTIAL EFFECTS OF SODIUM ON TWO TYPES OF OPIATE BINDING SITES[1]

Tai Akera, Cheng-Yi Lee and Theodore M. Brody

Department of Pharmacology, Michigan State University,
East Lansing, Michigan 48824

Effects of Na^+ on saturable naloxone binding were
studied in vitro using particulate fractions obtained from
rat brain homogenates. Na^+ stimulated the saturable naloxone
binding in thalamus-hypothalamus regions, but inhibited it in
cerebellum. These findings strongly support the hypothesis
that two types of naloxone binding sites exist in brain tissues.

High affinity binding of opiates to nervous tissue in vitro has been shown
with several opiate agonists and antagonists. In a previous study (1), we have
shown that naloxone has at least two saturable binding sites, one of which is
not available to an agonist, dihydromorphine. This naloxone-specific binding
site is the major fraction of opiate binding in the cerebellum but is a minor
fraction in the thalamus-hypothalamus in which a predominant fraction of the
opiate binding sites is capable of binding both naloxone and dihydromorphine.
These two types of opiate binding sites differ in their affinity for dihydromorphine and naloxone. In the present study, quantitative differences between
these two types of opiate binding sites were further explored by their response to Na^+, since the Na^+ effect is one of the distinguishing characteristics of opiate binding to brain tissue in vitro (2-4).

Methods

Brain homogenates obtained from various regions of male Sprague-Dawley
rats (200 grams) were centrifuged at 100,000 x g for 60 min and the resulting
sediment rehomogenized in 50 mM Tris-HCl buffer (pH 7.4). The binding of (^{3}H)-
naloxone (New England Nuclear, Boston, Mass.; specific activity, 23.6 Ci/mmole)
was assayed in the above buffer in the presence and absence of 20 μM nonlabelled naloxone. After a 15-min incubation at 35°C, tissue-bound (^{3}H)-na-
loxone was separated from unbound (^{3}H)-naloxone with a Millipore filter system
and the bound (^{3}H)-naloxone trapped on the filter was estimated using liquid
scintillation counting. The saturable binding is the difference in (^{3}H)-na-
loxone binding observed in the absence and presence of excess non-labelled
naloxone. Protein was assayed by the method of Lowry et al. (5).

Results

The saturable binding of (^{3}H)-naloxone to the particulate fraction obtained from the thalamus-hypothalamus region ranged from 62 to 24 percent of
the total naloxone binding with (^{3}H)-naloxone concentrations of 1 to 25 nM in
the incubation medium. The maximal binding calculated from the Scatchard plot
of the data was 0.383±0.025 pmoles/mg protein and the Km value was 8.95±0.81 nM

[1] This work was supported by the Department of the Navy, Office of Naval
Research, NR-305-958.

(n=14). The saturable naloxone binding was increased in the presence of 50 mM NaCl. With 5 and 10 nM (^{3}H)-naloxone, the increase was 54 and 33%, respectively. Since the maximal binding capacity was unchanged by Na$^+$, the enhancement of the saturable binding with Na$^+$ was greater at lower (^{3}H)-naloxone concentrations, but diminished at higher concentrations. When the concentration of NaCl was increased to 100 or 150 mM, the enhancement of the saturable naloxone binding became less, indicating the biphasic nature of the Na$^+$-effect. The saturable naloxone binding was significantly reduced with 50 mM KCl added to the incubation mixture. The inhibitory effect of KCl was shared by many other monovalent cations but not by sucrose, suggesting an ionic inhibition of the saturable naloxone binding. Thus, it appears that the biphasic effects of Na$^+$ on the saturable naloxone binding is due to a Na$^+$-specific enhancement of the binding and an inhibition due to the cationic property of Na$^+$. Scatchard plot analyses of the data revealed that 50 and 100 mM Na$^+$ increased the affinity of the saturable binding sites for naloxone. At 150 mM, however, the Na$^+$-induced increase in the affinity was not significant. Na$^+$ failed to affect the maximal naloxone binding at all concentrations studied. K$^+$ decreased the affinity for naloxone and also appears to decrease maximal naloxone binding. The change in the latter parameter, however, was not significant.

The results of similar experiments performed with particulate fractions obtained from cerebellar homogenate were different. With cerebellar particulate fractions, the saturable (^{3}H)-naloxone binding accounted for 13 to 10 percent of the total binding with (^{3}H)-naloxone concentrations ranging from 2 to 25 nM. Na$^+$, as well as K$^+$, markedly decreased the saturable naloxone binding. At no concentration, did Na$^+$ enhance the saturable naloxone binding to the cerebellum.

Discussion

The enhancement of (^{3}H)-naloxone binding by Na$^+$ in particulate fractions obtained from rat brain thalamus-hypothalamus homogenates is consistent with previous reports (2-4). The present data support the contention by Simon et al. (6) that the Na$^+$-induced increase in opiate antagonist binding is primarily due to an increased affinity but not due to the unmasking of new binding sites. In cerebellum, however, Na$^+$ reduced the saturable (^{3}H)-naloxone binding. The presence of relatively large non-saturable binding in cerebellar tissue precluded detailed kinetic analyses and hence it is not known if the effect of Na$^+$ or K$^+$ on the saturable naloxone binding in cerebellum is due to a change in affinity or maximal binding capacity. Nevertheless, it is clear from the present data that the properties of the saturable naloxone binding site in cerebellum are different from those of the binding site in the thalamus-hypothalamus region. These data strongly support the hypothesis that two qualitatively different binding sites exist in rat brain tissue.

References

1. C. Y. Lee, T. Akera, S. Stolman and T. M. Brody, J. Pharmac. exp. Ther. (in press).
2. C. B. Pert, G. Pasternak and S. H. Snyder, Science 182, 1359-1361 (1973).
3. C. B. Pert and S. H. Snyder, Mol. Pharmac. 10, 868-879 (1974).
4. R. J. Hitzemann, B. A. Hitzemann and H. H. Loh, Life Sic., 14, 2393-2404, (1974).
5. O. H. Lowry, N. J. Rosebrough, A. L. Farr and R. J. Randall, J. Biol. Chem. 193, 265-275 (1951).
6. E. J. Simon, J. M. Hiller, J. Groth and I. Edelman, J. Pharmac. exp. Ther. 1925, 531-537 (1975).

COMPETITIVE INHIBITION OF STEREOSPECIFIC OPIATE BINDING BY LOCAL ANESTHETICS IN MOUSE BRAIN[1]

Gale L. Craviso and José M. Musacchio[2]

Department of Pharmacology, New York University School of Medicine, New York, New York 10016

(Received in final form May 24, 1975)

Cationic local anesthetics inhibit competitively the stereospecific binding of naltrexone and etorphine on the mouse brain opiate receptor. In contrast, the inhibition produced by benzocaine, a non-cationic local anesthetic, is non-competitive. It is suggested that the cationic group of local anesthetics interacts with a specific anionic binding site on the opiate receptor and that there are certain structural similarities between the receptors for both types of drugs. It is evident from these studies that several drugs can unspecifically modify the pharmacologic effects of opiates and that they could be useful tools to further characterize the opiate receptor.

Stereospecific opiate binding sites have been described in the brain and in other tissues (1,2,3,4). The opiate receptors bind radioactive narcotics and narcotic antagonists with an affinity that correlates well to their relative potency in several pharmacological preparations and to their clinical effectiveness. There is considerable evidence indicating that sodium, through an allosteric mechanism, decreases the binding of opiate agonists and increases the binding of antagonists (4,5). Since several drugs and toxins are known to interfere with sodium movements through biological membranes and since the opiate receptor could be involved in the control of these sodium movements, we thought it would be interesting to test the effects of some of these drugs on the opiate receptor stereospecific binding. Additional drugs were tested either because they have local anesthetic properties in high concentrations or because they are known to interact with narcotic effects in some test systems.

Methods

The cortex from male Swiss Webster mice (24-30 g) was homogenized in 0.05 M Tris-Cl, pH 7.4 and diluted to a final concentration of 1 gm per 150 ml of buffer. Aliquots of the homogenate (1.9 ml) were preincubated in the presence of 10^{-7}M dextrorphan or levorphanol and the appropriate test drug for 10 min at 25°C; after the addition of the radioactive naltrexone or etorphine, samples were incubated for 30 min. The reaction was stopped by transfering the samples to an ice-water bath. Each sample was filtered essentially as described by Pert and Snyder (3) and the radioactivity retained in the glass-fiber filters was determined by liquid scintillation spectrometry.

---

[1] These studies were supported by PHS grant # DA-00351.
[2] Research Scientist awardee grant # 1-K5-MH-17785.

Drugs were donated by the following companies: Ayerst (d- and l-propranolol HCl, pronethalol HCl, practolol HCl); Abbott (pramoxine HCl); Astra (lidocaine HCl, prilocaine HCl, 6211); Lilly (piperocaine HCl); Roche (RO 20-1724); Winthrop (mepivacaine HCl); Squibb (procainamide HCl); Boehringer Sohn (dipyridamole); Smith, Kline and French (chlorpromazine, chlorpromazine sulfoxide). All other drugs were obtained from commercial sources. Etorphine-15,16-^{3}H (21 Ci/mmole) and naltrexone-15, 16-^{3}H (16.3 Ci/mmole) were obtained from the National Institute of Drug Abuse and they were used at the original specific activities.

Results

The effect of several drugs on the stereospecific binding of naltrexone-^{3}H (1 nM) is shown in Table 1. Procaine, at a local anesthetic concentration

TABLE I

Effect of Various Drugs on the Stereospecific Binding of Naltrexone-15,16-^{3}H

	Concen. (mM)	% Inhib		Concen. (mM)	% Inhib
Procaine	5.0	100	Dipyridamole	0.1	20
Diphenhydramine	2.0	97	RO 20-1724	0.1	5
Tripelennamine	1.0	95	Papaverine	0.1	75
Cyclizine	0.33	89	Chlorpromazine	0.01	22
d-Propranolol	0.1	52	"	0.1	97
l-Propranolol	0.1	55	Chlorpromazine sulfoxide	0.1	76
Practolol	0.5	52	Diphenylhydantoin	0.1	6
Pronethalol	0.2	87	"	0.8	29
Isoproterenol	0.1	0	Phenobarbital	5.0	3
Quinidine	0.01	77	Amiloride	0.001	0
Quinine	0.05	80	Tetrodotoxin	0.001	2
Theophylline	0.5	23			

(5 mM), produced a complete inhibition of stereospecific binding. Some antihistamines, β-blocking agents, chlorpromazine, chlorpromazine sulfoxide, etc., in concentrations at which they are known to produce local anesthesia, also produced a considerable degree of inhibition. Quinine and quinidine were effective inhibitors of stereospecific binding in concentrations at which they have antiarrhythmic effects. Of several phosphodiesterase inhibitors tested, only papaverine inhibited the binding of naltrexone. Diphenylhydantoin, phenobarbital, amiloride and tetrodotoxin were inactive in concentrations at which they exert their specific pharmacological effects.

The log probit analysis of inhibition of stereospecific naltrexone binding by some local anesthetics was compared with that of naloxone (Fig. 1) and levorphanol (not shown) and found to be parallel in most cases, indicating that the opiate ligand and the local anesthetic compete for the same population of binding sites. The reason why some of the local anesthetics show a slight deviation from a parallel log probit plot is not apparent at the present time.

FIG. 1

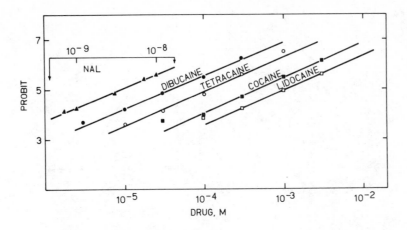

Log probit analysis of inhibition of stereospecific naltrexone binding by naloxone (NAL) and several local anesthetics. Naltrexone-3H (1 nM) was incubated in duplicate with the concentrations of different drugs indicated in the abscissa.

The parallel plots obtained for levorphanol, naloxone and most of the local anesthetics tested suggested that the interaction between the opiate ligands and the local anesthetics could be of a competitive nature. The competition between local anesthetics and opiate agonists and antagonists for the opiate binding sites was studied in experiments that could be analyzed with the aid of Klotz double reciprocal and Scatchard plots. Typical results are illustrated in Fig. 2. These results demonstrate that the interaction between tetracaine on one side, and naltrexone on the other side, is competitive in nature; similar results were obtained for etorphine.

In contrast, benzocaine, a local anesthetic of a different class that does not carry a positive charge, inhibited the binding of naltrexone non-competitively (Fig. 3).

The slopes and constants obtained from the regression lines of the double reciprocal plots were used to calculate the K_i's for the different local anesthetics (Table 2); it is apparent that in general, the most potent local anesthetics are more effective in competing with naltrexone-3H for the opiate receptor. It is also apparent from Table 2 that benzocaine is several fold less effective than the rest.

Discussion

As we have indicated, the interactions between sodium and narcotic agonists and antagonists at the opiate receptor level prompted us to test the effects of several compounds which are known to interfere with sodium movements through membranes. Tetrodotoxin, which is one of the most potent nonprotein poisons known, acts by blocking nerve membrane sodium channels (6); the toxin binds to the exterior opening of the channel and it is quite ineffective

FIG. 2

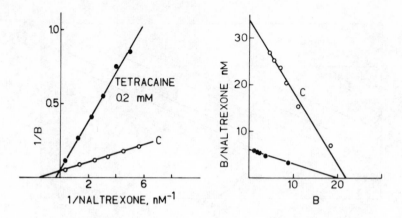

Effect of 0.2 mM tetracaine on the stereospecific binding of
naltrexone. Results were calculated from duplicate samples and
plotted according to Klotz at left, and to Scatchard at right.
B: pmoles of stereospecific bound naltrexone-^{3}H per g of brain
cortex.

FIG. 3

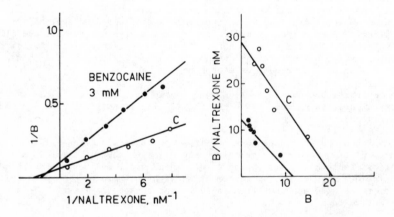

Effect of 3 mM benzocaine on the stereospecific binding of
naltrexone-[3]H. Experiment is similar to the one described in
Fig. 2.

TABLE 2

K_i (mM) of Some Local Anesthetics for the Inhibition of Naltrexone-^{3}H
Stereospecific Binding

Dibucaine	0.02	Procaine	0.17
Piperocaine	0.03	Mepivacaine	0.24
Tetracaine	0.04	Procainamide	0.37
Pramoxine	0.12	Lidocaine	0.52
Cocaine	0.15	6211 (Astra)	0.85
Prilocaine	0.16	Benzocaine	2.21

The K_i's for the different local anesthetics were calculated
from the slopes and constants obtained from the regression
lines of Klotz plots.

when applied inside the axon (7). As shown in Table 1, tetrodotoxin has no
effect on naltrexone binding; moreover, other experiments (not reported here)
demonstrated that tetrodotoxin does not block the sodium enhancement of
naltrexone binding. These findings indicate that the opiate receptor does not
have any tetrodotoxin binding site.

Local anesthetics have more than one mechanism of action (8). The most
effective local anesthetics carry a cationic charge and act at a receptor site
on the axoplasmic end of the sodium channel; this has been established by
studying the effects of quaternary ammonium local anesthetic analogs that block
sodium currents only when they are applied on the axoplasmic side of the membrane and not on the exterior of the nerve (10,11,12). This local anesthetic
binding site is different from the tetrodotoxin site as demonstrated by direct
competition studies (13,14).

In addition, there are several compounds that act as local anesthetics
and do not carry a positive charge at physiological pH. These compounds are
thought to block nerve conduction by disorganizing the membrane structure
around the sodium channels and in this way block sodium conductance (9). A
typical example of this kind of compound is benzocaine. It has been proposed
that the fraction of unionized molecules of local anesthetics that have an
amino group may also act by this mechanism (8).

The existence of certain similarities between the opiate and the local
anesthetic receptor is suggested by the following findings: 1) there is a
direct competition between local anesthetics and opioids for the opiate receptor binding sites; 2) this competition takes place with concentrations of
local anesthetics that produce nerve blockade; 3) the more potent local
anesthetics are also more potent inhibitors of opiate stereospecific binding;
and 4) other drugs such as antihistamines, antiarrhythmic drugs, tranquilizers,
etc. that have local anesthetic effects in high concentrations also interfere
with stereospecific opiate binding. The finding that cationic local anesthetics
act competitively with opioids suggests that the cationic group of local
anesthetics interacts with a specific anionic binding site on the opiate receptor. That the inhibition of naltrexone binding by benzocaine is non-
competitive is consistent with the disrupting effect that non-cationic local
anesthetics are thought to have on membranes.

Despite the existence of certain similarities between the opiate and the local anesthetic receptor, it is evident that they are two distinct structures. Regional distribution studies indicate that the opiate receptor is not uniformly distributed in nervous tissue (15,16) while all nerves are susceptible to the effects of local anesthetics. The cellular localization of both receptors also seems to be different. The local anesthetic receptor is intracellular while the opiate receptor should be extracellular in order to be accessible to the endogenous ligand, which is known to be a polypeptide of relatively large size (17,18) and therefore not expected to pass through cell membranes unless there is a specialized uptake system.

The finding that other drugs such as quinidine can interact with the opiate receptor at very low concentrations ($K_i = 0.73\,\mu M$) suggests that many drugs may interact with certain narcotic effects by other than their specific pharmacologic actions. This idea is supported by the report that eserine, in μM concentrations, can displace dihydromorphine from particulate fractions of rat brain homogenates (19). Therefore, it is recommended that when interactions between narcotics and other drugs are described, the possibility of unspecific interaction should be considered and ruled out by appropriate studies. It is evident from our studies that local anesthetics and other drugs that interact with opiate stereospecific binding could be useful tools to further characterize the opiate receptor.

References

1. A. Goldstein, L.I. Lowney, and B.K. Pal, Proc. Nat. Acad. Sci. USA 68: 1742-1747 (1971).

2. L. Terenius, Acta Pharmacol. Toxicol. 32: 317-320 (1973).

3. C.B. Pert and S.H. Snyder, Science 179: 1011-1014 (1973).

4. E.J. Simon, J.M. Hiller, and I. Edelman, Proc. Nat. Acad. Sci. USA 70: 1947-1949 (1973).

5. C.B. Pert and S.H. Snyder, Molec. Pharmacol. 10: 868-879 (1974).

6. C.Y. Kao and A. Nishiyama, J. Physiol. London 180: 50-66 (1965).

7. T. Narahashi, N.C. Anderson, and J.W. Moore, J. Gen. Physiol. 50: 1413-1428 (1967).

8. B.H. Takman, Br. J. Anaest. 47: 183-190 (1975).

9. P. Seeman, Pharmacol. Rev. 24: 583-655 (1972).

10. D.T. Frazier, T. Narahashi, and M. Yamada, J. Pharmacol. Exp. Ther. 171: 45-51 (1970).

11. T. Narahashi and D.T. Frazier, Neurosciences Res. 4: 65-99 (1971).

12. G.R. Strichartz, J. Gen. Physiol. 62: 37-57 (1973).

13. D. Colquhoun, R. Henderson, and J.M. Ritchie, J. Physiol. 227: 95-126 (1972).

14. R. Henderson, J.M. Ritchie, and G.R. Strichartz, J. Physiol. 235: 783-804 (1973).

15. M.J. Kuhar, C.B. Pert, and S.H. Snyder, Nature 245: 447-450 (1973).

16. J.M. Hiller, J. Pearson, and E.J. Simon, Res. Comm. Chem. Path. Pharmacol. 6: 1052-1061 (1973).

17. L. Terenius and A. Wahlstrom, Acta Pharmacol. Toxicol. 35 (Suppl):55(1974).

18. J. Hughes, Brain Res. 88: 295-308 (1975).

19. W.A. Klee and R.A. Streaty, Nature 248: 61-63 (1974).

ON THE USE OF TRYPTIC DIGESTION TO LOCALIZE NARCOTIC BINDING MATERIAL

Robert J. Hitzemann and Horace H. Loh

Langley Porter Neuropsychiatric Institute and
Department of Pharmacology, University of California,
San Francisco, California 94143

(Received in final form May 24, 1975)

Trypsin (EC 3.4.4.4) has been successfully used to determine the internal or external position of membrane proteins (1). Trypsin does not penetrate through the membrane and thus only those proteins which are partially or completely located on the external surface of the membrane will be susceptible to tryptic activity (1). The highest subcellular density of the narcotic receptor material or, more precisely, stereospecific narcotic binding material (SNBM) is located in the nerve ending particle (NEP) fraction and in particular in the synaptic plasma membrane (SPM) fraction (2,3). Furthermore, SNBM is exquisitely sensitive to degradation by trypsin (4). Since NEP may be considered miniature cells, it should be possible to localize the internal or external membrane location of the SNBM by incubating intact NEP with trypsin under various buffer conditions. In the present experiments, both purified NEP and a well-washed brain mitochondrial fraction (5) were used to assess trypsin's effects. The mitochondrial fraction gave no significantly different data than the purified NEP; this is not unexpected since a washed mitochondrial fraction contains 30 to 40% NEP (5) with the remainder of the fraction being primarily mitochondria and myelin fragments which have little, if any, SNBM (2,3).

Binding was measured by incubating 1 mg of brain mitochondrial or NEP protein in 2 ml of 5 mM tris buffer (pH = 7.4, 33° C) with either ^{3}H-levorphanol or ^{3}H-dextrorphan (specific activity 4 Ci/mmol) for 15 min, filtering the reaction mixture over GFC filters and washing the filter 3 times with ice-cold buffer. Stereospecific binding (SsB) was defined as ^{3}H-levorphanol bound minus ^{3}H-dextrorphan bound. In all experiments to be described, the NEP were lysed in 5 mM tris (pH = 8.2, 4° C) for 1 hr prior to the binding assay per se. After lysis, the mixture was centrifuged and resuspended in fresh 5 mM tris buffer (pH = 7.4, 33° C).

The binding of ^{3}H-levorphanol and ^{3}H-dextrorphan to normal lysed NEP suggested that there were only two types of binding sites present, namely, high affinity, low capacity stereospecific sites and low affinity, non-saturable sites. Maximal SsB occurred at 10^{-7} M drug concentrations. NEP were incubated with various amounts of trypsin in either 5 mM tris (pH = 7.4), Krebs-Ringer-Bicarbonate (KRB) buffer (pH = 7.4) or 0.32 M sucrose plus 5 mM tris (pH = 7.4). The mixture was incubated 15 min at 33° C before adding an equi-weight amount of trypsin soybean inhibitor and then centrifuging the mixture. The tissue pellets from all groups were then resuspended in cold 5 mM tris for lysis. In both the hypotonic tris buffer and the isotonic sucrose buffer groups as little as 1 ug of trypsin/mg protein significantly decreased SsB. However, in the

This investigation was supported in part by NIDA Grant DA-00564.

KRB buffer group, no decrease in binding was observed until the trypsin concentration reached 30 ug/mg protein. The inhibition of binding observed in the sucrose buffer group could be reversed by replacing sucrose with NaCl during the tryptic digestion. Some reversal was noted at 50 mM NaCl and complete reversal was observed at 125 mM NaCl. The ability of NaCl to reverse the effects of trypsin does not seem to be related to a decrease in enzyme viability. Using the artificial substrate BAFE, it was found that trypsin was at least twice as active in salt solutions as compared to 5 mM tris or the sucrose buffer.

At 10 ug/mg NEP protein trypsin had virtually no effect on SsB when KRB buffer was used but decreased binding 50 to 60 percent when the sucrose buffer was used. NEP digested with 10 ug of trypsin/mg protein in either KRB or sucrose buffer were analyzed for modifications in protein structure by means of SDS-disc gel electrophoresis. Trypsin significantly modified the protein patterns when either KRB or sucrose buffer was used. However, it was observed that there was a significantly greater reduction in high molecular weight material in the sucrose buffer gel. This data was of particular interest for the following reason. Previous studies in our laboratory have established that the high molecular weight gel region is particularly rich in SPM glycoproteins (unpublished observation). Since membrane glycoproteins extend into the external mileau and since they contain sulfate and carboxyl moieties which can bind cations, it is not unreasonable to consider that the narcotic receptor could be a glycoprotein. However, the role of glycoprotein carboxyl groups in binding is apparently not important since extensive neuraminidase treatment does not decrease SsB (4). The binding of narcotics to sulfated glycoproteins would be in many respects similar to the binding of narcotics to cerebroside sulfate previously demonstrated in our laboratory (6).

The present data demonstrate that the SNBM is probably located on the external surface of the NEP and that the ability of trypsin to digest the binding material is markedly dependent on the ionic conditions in the external mileau.

References

1. STECK, T.L., in Membrane Research (ed. FOX, C.F.) pp. 71-93, Academic Press, New York (1972).
2. HITZEMANN, R.J., HITZEMANN, B.A. AND LOH, H.H. Life Sci. 14, 2393,(1974).
3. PERT, C.B., SNOWMAN, A.M., AND SNYDER, S.H. Brain Res. 70, 184 (1974).
4. PASTERNAK, G.W., AND SNYDER, S.H. Mol. Pharmacol. 10, 183 (1974).
5. COTMAN, C.W., in Methods in Enzymology, Vol. 31, (eds. FLEISCHER, S., and PACKER, L.) p. 449, Academic Press, New York (1974).
6. LOH, H.H., CHO, T.M., WU, Y.C. AND WAY, E.L. Life Sci. 14, 2231 (1974).

OPIATE BINDING TO CEREBROSIDE SULFATE:
A MODEL SYSTEM FOR OPIATE-RECEPTOR INTERACTION

Horace H. Loh, T. M. Cho, Y. C. Wu, R. A. Harris and E. L. Way

Langley Porter Neuropsychiatric Institute
and
Department of Pharmacology
University of California
San Francisco, California 94143

(Received in final form May 24, 1975)

Summary

Cerebroside sulfate was shown to bind etorphine and levorphanol with high affinity. The relative potency of narcotic
analgesics in preventing the binding of levorphanol to cerebroside sulfate correlated well with their reported analgetic
activity. The data indicate similarities between cerebroside
sulfate and a purified opiate receptor from mouse brain which
has been reported to be a proteolipid. Some preliminary animal data also imply the involvement of CS in opiate action
We, therefore, propose that CS may serve as a useful "receptor" model for the study of opiate-receptor interaction in vitro.

Numerous attempts have been made to elicit the mechanism of action
of morphine and its surrogates in analgesia, tolerance and physical dependence. The central concern of recent reseach has been to identify
and isolate the "receptor(s)" with which opiates interact and to study its
pharmacologic properties. Initial attempts to identify selective opiate-
receptor interaction by comparing the distribution and binding characteristics of pharmacologically active and inactive isomers, or reduced binding of agonists in the presence of an antagonist, were unsuccessful (1-5).
Recently, Goldstein et al (6) elaborated a procedure for demonstrating
stereospecific binding and reported that mouse brain contains a fraction
that binds opiates stereospecifically. Subsequently, several groups of investigators, using an antagonist (7) and various agonists (8-11) with high
specific radioactivity, have unequivocally demonstrated stereospecific binding of narcotics to nerve membranes (12).

Stereospecific binding to membrane is a necessary, but not a sufficient, requisite for identifying the opiate receptor(s). Other criteria
which have been applied include saturability, target cell specificity and
demonstrating a correlation between affinities of various opiates with their
analgetic potency. Moreover, the affinity for the opiate should be compatible with the brain concentrations of the drug necessary for eliciting
pharmacologic action (12).

In our laboratory, we have been investigating membrane constituents

Supported in part by U.S. Army Research and Development Command Contract #DADA-17-73-C-3006.

of the brain which may serve as a binding site(s) for opiate agonists and antagonists. In exploring this avenue, we have examined a number of molecular models and have observed that parts of the structures of several membrane acidic lipids appear to exhibit structural complimentariness to opiates. As a consequence, an investigation of these substances as stereospecific binding sites for opiates was initiated (13, 14).

Structural complimentariness: Based on molecular models, it appears that one conformer of CS, as shown in Fig. 1, appeared to fulfill the requisites of the analgetic receptor postulated by Beckett and Casy (15). Fig. 1 shows that several parts of the structure of CS exhibit structural complimentariness to opiates and the interactions between opiates and CS may involve electrostatic attraction, hydrogen bonding and hydrophobic interactions. Our subsequent studies have indicated that the SO_4 moiety of CS is an important anionic site for the interaction with the protonated N in the opiate molecule. This is in agreement with the concept of receptor postulated by Portoghese (16).

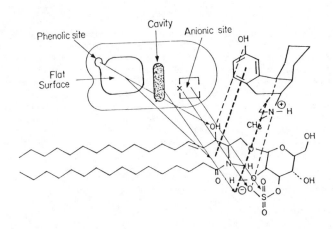

Fig. 1 - A comparison between the molecular model of CS and the postulated opiate receptor (15) and their possible sites of interaction with a narcotic.

Properties of opiate binding to cerebrosides: Initially, the binding of opiates to liposomes prepared from commercial cerebroside (13) was studied according to a modification of the method of Goldstein et al (6). Using this system, substantial amounts of ^{3}H-naloxone and ^{3}H-etorphine were shown to be bound (13) and about 20-30% of the total binding was stereospecific. However, the commerical source of cerebroside consists of 4 different compounds: cerebroside, hydroxycerebroside, cerebroside sulfate, and hydroxycerebroside sulfate. The latter two sulfated derivatives comprise about 10-15% of the total material (unpublished data). Thus, when concentration binding curves were made (Fig. 2), four plateaus were observed indicating multiple binding affinities. With ^{3}H-etorphine, the highest affinity binding appeared to reach saturation at about 10 nM and this was attributed to binding to hydroxycerebroside sulfate; another binding plateau at 40 nM was found to be due to the binding to cerebroside sulfate. The other two sites of lesser affinity but higher capacity were related to ^{3}H-etorphine binding to hydroxy and non-hydroxycerebroside.

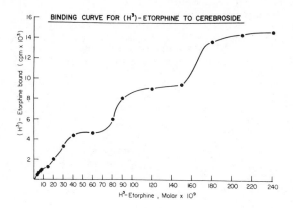

Fig. 2 - H^3-etorphine binding to cerebrosides. One mg of cerebroside liposome was incubated at 37° C for 1 hr with increasing concentrations of H^3-etorphine (3.4 CimM) in 50 mM sodium phosphate buffer. Data obtained from (13).

The binding affinities of other opiates to cerebrosides were also determined. Morphine had an affinity of approximately 5 μM, about the same as levorphanol, while dextrorphan had an affinity of about 1 to 5 mM. Since etorphine had an affinity of 10 nM, it was, therefore, about 200 times more potent than morphine. When radioactive naloxone was compared to morphine (13), the two drugs differed in affinity by only a factor of 10.

We now realize that the liposome method for studying binding presents two major difficulties: (1) controlling the particle size and (2) differentiating binding of the drug from solubility of the drug in the liposomes. Furthermore, the total binding and solubility of the drug to the liposomes represented only a small portion of the radioactivity added (≈10%). Therefore, in subsequent studies, we have used cerebroside sulfates and have measured binding to it in an organic solvent/water partition system as described by Weber et al (17) and by Goldstein et al (6). For a typical experiment, a 1 ml aqueous solution containing 5×10^{-8} M ^{3}H-levorphanol and varying concentrations of an unlabelled narcotic was adjusted to pH 6.0 and vortexed with 1 ml of organic solvent containing 4 μg of CS. The organic solvent consisted of heptane, chloroform and methanol in the proportion of 1500: 2:1.

In our hands, 80% of the levorphanol was bound to CS at 5 x 10 M concentration. The saturable component of the binding was distributed with 96% at the interface and 4% in heptane phase. Based on the drug concentration added to the partition system, dissociation constants of 9.1 x 10^{-8} M (capacity 0.45 nmole) and 1 x 10^{-6} M (capacity 1.4 nmole) were obtained. The former is for hydroxycerebroside sulfate while the latter is for non-hydroxycerebroside sulfate. The concentration of non-radioactive drug required to displace 50% of the ^{3}H-levorphanol from CS (ID50) was determined for over 20 narcotics including the complete series of 10 N-alkylnorketobemidones. The results, shown in Fig. 3 and 4, indicate that the ID50 of each of these drugs for binding to CS closely correlates with their pharmacologic potencies in both humans and other animals (18, 19).

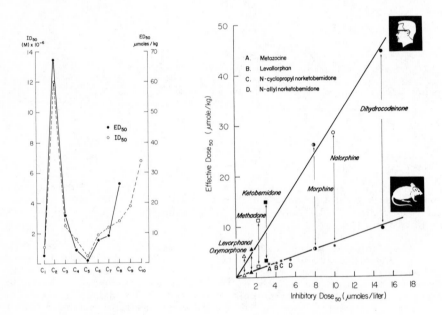

Fig. 3 - Comparison of ID50 with pharmacological potency (ED50) of N-alkylnorketobemidones. The inhibition of 1 µM H^{3}-levorphanol (26 mCi/mmole) binding to 10 µg cerebroside sulfate by N-alkylnorketobemidones was determined with increasing concentrations of the homologs by the heptane-water partition method. The ID50 is defined as the concentration of the homologs required to inhibit H^{3}-levorphanol binding to cerebroside sulfate by 50%.

Fig. 4 - Correlation between the ID50 and analgetic activity (ED50). The ID50 is the concentration of the narcotic analgetics required to inhibit the binding of 5 x 10^{-8} M, H^{3}-levorphanol (3 Ci/mmole) with 4 µg of cerebroside sulfate by 50%. The analgetic activities (ED50's) of the drug were taken from E. L. May et al (19) and converted into µmoles/kg.

Comparison of cerebroside sulfate to a partially purified opiate receptor: While the identification of opiate receptor(s) in the CNS have been reported by several laboratories (7-11), only Lowney et al (20) have described attempts to purify the receptor. In 1974, they isolated from mouse brain a partially purified opiate receptor which they reported to be a proteolipid. However, we have established by chemical and chromatographic analyses, and by its narcotic binding properties that the opiate receptor is virtually identical to cerebroside sulfate (13). Further attempts to determine the extent to which cerebroside sulfate could mimic the behavior of the purified opiate receptor involved comparison of the elution pattern of cerebroside sulfate and its levorphanol complex with that of the opiate receptor and its levorphanol-complex on a Sephadex LH-20 column as described by Soto et al (21) and by Lowney et al (20).

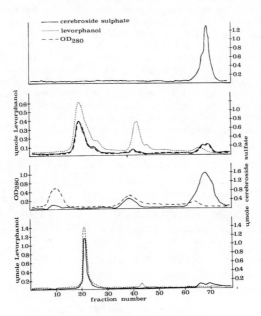

Fig. 5 - Elution behavior on Sephadex LH-20 of:
    A. Pure CS (5 mgm)
    B. CS-levorphanol complex
    C. Purified opiate receptor from mouse brain (20)
    D. Opiate receptor-levorphanol complex

Fig. 5 shows that a mixture of hydroxy and non-hydroxy CS is eluted in the same fractions as the Lowney receptor. Moreover, when CS is complexed with levorphanol, the complex also migrates on the column to a more lipophilic region. Various chemical determinations of these purified fractions were also used to further establish the similarity between CS and the purified opiate receptors. Thus, CS appears to be at least the major, if not entire, constituent of the opiate receptor reported by Lowney et al (20). Explanations for the apparent proteo-like behavior of the opiate receptor have been provided and were discussed in our previous publications (13).

Evidence for involvement of cerebroside sulfate in the actions of morphine: In addition to the in vitro experiment discussed above, we have carried out several in vivo experiments in which we have attempted to alter the availability of brain CS and to determine the effects of this alteration on the antinociceptive effects of morphine. In the first experiment, we evaluated the effects of morphine on Jimpy mutant B6CBA mice and their normal littermates. These mutants were used as they are known to have low levels of brain cerebrosides but normal levels of brain phospholipids and gangliosides in comparison to their normal littermates (22). The jimpy mice were found to be quite resistant to morphine as the median analgetic dose (AD50) was 11-fold higher in the jimpy mutants than in the normal controls (Table 1). In the next experiments, we reduced the availability of CS in normal mice by injecting agents which have been found (Loh et al, unpublished, 23) to bind strongly to CS. These agents, Azure A and cetylpyridinium chloride (CPC), were found to antagonize the effects of morphine as they increased the AD50 by 3X and 8X, respectively (Table 1). CPC was found to be quite toxic when injected intracerebrally (i.c.) but this toxicity was reduced by complexing CPC with chondroitin sulfate and injecting this mixture. Thus, three different conditions which reduced the availability of brain CS also reduced the effectiveness of morphine. Although these experiments cannot be considered conclusive, they do suggest that the interaction of narcotic drugs with CS may be an important step in the production of the pharmacological effects of these drugs.

Table I
EFFECTS OF REDUCED AVAILABILITY OF BRAIN SULFATIDE
ON MORPHINE ANALGESIA

Strain of mice	Pretreatment	Morphine AD50, mg/kg (tail-flick test)[1]
B6CBA 21-25 days old		
Jimpy mutants	None	43.0[2]
Normal littermates	None	3.9
Simonsen ICR	Saline (200 μl/kg) i.c. 20 hr before morphine	5.8
	Azure A (15 μmole/kg) i.c. 20 hr before morphine	14.2[2]
Simonsen ICR	Chondroitin sulfate (8 mg/kg) i.c. 5 hr before morphine	3.0
	CPC (11 μmole/kg) + Chondroitin sulfate (8 mg/kg) i.c. 5 hr before morphine	24.0[2]

[1] Morphine sulfate was injected s.c. 30 min before testing.
[2] Significantly different from appropriate control, $p < 0.05$.

Discussion: The fact that CS exhibits high affinity, stereoselective binding to a number of narcotic drugs and the affinity of this binding can be correlated with the analgetic potency of these drugs in both man and rodents indicate that CS demonstrates many of the properties which are thought to be necessary, if not sufficient, for the identification of an "opiate receptor." Cerebroside sulfate appears to fulfill many of the structural requirements of a hypothetical opiate receptor. It is an endogenous component of brain tissue and, in fact, a partially purified opiate receptor from mouse brain has now been shown to be CS. Other animal experiments indicate that reduced availability of brain CS decreases the analgetic effects of morphine, suggesting that the interaction of opiates with CS observed in vitro may also have importance in vivo. We suggest that CS can serve as a heuristically useful model which will allow more rigorous determination of conditions which are both necessary and sufficient for the identification of drug receptors.

References

1. Chen-Yu Sung and E. Leong Way, J. Pharmac. exp. Ther. 109, 244 (1953).
2. N. A. Ingoglia and V. P. Dole, J. Pharmac. exp. Ther. 178, 84 (1970).
3. S. J. Mule, L. A. Woods and L. B. Mellett, J. Phramac. exp. Ther. 136, 242 (1962).
4. D. Van Praag and E. Simon, Proc. Soc. Exp. Biol. Med. 122, 6 (1966).
5. K. D. Wuepper, S. Y. Yeh and L. D. Woods, Proc. Soc. Exp. Biol. Med. 124, 1146 (1967).
6. A. Goldstein, L. I. Lowney and B. K. Pal, Proc. Natl. Acad. Sci. 68, 1742 (1971).
7. C. B. Pert and S. H. Snyder, Science 179, 1011 (1973).
8. E. J. Simon, J. M. Hiller and I. Edelman, Proc. Natl. Acad. Sci. U.S.A. 70, 1947 (1973).
9. D. T. Wong and J. S. Horng, Life Sci. 13, 1543 (1973).
10. L. Terenius, Acta Pharmacol. Toxicol. 32, 317 (1973).
11. C. Y. Lee, S. Stolman, T. Akera and T. M. Brody, Pharmacologist 15, 202 (1973).
12. S. H. Snyder and S. Matthysse, Opiate Receptor Mechanisms, Neuroscience Research Program Bulletin, 1975.
13. H. H. Loh, T. M. Cho, Y. C. Wu and E. L. Way, Life Sci. 14, 2233 (1974).
14. H. H. Loh, T. M. Cho and Y. C. Wu, Fed. Proc. 34, 3368 (1975).
15. A. H. Beckett and A. F. Casy, J. Pharm. Parmac. 6, 986 (1954).
16. P. S. Portoghese, J. Med. Chem. 8, 609 (1965).
17. G. Weber, D. P. Borris, E. De Robertis, F. J. Barrantes, J. L. LaTorre and Mo De Carlin, Mol. Pharmacol. 7, 530 (1971).
18. Tokuro Oh-ishi and E. L. May, J. Med. Chem. 16, 1376 (1973).
19. E. L. May and L. J. Sargent, in Medicinal Chemistry (Ed. de Stevens) Chap. IV, p. 123, Academic Press, N.Y. (1965).
20. L. I. Lowney, K. Schulz, P. J. Lowery and A. Goldstein, Science 183, 749 (1974).
21. E. F. Soto, J. M. Pasquini, R. Placido and J. L. La Torre, J. Chromat. 41, 400 (1969).
22. P. Mandel, in Glycolipids, Glycoproteins and Mucopolysaccharides of the Nervous System (Eds. V. Zambott, G. Tettamanti and M. Arrigoni) Plenum Press, N.Y. 1972.
23. E. L. Kean, J. Lipid Res. 9, 319 (1968).

Contribution #75-5, Department of Pharmacology, University of California, San Francisco, California 94143.

POSSIBLE MOLECULAR FORMS OF THE OPIATE RECEPTOR

J. R. Smythies

Department of Psychiatry and Neurosciences Program,
University of Alabama, Birmingham, Alabama

(Received in final form May 24, 1975)

In a previous communication (1) the hypothesis was presented, based on
binding experiments, that a stereochemically possible 'opiate receptor' could
be constructed from a stack of CMP molecules complexed to acetylcholine (1:1).
Predictions from this model were that (i) the agonist/antagonist ratio binding
at the receptor would be 2:1 and (ii) the amino acid sequence of the endogenous
ligand would be based on an $(AB)_n$ sequence where A is a lipophilic and B a basic
amino acid. However, since recent work suggests that the agonist/antagonist
ratio binding is 1:1 and not 2:1, a search was made for another molecular form
(using protein only). A general theory of receptors has been published (2,3)
suggesting that the molecular basis for transmitters such as ACh, GABA, catecholamines, glycine, etc. is a Kusnetsov-Ghokov grid [two parallel β-chains (primary
chains)]cross linked by the complementary binding of their apposed amino acids
(i.e. acidic to basic; lipophilic to lipophilic; hydrogen bonding to hydrogen
bonding). This grid can most simply be converted into a receptor 'cup' by adding
two further segments of polypeptide chain (secondary chains) each of which forms
a formal β-pleated sheet with one of the primary chains. Experiments using CPK
models and a variety of opiate agonists and antagonists led to the following
specification of a model 'opiate receptor' capable of explaining structure-
activity relationship data. The two primary chains have the sequence (1) -met-
x-glu-x-A- and(2)-met-x-leu-x-A-(where A is small). These could bind by [met-
met] lipophilic binding but the middle terms glu and leu are incompatible in
the absence of the agonist. The sequence of the secondary chains suggested is
(3)-met-x-ala (or conservative substitution)-x-arg- (β-sheet with (1)) and (4)-
met-x-asp-x-glu-(β-sheet with (2)). These can bind by [met-met] lipophilic
binding and [arg-glu] double resonating ionic bonding but the middle terms
(ala and asp) are again incompatible in the absence of the agonist. Less good
but still possible fits would be provided by replacement of the arg-glu pair
by gln-gln or even a second met-met pair.

This protein structure would have two conformations - "closed" or R (with
the met-met and arg-glu links made) and "open" or R_1 (with the two sides some
1A further apart and the met-met and arg-glu links broken). It is suggested
that opiate agonists bind preferentially to R. In the case of levorphanol the
basic N (protonated) binds ionically to glu and the phenolic hydroxyl hydrogen
bonds to asp. Thus the incompatibilities are cancelled. There are also close
lipophilic bonds to the mets, ala and leu. It is also suggested that antagonists bind preferentially to R_1 as the bulkier (and rigid) N substitution characteristic of antagonists fits into the lipophilic slot on chain (3) between
met and ala and prevents the 1A 'closing' movement necessary to convert R_1 into
R.

The hypothesis was illustrated by a number of CPK models of the 'receptor' and the binding thereto of phenyletorphine, dextrorphan (which fails to
bind to asp by its phenolic OH), etonitazine and the steroid agonist 6-dimethyl-

aminomethyl-1-3-ethoxy-21-fluoro-3,5-pregnadiene 20-one-17α-ol acetate (the later two as examples of opiate agonists of widely differing chemical structure to morphine).

References

1. J. R. Smythies, F. Antun, G. Yank, and C. York, Nature 231 185–188 (1971).
2. J. R. Smythies, Ann. Rev. Pharmacol. 14 9–21 (1975).
3. J. R. Smythies, Intern. Rev. Neurobiol. 17 131–187 (1975).

PLASMA CHOLINESTERASE AND THE MORPHINE RECEPTOR

Alexander Gero and Robert J. Capetola

Department of Pharmacology, Hahnemann Medical College,
Philadelphia, Pennsylvania 19102

(Received in final form May 24, 1975)

When thinking of narcotic analgesics, most pharmacologists are concerned
with them only as narcotics or as analgesics. That, however, is a clinical
attitude which disregards the many other actions that opiates also have;
neither their analgesic action nor the development of dependence may be best
suited to help understand the interaction of opiates with their receptors.

Over the past 12 years we have studied one of these other opiate actions,
namely, their effect on the nonspecific esterase in human blood (pseudo-
cholinesterase, acylcholine acyl-hydrolase, E.C.3.1.1.8.). This enzyme is com-
mercially available, if not in a pure, at least in a reproducible state in
which its enzymatic activity is measureable with exquisite accuracy (1,2).
The enzyme obeys Michaelis-Menten kinetics (3,4); and it contains a morphine
receptor, that is, a site separate from its active site, for which both
natural and synthetic opioids and their specific antagonists have affinity;
some also have efficacy or intrinsic activity, manifested in an increase of the
rate constant of enzymatic activity. Because of the great accuracy with which
the rate of this enzymatic reaction can be measured, we have obtained exact
numerical values for the affinity constants and efficacies of a number of such
compounds (5,6), something not easily done with other opiate actions. We have
also been able to propose a hypothesis on the interaction of opiates with this
receptor (7) which fits all experimental results and which makes both their
affinity for the receptor and their efficacy intelligible. The hypothesis considers affinity to the receptor to depend on an N-alkyl group and a benzene
ring at about $6 \overset{\circ}{A}$ from each other, with other groups supplying assistance by
hydrogen bonds and hydrophobic binding, while efficacy results when a drug
molecule rigidly holds the N-methyl and phenyl group at about $4 \overset{\circ}{A}$ from each
other, distorting the receptor and forcing it to conform to the drug rather
than the reverse. It is the stress of this enforced conformational change in
the receptor which manifests itself in accelerated enzymatic activity.

We do not claim that the morphine receptor in plasma esterase is the morphine receptor. For years it has been known (8,9) that there are several morphine receptors which may differ in both their affinity and their responsiveness to opiates, and the esterase receptor does differ in various ways from the
analgesic receptor(s): for instance, methadone and meperidine have only
affinity for the receptor in the enzyme but no efficacy, that is, they competitively antagonize morphine, as does nalorphine. On the other hand, naloxone does have efficacy in the enzyme, in fact, it is one of the most potent
agonists we have found. At the same time, we also find many parallels between
the actions of drugs on the enzyme and on the analgesic receptor: for
instance, the sequence of decreasing affinities to the enzymatic receptor of
some commonly used drugs is methadone - dihydromorphinone - levorphanol -
morphine - codeine, which is also the sequence of their analgesic potencies; so
that it would be wrong to dismiss the parameters obtained with the enzyme as

irrelevant for understanding analgesic opiate action.

The fact has perhaps not received adequate attention that the opiate receptor is an oddity in that it is the only receptor that plays no known role in the physiology of the organism but responds to an exogenous chemical structure. That this structure has such a great variety of actions in the organism suggests to us that it can complex with a grouping that must be a rather commonplace feature of many proteins; and if such proteins happen to have a physiological function, the attachment of an opiate molecule may have a pharmacological effect. This view implies some correlation between the relative affinities of different opiates for the various organs in which they find sites of attachment, but not necessarily any correlation between their efficacies.

If there is any merit in this view, then our studies on the interaction of opioid drugs with human plasma esterase may give us some insight into the interactions of these drugs with other receptor sites, including the analgesic receptor. Furthermore, since pure plasma cholinesterase has been prepared (10), we may hope eventually to be able to establish its complete structure; and, combined with our findings on structure-activity relationships in the binding of drugs to the receptor site on the enzyme and in their agonistic efficacy, we may hope that we shall be able to identify that portion of the protein structure which functions as the morphine receptor, and perhaps also to understand the details of the allosteric change in the enzyme which we postulated for efficacy (7).

References

1. M.J. ETTINGER and A. GERO, Arch. int. Pharmacodyn. 164 96-110 (1966).
2. M.J. ETTINGER and A. GERO, Arch. int. Pharmacodyn. 164 111-119 (1966).
3. A. GERO, Enzymologia 38 283-307 (1970).
4. A. GERO, Enzymologia 43 261-269 (1972).
5. A.P. FERKO and A. GERO, Arch. int. Pharmacodyn. 187 213-235 (1970).
6. A. GERO and R.J. CAPETOLA, Arch. int. Pharmacodyn. 213 274-283 (1974).
7. A. GERO, Arch. int. Pharmacodyn. 206 41-46 (1973).
8. T.K. ADLER, J. Pharmacol. Exp. Ther. 140 155-161 (1963).
9. P.S. PORTOGHESE, J. Med. Chem. 8 609-616 (1965).
10. P.K. DAS and J. LIDDELL, Biochem. J. 116 875-881 (1970).

COMPARISON OF IN VIVO AND IN VITRO PARAMETERS OF OPIATE
RECEPTOR BINDING IN NAIVE AND TOLERANT/DEPENDENT RODENTS.

V. Höllt, J. Dum, J. Bläsig, P. Schubert and A. Herz

Department of Neuropharmacology, Max-Planck-Institut
für Psychiatrie, Munich, Germany.

(Received in final form May 24, 1975)

Summary

In vivo and in vitro approaches were used to investigate a possible change in the opiate receptors during the development of to-
lerance/dependence. With the pAx method no significant change in
the apparent pA_2 of naloxone in tolerant rats in vivo could be
found, indicating that no substantial change in the affinity for
the receptors takes place. Comparison of receptor binding of [3]H-
etorphine and ^{3}H-naloxone to rat brain homogenate in vitro showed
no difference in binding between naive and tolerant rats. The displacement of small amounts of high labeled antagonist or agonist
by increasing amounts of unlabeled antagonist in mouse brain in
vivo offered the possibility of characterizing properties of receptors in the intact animal. This technique revealed no indication
of a change in the number of receptor sites in tolerant animals.
An apparently lower affinity in the tolerant animals could be explained by the morphine present in these animals. Displacement of
[3]H-etorphine from receptors by a high amount of unlabeled naltrexone in vivo could also be demonstrated by autoradiography.

Some theories try to explain opiate tolerance and dependence
with changes at the receptor level (1). From experiments in which
the "apparent affinity constant" was calculated in vivo it was
concluded that acute and chronic opiate administration increases
the sensitivity for opiate antagonists, implying a structural
change in the receptors (2,3,4). Studies of possible changes in
the stereospecific opiate binding in vitro by morphine pretreatment had ambigeous results (5,6,7,8,9). In order to get more data
on these problems we employed several techniques. The main emphasis was put on in vivo investigations, as one has to consider that
changes in the receptors might be lost during the killing and processing of brain tissue for in vitro assay.

Methods

For the evaluation of the apparent pA_2 values (10) dose response curves of morphine (s.c. inj.) alone and in combination with
logarithmically increasing doses of naloxone (i.p.) were established. As antinociceptive test, vocalization induced by electrical
stimulation of the tail root was used. Experiments were performed
at a time, when the effects of both drugs were maximum. Stereospecific binding of opiates to rat brain homogenates in vitro was tested using the filtration technique (5). The homogenates (final
dilution 1:100) were washed 4 times with sodium phosphate buffer
(pH 7.4, 50 mM).- In vivo displacement experiments were performed
in mice. Labeled morphine antagonists and agonists were injected

71

i.v. together with increasing amounts of unlabeled compound. The animals were killed 15 min. after injection, the brains removed and the radioactivity determined after combustion by scintillation counting.- Rats were implanted repeatedly with morphine pellets (75 mg morphine base), according to various implantation schedules to induce tolerance/dependence (11). Mice were implanted with two morphine pellets (37 mg), one three days after the other.

Labeled substances used:
[3]H-naltrexone (15.3 Ci/mmole, kindly supplied by Prof. E. Simon, New York),
[3]H-naloxone (23.6 Ci/mmole, New England Nuclear Cooperation),
[3]H-etorphine (41 Ci/mmole, The Radiochemical Center, Amersham).

In Vivo Determination of the Apparent pA_2 Value of Naloxone

The apparent pA_2 value of naloxone, as calculated in naive and three groups of rats with increasing degrees of tolerance, was about 6.8 in all animals. Thus there is no indication that the affinity of the antagonist to the receptor is changed in tolerant animals. These experiments were performed without first removing the morphine pellets in order to avoid any interference from withdrawal. When the morphine present in the tolerant animals is taken into account, a small tendency of the pA_2 lines of the tolerant animals to the right is compensated for. The pA_2 line obtained in experiments, done after pellet removal, had a slope different from -1 and could therefore not be interpreted using the simple pA_2 model.

In Vitro Displacement in Rat Brain Homogenates

The binding of an agonist and an antagonist to brain homogenates obtained in naive and tolerant rats is represented in Fig.1.

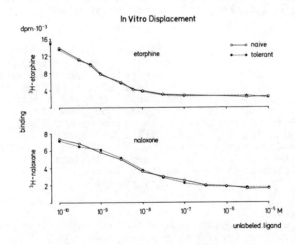

Fig.1 Displacement of ^{3}H-etorphine (0.6 nM) and of ^{3}H-naloxone (2.5 nM) by increasing amounts of the unlabeled ligand in brain homogenates obtained from naive and tolerant rats. Each point represents the mean of 4-6 independent experiments.

Addition of increasing amounts of the unlabeled ligand to the homogenate induces increasing displacement of the labeled ligand. No difference between naive and tolerant rats was found for either substance.

This result accords in principle with other investigations (8,9). Other studies (5,6,7) which revealed some differences in binding between naive and morphine pretreated animals can hardly explain the phenomenon of tolerance/dependence as either the changes were rather small and/or had a time course other than that of the development of chronic opiate effects.

In Vivo Displacement in Mice

When increasing amounts of unlabeled naltrexone were injected i.v. together with a constant dose of ^{3}H-naltrexone (2 pmole/g), radioactivity in brain declined and reached a plateau at about 1000 µg/kg (Fig.2). About 60 % of the total radioactivity proved to be displaceable by high doses of the unlabeled compound in the case of the naive animals.

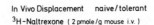

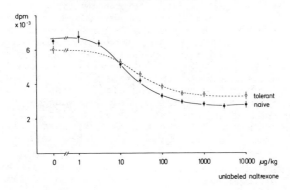

Fig.2 In vivo displacement of ^{3}H-naltrexone from the brain by unlabeled naltrexone after i.v. injection in naive and tolerant mice. Mixtures of ^{3}H-naltrexone and unlabeled naltrexone were injected and the animals killed 15 min. later. Each point represents the mean value and standard error of 10-40 mice.

The interpretation of these results in terms of a displacement of the labeled compound by the unlabeled ligand from the opiate receptor is supported by experiments in which the effect of the morphine antagonist (-)-hydroxy-N-allyl-morphinan (levallorphan) is compared to that of its detrorotatory isomere (+)-hydroxy-N-allyl-morphinan (dextrallorphan), which lacks antagonistic activity (Fig.3). While in the case of dextrallorphan, ^{3}H-naltrexone binding was not affected, levallorphan displaced ^{3}H-naltrexone in a dose-dependent manner.

Results similar to those found with naltrexone were also obtained with naloxone. The displaceable portion of naloxone was

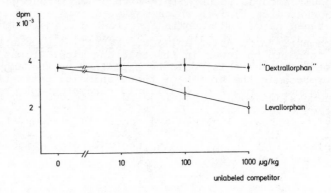

In Vivo Displacement
^{3}H-Naltrexone (1 pmole/g mouse i.v.; spec.act. 15,3 Ci/mmole)

Fig.3 In vivo displacement of ^{3}H-naltrexone from the brain
of mice by injection of levallorphan and the lack of this
effect in the case of dextrallorphan. Mixtures of ^{3}H-nal-
trexone and levallorphan or dextrallorphan were injected
i.v. and animals killed 15 min. later. Each point represents the mean value and standard deviation of 6 mice.

smaller, however. This demonstrates that the affinity of the drug
used is important for the magnitude of the displacement effect obtained. It explains the failure of earlier studies in which no or
only minor changes in brain concentration of opiates were observed when compounds with lower affinity were used (12); clear displacement effects, however, could be obtained with etorphine
(13,14).

These experiments were analysed by means of Scatchard plots.
The number of binding sites calculated amounted to about 8 pmoles/
g for naltrexone and naloxone. For both substances the measured
points fit the regression line rather well, pointing to one type
of receptor. A dissociation constant of $5 \cdot 10^{-9}$ was obtained for
naltrexone and of $1.6 \cdot 10^{-8}$ for naloxone. This means that naltrexone shows about a 3-fold greater affinity than naloxone. A similar
difference between the antagonists was found in in vitro experiments. Furthermore, the Scatchard plots for naloxone displacement
in vivo and in vitro were compared. About 20 pmoles binding sites/
g brain and a dissociation constant of $6.4 \cdot 10^{-9}$ M was calculated
for the in vitro experiment. Having in mind the differences in experimental approach between the two investigations, the estimations of the number of binding sites calculated from the in vivo and
in vitro experiments are quite close.

On the basis of these results the displacement of antagonists
in tolerant mice was studied. The results obtained for naltrexone
in comparison to naive mice are shown in Fig.2. There are some significant differences between the two displacement curves. A significantly lower displaceable activity was found in tolerant mice
and the plateau of indisplaceable labeled compound was found to be
higher than in the naive animals. The former difference may be due
to morphine - which also competes for the receptors - present in

the brain of the tolerant animals (see next paragraph). The somewhat higher level of the plateau when higher dosages of unlabeled naltrexone are given indicates that the portion of indisplaceable naltrexone is higher than in naive animals. Presently an explanation for this finding cannot be given.

Scatchard plots of the data obtained for naltrexone in tolerant mice revealed no significant changes in the number of the binding sites in comparison to naive animals. The affinity constant, however, was found to be lower in the tolerant mice. It was checked to see whether or not this could be explained by the amount of morphine present in the brains of these animals. Estimation of the morphine content by means of gas liquid chromatography revealed morphine concentrations between $1-3 \cdot 10^{-6}$ M. In in vitro measurements the affinity of naltrexone in sodium phosphate buffer was found to be about 400 times higher than that of morphine. When this data was taken into account, the lower apparent affinity found for the tolerant mice could be largely explained. This would indicate that not only does the number of binding sites not change during the development of tolerance, but also that the affinity for the receptor remains nearly the same.

These studies offer the possibility of correlating the receptor occupation with the pharmacological effects. In Fig.4 naltrexone displacement by increasing amounts of unlabeled ligand in tolerant/dependent mice is compared to the withdrawal jumping precipitated by the same dose of antagonist. The small amounts of ^{3}H-nalt-

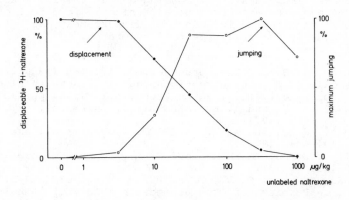

Comparison:
In Vivo Displacement of ^{3}H-Naltrexone / Jumping

Fig.4 In vivo displacement of ^{3}H-naltrexone from the brain by increasing amounts of unlabeled naltrexone injected i.v. into tolerant mice, in comparison to withdrawal jumping precipitated by the same doses of naltrexone. The mice in which displacement of ^{3}H-naltrexone was studied were killed 15 min. after injection. The number of jumps precipitated 0-30 min. after injection was counted. The maximum jumping (mean of 155 jumps/30 min.) observed after 300 μg/kg naltrexone was taken as 100 %. The displaceable amount of ^{3}H-naltrexone, obtained from the data represented in Fig.2, are taken as 100 %.

rexone (2 pmoles/g) are ineffective in inducing jumping. Application of increasing amounts of unlabeled naltrexone starts to precipitate jumping at doses at which labeled naltrexone is also displaced. The maximum displacement of naltrexone occurs in a similar dose range, when jumping is also at its peak.

In vivo displacement experiments, as presented for naltrexone and naloxone, were also performed with agonists and combinations of agonists and antagonists. Highly labeled etorphine (1 pmole/g i.v.) could be displaced by naltrexone. Doses between 10-100 μg/kg naltrexone caused a steep decline in radioactivity, tending to plateau at about 50 % replacement of etorphine.

The displacement of ^{3}H-etorphine by naltrexone could also be shown by means of autoradiography. When 50 μCi/kg ^{3}H-etorphine were injected in mice i.v., considerable differences in the density of silver grains between various brain areas became obvious, e.g. a low labeling in the cerebellum and a rather high labeling in some nuclei of the adjoining brain stem. (The results of such mapping to be described elsewhere.) In mice, which received, besides the same dose of etorphine, 1000 μg/kg cold naltrexone, the high labeling of some structures seemed to be reduced; thus the differences between labeling of the brain stem and the cerebellum became less obvious than when etorphine was applied alone.

While a displacement of etorphine by naltrexone with both methods - scintillation counting and autoradiography - was quite obvious, an effect was not demonstrable when, instead of naltrexone, increasing amounts of unlabeled etorphine were applied. On the contrary, the radioactivity measured increased. In tolerant mice such an increase was observed only at considerably higher dosages of etorphine. From this it is concluded that the increase observed in case of agonists results from a pharmacologic effect of the opiate, counteracting the influence of displacement, an effect which seems to underly the development of tolerance.

References

1) COLLIER, H. O. J., Adv. Drug Res. <u>3</u>, 171-188 (1966).
2) TAKEMORI, A. E., In: Narcotic Antagonist, Adv. in Biochem. Psychopharmacol.Vol.<u>8</u>, Raven Press, N.Y. 1974, pp. 335-344.
3) TULUNAY, F. C. and A. E. TAKEMORI, J. Pharmacol. exp. Ther. <u>190</u>, 395-400 (1974).
4) TULUNAY, F. C. and A. E. TAKEMORI, J. Pharmacol. exp. Ther. <u>190</u>, 401-407 (1974).
5) PERT, C. B., G. PASTERNAK and S. H. SNYDER, Science <u>182</u>, 1359-1361 (1973).
6) FREDERICKSON, R. C. A., J. S. HORNY, V. BURGIS and D. T. WONG, Comm. on Problems of Drug Dependence (NAS-NRC) 36th Ann. Scientific Meeting, Mexico City, March 1974, 411-434.
7) WEBER, N. E., L. de BAARE and B. P. DOCTOR, Fed. Prod. <u>33</u>, 1527 (1974).
8) KLEE, W. A. and R. A. STREATY, Nature <u>248</u>, 61-63 (1974).
9) HITZEMAN, R. J., B. A. HITZEMAN and H. H. LOH, Life Sci. <u>14</u>, 2393-2404 (1974).
10) SCHILD, H. O., Brit. J. Pharmacol. <u>4</u>, 277-280 (1949).
11) BLÄSIG, J., Phsychopharmacologia <u>33</u>, 19-38 (1973).
12) MULE, S. J., J. Pharmacol. exp. Ther. <u>148</u>, 393-398 (1965).
13) DOBBS, H. E., J. Pharmacol. exp. Ther. <u>169</u>, 407-414 (1968).
14) CERLETTI, C., L. MANARA and T. MENNINI, Brit. J. Pharmacol. <u>54</u>, 606 (1974).

ANTAGONIST DISPLACEMENT OF BRAIN MORPHINE DURING PRECIPITATED ABSTINENCE

Jeanne W. Shen & E. Leong Way

Department of Pharmacology, School of Medicine,
University of California, San Francisco, CA 94143

(Received in final form May 24, 1975)

Summary

In mice rendered physically dependent on morphine, naloxone elicited a brief precipitous fall in brain levels of morphine. The effect was maximal at about 15 minutes, lasted about 1 hour, and appeared to coincide with the time course of naloxone precipitated withdrawal.

Since the initial report by Wikler et al., in 1953 (1), it has been well established that the administration of a narcotic antagonist in a subject dependent on morphine precipitates a marked abstinence-like syndrome. The precipitated signs resemble those seen during abrupt withdrawal, but are more rapid in onset, shorter in duration and more severe in intensity. Although the mechanism of precipitated withdrawal is unknown, many believe that the syndrome is due to the sudden displacement of morphine from its receptor site. However, evidence to this effect has not been established and the present studies were initiated to investigate the effects of the antagonist, naloxone, on brain levels of morphine during the course of precipitated withdrawal.

Male ICR mice weighing 25-30 grams and male Sprague-Dawley rats weighing 180-200 grams (both from Simonsen Laboratories, Gilroy, California) were rendered dependent on morphine by subcutaneous implantation with a specially formulated pellet containing 75 mg of morphine alkaloid as described previously (2). After 72 hours, the pellet was removed and the animals were divided randomly into two groups. At 6 hours after pellet removal, one group was subdivided and injected with either physiological saline or naloxone, 10 mg/kg intraperitoneally. The animals were sacrificed 15 and 60 minutes later. The second group received an additional dose of either naloxone or saline 1 hour after the first administration and was sacrificed after 30 and 60 minutes. The brains were removed and morphine was extracted by the method of Kupferberg et al., (3). An aliquot of 0.1 ml of acid extract was subjected to radioimmunoassay using the rabbit antiserum developed by Catlin et al., (4).

Six hours after removal of the morphine pellet, the brain concentration of morphine was approximately 100 ng/gm. Injection of naloxone elicited a precipitous fall in the levels of brain morphine. As shown in Figure 1, the level of morphine 15 minutes after saline was 75 ng/gm whereas after naloxone the level was only 1/10 that of the control group. The effect of naloxone was short-lived as evidenced by the nearly comparable levels in

Supported by Grant DA-00037 from the National Institute of Drug Abuse.
Contribution number 75-6

the control and test animals 1 hour after challenge. In the 7 hour group, naloxone also produced a marked decline in brain concentration of morphine; the level 30 minutes following challenge was 23 ng/gm for the saline group and 2.6 ng/gm for the naloxone group. Again, rapid recovery was indicated by the fact that 1 hour after naloxone, the brain concentration noted was not significantly different from that of the control group given saline. The time course and duration of the decline in brain morphine appeared to coincide closely with the reported onset, peak and duration of the precipitated withdrawal syndrome (2).

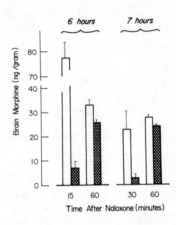

Fig. 1. Displacement of brain morphine by naloxone in
morphine dependent mice

In morphine-dependent rats, a similar rapid and extensive displacement of morphine from the brain was effected by naloxone. Among several brain regions examined, the decrease appeared to be greatest in thalamus, hypothalamus, brain stem and midbrain, whereas cortex showed the least displacement of morphine by naloxone.

The present study provides strong evidence compatible with the hypothesis that antagonist precipitated withdrawal is a result of the displacement of morphine from its receptor sites and also (5) that the affinity of the brain for morphine (or naloxone) is altered in the physical dependent state.

References

1. Wikler, A., Fraser, H.F. and Isbell, H. J. Pharmac. exp. Ther. 109, 8, (1953).
2. Way, E.L., Loh, H.H. and Shen, F.H. J. Pharmac. exp. Ther. 167 1 (1969).
3. Kupferberg, H., Burkhalter, A. and Way, E.L. J. Pharmac. exp. Ther. 145, 247 (1964).
4. Catlin, D., Cleeland, R. and Grunberg, E. Clin. Chem. 19, 216 (1973).
5. Brase, D.A., Tseng, L.F., Loh, H.H. and Way, E.L. Europ. J. Pharmacol. 26, 1 (1974).

MORPHINE TOLERANCE AND NALOXONE RECEPTOR BINDING

Joseph Harris and Dolores T. Kazmierowski

Division of Neurobiology, Barrow Neurological Institute of
St. Joseph's Hospital & Medical Center, Phoenix, Arizona 85013.

(Received in final form May 24, 1975)

^{3}H-naloxone specific binding studies have confirmed the induction of receptor expansion after an
acute injection of morphine, as reported by Pert et al
(3) as well as the lack of expansion in chronically
morphinized rats shown by Klee and Streaty (4) using
dihydromorphine. With a challenging test dose of morphine given to rats maintained drug free after acute
and chronic regimens of morphine, the lack of expansion as measured by 3H-naloxone specific binding per-
sisted up to at least 4 weeks. Between 4-8 weeks receptor expansion can be re-induced with a challenging test
dose. This "physical binding tolerance" is dose related. That this persistant "tolerance" is not attributable to the presence of dissociable morphine
remaining after the drug regimen or challenge dose can
be shown by detergent extraction and exhaustive dialysis of the standard buffer homogenate preparation as
well as with fresh excised tissue.

Many investigators of opiate receptors base their approach
on the principle of stereospecificity of opiate-receptor binding,
laid down by Goldstein et al (1), and the procedure of Pert and
Snyder (2) which uses ^{3}H-naloxone for studying receptor binding.
Pert et al (3) reported that acute in vivo administration of opiates of their antagonists produced enhanced receptor binding,
that is, the number of opiate binding sites appeared to have increased, an increase they consider not related to the phenomena
of tolerance and dependence. Klee and Streaty (4) did not find a
comparable enhancement of receptor binding to ^{3}H-dihydromorphine
in morphine-dependent rats, an observation they believe, "provide
(s) evidence that morphine dependence (and therefore also tolerance) is not the result of an alteration in the number, or the
nature of, the specific receptor sites." In accordance with Klee
and Streaty we have observed, using ^{3}H-naloxone, a lack of expansion of receptor binding in brains of rats chronically treated
with morphine over a period of seven days, but we have also confirmed the increase in naloxone receptor binding after an acute
single opiate injection in the naive rat. In addition we have
used challenging dose injections to test for receptor expansion
under conditions of 1) a single acute injection previously administered 2) chronic morphinization and 3) post-drug free state up
to 8 weeks after the last dose of opiate.

We now present data showing that: a) The lack of expansion
in a chronically morphinized animal when assayed by the Pert et

al (3) technique reflects the presence of induced tolerance; b)
This "physical binding tolerance" is induced after injection of
morphine and persists for a period of time; c) In situations
showing a lack of receptor expansion tolerance may be demonstrated by the acute injection of a higher dose of the drug; d) The
physical binding tolerance is dose related.

Methods

Preparation of Animals

Groups of 10 adult Long-Evans male rats with an initial
weight 150-200 gms were used. Acute experiments were performed
employing a single intra-peritoneal injection of morphine sulfate
20 mg/Kg. For chronic experiments two injections were given per
day. The initial dose was 5 mg/Kg/day, doubling progressively to
20 mg/Kg/day and maintained at the 20 mg/Kg level for an additional 4 days. In experiments to test for persistence of tolerance,
groups of 10 rats were placed on the acute or chronic regimen respectively, then maintained for 8 weeks without further treatment.
At weekly intervals after drug withdrawal, the rats were challenged with an acute intra-peritoneal injection of morphine sulfate, 20 mg/Kg, and decapitated 15 minutes after the acute drug
test treatment. For experiments designed to show a dose relationship to physical binding tolerance, groups of naive and chronically morphinized rats were injected with increasing concentrations
of morphine sulfate; 15 minutes later the animals were sacrificed
and binding assays performed.

Preparation of Tissue

Brains without the cerebellum, were homogenized with cold 10
volumes of 0.05 M Tris-HCl buffer, (pH 7.4 at 35°C) using a Teflon
glass homogenizer (1800 rpm). Before assaying for "naloxone receptor binding", the injected morphine was removed by the exhaustive washing procedure of Pert et al (3). The homogenates were
centrifuged at 18000g for 10 minutes; the supernatants discarded
and the pellets re-suspended in 14 ml of cold Tris-buffer. This
washing procedure was repeated three times and, as shown by Pert
et al (3), removed virtually all of the opiate present. The
washed homogenate was diluted to 120 volumes of original brain
weight with cold Tris-buffer.

A detergent extraction and exhaustive dialysis was used to
assure removal of any dissociable morphine. Goldstein et al (1)
reported that stereospecific-binding capacity is retained after
extraction by 0.5% Triton X-100 or 0.1% sodium dodecyl sulfate,
provided the detergent is removed by dialysis. A modified procedure of Swislocki and Tierney (5) was used. Excised tissue (10
gm/100ml) was homogenized in 0.2M Tris-Hcl (pH 7.4) containing
0.2M sucrose and Lubrol-PX (0.1M). The homogenate was centrifuged
at 27,000g for 10 min. The supernatant was recentrifuged at
165,000g for 2 hr. and the non-sedimentable fraction was recentrifuged at 165,000g for 2 hr. resulting in a soluble clear preparation. Tissue homogenates (1:10) prepared by the standard Tris-HCl
(pH 7.4) buffer method (3) were subjected to extraction with detergent (1:10), centrifugation and dialysis (5). Protein determinations were made by the method of Lowry et al (6).

3-Naloxone Receptor Binding

Specific binding of ^{3}H-naloxone (23.6 Ci/mM, 98% purity, New England Nuclear Corp.) was assayed as described by Pert and Snyder (2). Aliquots of homogenate were incubated in triplicate at 35°C for 10 minutes in the presence of dextrorphan (0.1 uM) or levorphanol (1.0 uM), followed by the addition of varying concentrations to give saturation levels of ^{3}H-naloxone (16 nM/mg protein, 120,000 cpm). The incubation was terminated by filtration of the chilled samples through Whatman GF/B paper pads and washed 3 times with 4 ml cold Tris buffer. The filter pads, transferred to counting vials containing 1 ml of 10% sodium dodecyl sulfate, were shaken for 30 minutes; 10 ml of Packard "Insta-gel" was then added. After standing overnight, radioactivity was measured in a Tri-Carb Liquid Scintillation Spectrometer with counting efficiency at 30%. Specific naloxone binding was taken to be the difference between the amount of ^{3}H-naloxone bound in the absence and in the presence of excess levorphanol. Student's T-test (two-tailed) was used when applicable to analyze the data. All values shown represent the mean $\pm$ S. E. M.

Results and Discussion

We confirm the expansion of receptor after an acute injection of morphine as reported by Pert et al (3) as well as the lack of expansion in the chronically morphinized animal as shown by Klee and Streaty (4). We also show the absence of any effect on specific binding in both the acute and chronic rats when challenged by a 20 mg/Kg dose of morphine.

Enhanced receptor binding, seen by Pert et al (3) as early as 5 minutes after morphine administration, disappeared after 2 hours (Fig. 1).

FIG. 1

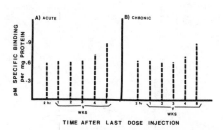

Specific binding of ^{3}H-naloxone to brain homogenates prepared from rats given a 20 mg/Kg challenge dose under conditions of a) a single acute injection of morphine and maintained drug-free up to 8 weeks; b) chronically morphinized rats maintained drug-free up to 8 weeks after the last dose of morphine.

Further, if acute or chronically morphinized rats are tested with the same challenging dose of morphine up to 4 weeks after their last drug administration, no receptor expansion is obtained until 4-8 weeks. This condition, we believe, reflects a physical binding tolerance related to pharmacological tolerance rather than to behavioral tolerance, since our animals have not been subjected to any test procedure. The question remains whether a single dose of opiate can induce tolerance. While Cochin and Kornetsky (7) as well as Goldstein and Sheehen (8) have demonstrated pharmacological tolerance after a single injection of opiate, Kayan and

Mitchell (9) consider this to be behavioral tolerance, despite evidence of Misra et al (10) of a prolonged, firm and persistent association of morphine after a single injection.

The physical binding assay of homogenates from an animal, previously acutely or chronically morphinized, exhibiting no receptor enhancement at a challenging acute test dose of 20 mg/Kg, will do so at a higher acute challenging doses (Fig. 2).

FIG. 2

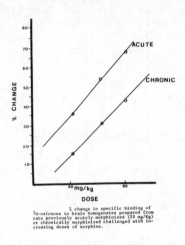

% change in specific binding of
³H-naloxone to brain homogenates prepared from
rats previously acutely morphinized (20 mg/Kg)
or chronically morphinized challenged with increasing doses of morphine.

That our results are not attributable to the presence of dissociable morphine are supported by data obtained with detergent extraction and exhaustive dialysis of a standard buffer homogenate preparation or of freshly excised brain tissue (Fig. 3). Rats tolerant to morphine gave specific binding measurements similar to their naive counter-parts.

FIG. 3

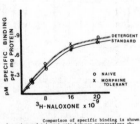

Comparison of specific binding is shown
for naive and tolerant rats between preparations obtained by the usual Tris-HCl (pH 7.4) buffer homogeni-
zation according to Pert et al (3) and by a detergent
extraction dialysis procedure (5).

We have observed that the injection of a single dose of morphine did not prevent receptor expansion induced by naloxone given one week later nor did an injection of naloxone prevent the induced receptor expansion when morphine was given a week later. Independent action thus appear to exist between naloxone and morphine. In this connection, we previously obtained differences between morphine and naloxone in their respective effects on calcium and catecholamine uptakes in rat brain striatal slices (11), differences suggesting that morphine and naloxone may react with a receptor at adjacent but overlapping sites. Such differences in binding sites on the opiate receptor for agonist and antagonist have been found recently by Wilson et al (12). This may contribute to the increased pharmacological sensitivity to naloxone that has been reported to occur with the development of dependence (13, 14). That morphine has induced some type of structural change in the analgesic receptor or that two types of analgesic receptors are present, has been discussed by Takemori and his group (15). Further support for structural changes come from our detergent-dialysis treatment of brain preparations and in liver tissue used as a control. The detergent treatment of brain tissue slightly increased ^{3}H-naloxone specific binding over that of the standard brain preparation to a degree suggestive of induced receptor expansion. The detergent treatment of liver converted the standard liver homogenates from one lacking in binding into one possessing specific naloxone binding characteristics.

Detergents alter membrane structure by removal of phospholipids (16), which could account for the transformation of liver having specific receptor binding properties. A possible role of phospholipid in the naloxone receptor binding is in keeping with the phospholipid changes produced by morphine (17). The possibility of an artifact resulting from the detergent treatment cannot be discounted although retention of specific binding properties of brain preparation has been shown by Goldstein and Sheehan (1) also. Artifactual receptor-ligand binding does occur under certain circumstances as has been reported in experiments using the lipophilic Sephadex LH-20 in the isolation and purification of acetylcholine receptors (18). Loh et al (19) found cerebroside sulfate devoid of protein to resemble the opiate receptor with respect to its elution pattern on Sephadex LH-20 with chloroform-methanol solvents.

Our in vitro decreased responsiveness of the naloxone receptor system to morphine and the persistence of this does not fit current notions on tolerance and dependence. We, therefore, suggest a modified view of these phenomena. If the pharmacological receptor is considered as a subunit of a membrane system of enzymes (20), then opiate interaction with the drug receptor site initiates allosteric conformation changes significantly modulating the activity of the pharmacological subunit (receptor) which may be reflected in a dose-response relationship. The initial drug effect on the subunit produces a change as well in adjacent components of the system, which then leads to a number of secondary changes in metabolic processes. Among these changes are alterations in level of neurotransmitter, ion transport, adenine nucleotide derivatives, energy transduction, oxidative metabolism, etc. Any or all of these changes, some probably acting in concert, are capable of effecting a stable configurational change in the receptor.

Our data on the binding of morphine antagonists are compatible with Collier's hypothesis for the drug-induced changes in the number or kinds of receptors (21). The significance of our results is that we have shown tolerance by means of a physical binding procedure, which persists for longer periods of time than is

83

currently believed. We note that the disappearance of this physical binding tolerance between 4-8 weeks follows a time course similar to the disappearance of the morphine-induced repression of brain RNA transcriptase reported by Hodgson et al (22).

Acknowledgement

This work was supported in part by a grant from the US Public Health Service. We thank Arthur Schwartz, Patricia Marchok and Jay Davies for technical assistance.

References

1. A. GOLDSTEIN, L. L. LOWNEY, and B. K. PAL, Proc. U.S. Nat. Acad. Sci. 68 1742 (1971).
2. C. B. PERT, and S. H. SNYDER, Proc. U.S. Nat. Acad. Sci. 70 2242 (1973).
3. C. B. PERT, G. PASTERNAK, and S. H. SNYDER, Science 182 1359 (1973).
4. W. A. KLEE, and R. H. STREATY, Nature 248 61 (1974).
5. N. SWISLOCKI and J. TIERNEY, Biochem. 12 1862 (1973).
6. O. H. LOWRY, N. J. ROSEBROUGH, A. L. FARR, and R. J. RANDALL, J. Biol. Chem. 193 765 (1951).
7. J. COCHIN and C. KORNETSKY, J. Pharmac. exp. Ther. 145 1 (1964).
8. A. GOLDSTEIN and P. SHEEHAN, J. Pharmac. exp. Ther. 169 175 (1969).
9. S. KAYAN and C. L. MITCHELL, Arch. int. Pharmacodyn. 199 407 (1972).
10. A. L. MISRA, C. L. MITCHELL, and L. A. WOODS, Nature 232 48 (1971).
11. S. L. MILLER and J. HARRIS, Trans. Soc. for Neurosci. 4 340 (1974).
12. H. A. WILSON, G. W. PASTERNAK, and S. H. SNYDER, Nature 253 448 (1975).
13. E. L. WAY, H. H. LOH, and R. H. SHEN, J. Pharmacol. exp. Ther. 167 1 (1969).
14. R. J. HITZMANN, B. A. HITZMANN, and H. H. LOH, Life Sci. 14 2392 (1974).
15. A. E. TAKEMORI, G. HAYASKI, and S. E. SMITS, Eur. J. Pharmacol. 20 85 (1972).
16. R. TANAHA and K. P. STRICKLAND, Arch. Biochem. Biophys. 111 583 (1965).
17. S. J. MULE, Biochem. Pharmacol. 19 581 (1970).
18. S. R. LEVINSON and R. D. KEYNES, Biochem. Biophys. Acta. 288 241 (1972).
19. H. H. LOH, T. M. CHO, Y. C. WU, and E. L. WAY, Life Sciences 14 2231 (1974).
20. B. LIBET and T. TOSAKA, Proc. U. S. Nat. Acad. Sci. 67 667 (1970).
21. H. O. J. COLLIER, Nature 205 181 (1965).
22. J. R. HODGSON, R. L. BRISTOW, and T. R. CASTLES, Nature 248 671 (1974).

DISCRIMINATION BY TEMPERATURE OF OPIATE AGONIST AND ANTAGONIST RECEPTOR BINDING

Ian Creese, Gavril W. Pasternak, Candace B. Pert and Solomon H. Snyder

Departments of Pharmacology and Experimental Therapeutics and Psychiatry and the Behavioral Sciences, Johns Hopkins University School of Medicine, Baltimore Maryland 21205

(Received in final form May 24, 1975)

Variations in incubation temperature can markedly differentiate opiate receptor binding of agonists and antagonists. In the presence of sodium increasing incubation temperatures from $0°$ to $30°$ reduces receptor binding of ^{3}H-naloxone by 50% while tripling the binding of the agonist ^{3}H-dihydromorphine. Lowering incubation temperature from $25°$ to $0°$ reduces the potency of morphine in inhibiting ^{3}H-naloxone binding by 9-fold while not affecting the potency of the antagonist nalorphine. At temperatures of $25°$ and higher the number of binding sites for opiate antagonists is increased by sodium and the number of sites for agonists is decreased by sodium with no changes in affinity. By contrast, in the presence of sodium lowering of incubation temperature to $0°$ increases opiate receptor binding of the antagonist naloxone by enhancing its affinity for binding sites even though the total number of binding sites are not changed.

The binding of opiate agonists and antagonists to the opiate receptor (1, 2,3) can be differentiated by a number of experimental manipulations. Sodium selectively enhances the binding of antagonists and decreases the binding of agonists (4,5,6,7). Protein modifying reagents (8,9) and some enzymes also selectively decrease the binding of opiate agonists (10). By contrast, manganese and certain other divalent cations, increase the binding of opiate agonists (11). In this study we report that temperature variations differentially affect opiate receptor binding of agonists and antagonists and interact with the influence of sodium on the opiate receptor.

METHODS

Brains, minus cerebella, from male Sprague-Dawley rats were homogenized in 20 volumes (w/v) of buffer for 20 secs, centrifuged and the pellets resuspended in 100 volumes of 0.02M Ammonium phosphate buffer (pH 7.4) which was used in preference to Tris-HCl as its pH is less temperature dependent. In some experiments (detailed in tables) 0.05M Tris-HCl buffer was used (pH 7.4 at $37°C$) so that data would be comparable to previous results. The homogenate was then used directly for assay or preincubated at $37°C$ for 40 min, centrifuged and resuspended in 100 volumes of buffer and then assayed. Aliquots of homogenate were incubated in triplicate $\pm$ 1μM levallorphan with the ^{3}H-opiate. When studying the inhibition of ^{3}H-naloxone binding by unlabeled opiates, six concentrations of the drug were included in the incubation. Samples were incubated at various temperatures to equilibrium: $37°C$-20min, $30°C$-30min, $25°C$-40 min, $20°C$-1 hr, $15°C$-2 hr, $10°C$-2 hr, $0°C$-3 hr. After incubation, samples were either immediately filtered at their incubation temperature or immersed in an ice bath for 15min [our previous standard assay technique (1,4,5)], and then filtered as previously described (12). Specific opiate receptor binding was defined as the difference between the binding of the labeled ligand in the presence and absence of 1μM levallorphan.

In the absence of sodium the binding of the pure antagonist ^{3}H-naloxone and the agonist ^{3}H-dihydromorphine display a similar temperature dependence (Fig. 1a). By contrast, in the presence of sodium ^{3}H-naloxone binding declines by 50% between 0° and 30° while ^{3}H-dihydromorphine binding increases about four-fold over the same range (Fig. 1b). As reported previously (5,6) sodium enhances the binding of ^{3}H-naloxone and decreases the binding of ^{3}H-dihydromorphine. The influence of sodium is markedly temperature dependent (Fig. 2). The augmentation of naloxone binding by sodium is more than 4 times greater at 0° than at 25°. The maximal reduction of ^{3}H-dihydromorphine binding by sodium is less markedly influenced by temperature but its binding is more sensitive to sodium at 0° than at 25° with respective EC_{50} values for sodium inhibition of 32mM and 70mM. Thus, in the presence of sodium, the binding of the antagonist, naloxone, is greatest at 0° compared to other temperatures while the binding of the agonist, dihydromorphine, is lowest at 0°. Accordingly, temperature alters the potency of the agonist morphine, but not the antagonist nalorphine, to inhibit ^{3}H-naloxone binding. Morphine becomes almost 9-fold weaker in inhibiting ^{3}H-naloxone binding at 0° (EC_{50} 130nM) than at 25° (EC_{50} 15 nM) while the ability of nalorphine is the same at 0° (EC_{50} 8nM) and at 25° (EC_{50} 10nM), all assayed in the presence of 100mM NaCl.

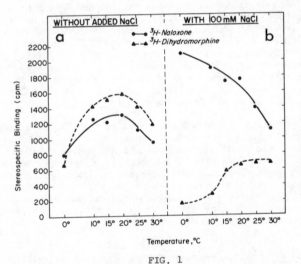

FIG. 1

Effect of incubation temperature on the stereospecific binding of ^{3}H-naloxone and ^{3}H-dihydromorphine ±100mM NaCl. Preincubated homogenate was incubated with either ^{3}H-naloxone (0.8nM) or ^{3}H-dihydromorphine (0.45nM) at each temperature, to equilibrium, and filtered immediately.

In previous experiments in which tissue was not preincubated and incubations with ^{3}H-naloxone were at 25° and then cooled to 0° prior to filtering, the enhancement of ^{3}H-naloxone binding appeared to result from an increase in the number of binding sites with no change in their affinity (5,6). When tissue is preincubated prior to a 25° incubation and cooled to 0° for 15 min, increased ^{3}H-naloxone binding elicited by sodium is also associated with an augmentation in the number of binding sites with no change in affinity. This is still true when tissue is preincubated and incubations are conducted at 25°

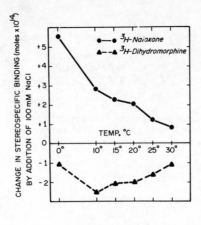

FIG. 2

Effect of incubation temperature on the increase in stereospecific
[3]H-naloxone binding and the decrease in stereospecific ^{3}H-dihydro-
morphine binding caused by 100mM NaCl. Preincubated homogenate was incubated at each temperature, to equilibrium, with either ^{3}H-naloxone
(0.8nM) or ^{3}H-dihydromorphine (0.45nM), and filtered immediately.
The change in stereospecific binding (moles x 10^{14}) caused by 100mM
NaCl is plotted against temperature.

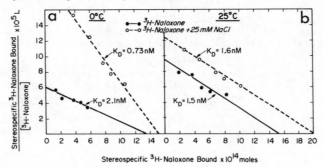

FIG. 3

Scatchard plots of ^{3}H-naloxone stereospecific binding ±25mM NaCl at
0°C or 25°C. Preincubated homogenates in ammonium phosphate buffer
were incubated to equilibrium with various concentrations of [3]H-
naloxone ±25mM NaCl, and filtered immediately.

and tissue is not cooled down prior to filtering (Fig. 3b). By contrast, the
more marked increase in ^{3}H-naloxone binding induced by incubation with sodium
at 0° compared to 25° in preincubated tissue (Fig. 2) appears to derive from a
2-3 fold greater affinity of binding sites for naloxone with no significant
difference in the total number of sites at 0° and 25° (Fig. 3a). Thus while
the ability of sodium per se to enhance opiate antagonist binding is due to an
increased number of binding sites, the distinct added increment of ^{3}H-naloxone
binding at 0° derives from enhanced affinity.

TABLE 1
Effect of Incubation and Filtration Temperatures on ^{3}H-Naloxone Binding in Nonpreincubated and Preincubated Tissue

Incubation Temperature °C	Filtration Temperature °C	Stereospecific ^{3}H-Naloxone Binding 0mM NaCl	100mM NaCl	Percent Increase in Stereospecific Binding
		Nonpreincubated Tissue		
37°	37°	1596	1517	-5
25°	25°	1831 _cpm_	2680	+46
25°	0° (15min)	1479	3102	+110
0°	0°	970	3495	+260
		Preincubated Tissue		
25°	25°	2153	2337	+8
25°	0° (15min)	1972 _cpm_	3618	+84
0°	0°	1504	3199	+113

Nonpreincubated or preincubated homogenate in Tris buffer was incubated with ^{3}H-naloxone (1.5nM) $\pm$100mM NaCl. Samples were then filtered at the incubation temperature except for the 25°C-0°C condition where the samples were cooled in an ice bath for 15 min before filtering.

The influence of preincubation, incubation and filtration temperature on the effect of sodium on opiate receptor binding is shown in Table 1. Preincubation enhances the binding of both agonists and antagonists in the absence of sodium, through an increase in the number of binding sites (9). Sodium maximally enhances ^{3}H-naloxone binding if tissue is not preincubated and if incubation and filtration are both carried out at 0°. As incubation and filtration temperatures are increased the ability of sodium to increase ^{3}H-naloxone binding is decreased. Under all conditions, preincubation decreases the extent of the sodium effect. Just as preincubation decreases the ability of sodium to

TABLE 2
Effect of Incubation and Filtration Temperature on the Ability of Morphine to Displace ^{3}H-Naloxone Binding

Incubation Temperature °C	Filtration Temperature °C	Inhibition of Stereospecific ^{3}H-Naloxone Binding EC_{50} nM 0mM NaCl	EC_{50} nM +100mM NaCl	$\dfrac{EC_{50}\ 100\text{mM NaCl}}{EC_{50}\ \ 0\text{mM NaCl}}$
		Nonpreincubated Tissue		
37°	37°	5	70	14
25°	25°	4	45	11.3
25°	0° (15min)	7	300	43
0°	0°	4.5	170	38
		Preincubated Tissue		
25°	25°	14	110	7.9
25°	0° (15min)	15	300	20
0°	0°	7	200	29

Nonpreincubated or preincubated tissue in Tris buffer was incubated with ^{3}H-naloxone (1.5nM) $\pm$100mM NaCl with six concentrations of morphine. Samples were filtered as indicated and the EC_{50} for inhibition of ^{3}H-naloxone binding was determined by log probit analysis.

enhance ^{3}H-naloxone binding, so in preincubated tissue sodium is less capable of decreasing morphine's ability to inhibit ^{3}H-naloxone binding (Table 2). Sodium maximally decreases the potency of morphine in inhibiting ^{3}H-naloxone binding when incubation and filtration are both conducted at 0° or when incubation at 25° is followed by filtration at 0°, the condition previously used to measure "sodium shifts" (4,5). Incubation and filtration at higher temperatures is associated with a lesser ability of sodium to reduce morphine's apparent affinity for the opiate receptor.

DISCUSSION

Lower temperatures clearly discriminate agonist and antagonist opiate receptor binding. At low temperatures, sodium increases antagonist and reduces agonist binding. If incubations are continued to equilibrium at $0°$, sodium increases ^{3}H-naloxone binding by an increase in affinity without a change in the number of binding sites. Since low temperature, like sodium, increases antagonist and decreases agonist binding, the low temperature effect synergizes with sodium in differentiating receptor binding of agonists and antagonists. However, because low temperature acts by a change in affinity of naloxone for binding sites rather than an alteration in their number, its influence appears to derive from a different mechanism than that of sodium, perhaps through a membrane transition known to occur at these temperatures (13). We have hypothesized that the influence of sodium on opiate receptors (4,5) may derive from two actions: 1) sodium exerts a specific influence on the conformation of the opiate receptor itself (5,7,8) and 2) sodium apparently speeds the dissociation of an endogenous factor from the opiate receptor, thereby increasing opiate receptor binding (9). The use of preincubated tissue, in order to remove the endogenous factor, allows the influences of sodium and temperature on the opiate receptor to be studied directly. Preincubation reduces the degree of sodium induced enhancement of ^{3}H-naloxone binding. The removal of the endogenous factor may enable naloxone itself to transform receptors into the antagonist state, even without the presence of sodium. The influence of sodium on agonist binding is not reduced by prior preincubation. An important conclusion to derive from these studies is that variations in incubation or filtration temperature and preincubation can exert marked influences upon opiate receptor binding of agonists and antagonists and the effect of sodium on this binding. Considerable attention should be devoted to these conditions in designing investigations of the opiate receptor.

ACKNOWLEDGEMENTS

We thank Adele Snowman for her inspired technical assistance. This work was supported by USPHS grant DA-00266. G.W.P. and C.B.P. are recipients of USPHS Postdoctoral Fellowships. S.H.S. is the recipient of an RSDA award.

REFERENCES

1. C.B. Pert and S.H. Snyder, Science 179:1011-1014 (1973).

2. E. Simon, J. Hiller and I. Edelman, Proc. Nat. Acad. Sci., USA 70:1947-1949 (1973).

3. L. Terenius, Acta Pharmacol. Toxicol. 33:377-384 (1973).

4. C.B. Pert, G. W. Pasternak and S.H. Snyder, Science 182:1359-1361 (1973).

5. C.B. Pert and S.H. Snyder, Mol. Pharmacol. 10:868-879 (1974).

6. G.W. Pasternak and S.H. Snyder, Nature 253:563-565 (1975).

7. E. Simon, J. Hiller, J. Groth and I. Edelman, J. Pharm. Exp. Ther. 192:531-537 (1975).

8. H.A. Wilson, G.W. Pasternak and S.H. Snyder, Nature 253:448-450 (1975).

9. G.W. Pasternak, H.A. Wilson and S.H. Snyder, Mol. Pharmacol. in press (1975).

10. G.W. Pasternak, and S.H. Snyder, Mol. Pharmacol. in press (1975).

11. G.W. Pasternak, A.M. Snowman and S.H. Snyder, Mol. Pharmacol. in press (1975).

12. I. Creese and S.H. Snyder, J. Pharm. Exp. Ther. in press (1975).

13. H. McConnell, P. Deveaux and C. Scantella, in Membrane Research, ed. C.F. Fox, p. 27-37, Academic Press, N.Y. (1972).

IRREVERSIBLE ALTERATION OF OPIATE RECEPTOR FUNCTION BY A

PHOTOAFFINITY LABELLING REAGENT

Rudiger Schulz and Avram Goldstein

Addiction Research Foundation, Palo Alto, California 94304

(Received in final form May 24, 1975)

Summary

A newly synthesized azido opiate derivative was studied
in the guinea pig myenteric plexus-longitudinal muscle preparation. In the dark this drug reversibly inhibits electrically
evoked acetylcholine output, a typical opiate action in this
tissue. After ultraviolet irradiation this opiate effect
becomes persistent and irreversible.

Winter and Goldstein (1) described the synthesis of an opiate derivative,
N-β(p-azidophenyl)ethylnorlevorphanol (APL), designed as a photoaffinity
label for opiate receptors. They demonstrated that this reagent was irreversibly bound to biologic material upon irradiation, but found no stereospecific
attachment such as would be required in the labelling of opiate receptors
(2,3). A likely reason for the extensive nonspecific labelling is the high
lipid solubility of APL. In order to reduce lipophilicity, the N-methyl
quaternary derivative of APL (MAPL) was synthesized. This new reagent behaved
like an opiate with about the same potency as levorphanol in inhibiting electrically induced twitches of the guinea pig ileum myenteric plexus-longitudinal muscle preparation (4). Since twitch inhibition by opiates is known to
be caused by a reduction of acetylcholine (ACh) release from the myenteric
plexus (5-7), we chose to measure the effect of MAPL on ACh release in the
dark and after ultraviolet irradiation. We shall report elsewhere on the
corresponding effects upon electrically induced twitches.

Methods

Myenteric plexus-longitudinal muscle strips of about 40 mg wet weight
were prepared from the guinea pig ileum according to Kosterlitz et al (8),
mounted in 5 ml Krebs-Ringer solution[1] as described previously (9) but equili-
brated without electrical stimulation. For measuring ACh release, eserine
(10 μM) was added to the bath fluid, and electrical field stimulation (0.1 Hz,
0.5 msec square wave, 80 V) was applied. These conditions were established
10 min before and maintained during each 20 min collection period. The first
collection period (A) was carried out 40 min after setting up the preparations. Subsequently, the strips were incubated for 5 min with the drug under
investigation. When the narcotic antagonist naloxone was tested, it was preincubated with the tissue for 3 min. For irradiation the preparations were

---

[1]The Krebs-Ringer solution consisted of (in mM): NaCl, 118; KCl, 4.75;
CaCl$_2$, 2.54; KH$_2$PO$_4$, 1.19; MgSO$_4$, 1.20; NaHCO$_3$, 25.0; glucose, 11.0; choline
chloride, 0.02; and 0.125 μM mepyramine maleate; it was bubbled with 95%
O$_2$/5% CO$_2$, at 37° C.

transferred into Corex tubes containing the same drug concentration in freshly
mixed Ringer solution, placed in a water bath (18°C), and irradiated for
20 min.[2] Thereafter, the strips were remounted in their organ baths. Control
preparations were treated identically but not irradiated. Some control strips
were kept in their baths and the ACh output was measured in presence of the
drugs for 20 min (collection period B) instead of the 20 min period of
irradiation. Regardless of which procedure was used, all preparations were
subsequently washed for 110 min at 5-10 min intervals, without eserine or
electrical stimulation. Finally, all strips were subjected to a further 20
min collection period (C). In unirradiated control preparations, the long
washing procedure removed MAPL or the other drugs tested, as indicated by the
recoevery of the twitch tension and the lack of response to naloxone
challenge.[3] At the end of the experiment the strips were blotted and weighed.
Whenever MAPL was under investigation, the experiments were carried out in the
dark except during irradiation.

To assay the ACh released, the collected Ringer samples (5 ml) were
adjusted to pH 4 with acetic acid. ^{14}C-ACh[4] was added to each sample to
correct for loss (about 25%) during the analytic procedure. After lyophi-
lizing the samples, each residue was extracted with 5 ml of a 100:1 mixture
of acetone with formic acid (88% w/v). The clear supernatant was dried under
a stream of nitrogen and the residue was taken up in 1 ml Ringer solution.
Employing the myenteric plexus-longitudinal muscle strip preparation and
standard solutions of ACh, each sample was assayed twice. The contractions
induced are considered to be due to ACh, since they were blocked by atropine
$(10^{-6}M)$ and not affected by morphine $(5 \times 10^{-7}M)$, and the activity of the
material collected in the presence of eserine was destroyed by boiling at
pH 10. Samples collected in the absence of eserine did not cause twitches.
The data for the released ACh are expressed as ng ACh/100 mg strip per 20 min.

Results

The results obtained without irradiation are given in the first part of
Table 1.   1: In the absence of any drug, the duration of the experiment
(about 4 h) and the handling of the preparations (removal from tissue bath and
holding for 20 min at 18° C in Ringer solution) had very little effect on ACh
release.   2: Levorphanol (a typical morphine-like narcotic) strongly inhibited ACh output (period B) and this effect was reversed by washing (period C).
3: Preincubation of strips with naloxone prevented the levorphanol effect.
4: In strips exposed continuously to levorphanol throughout the experiment,
naloxone reversed the inhibition of ACh output; indeed, there was an interesting "overshoot" above the initial output, which could represent an adaptation
to prolonged exposure to the opiate.   5: MAPL reduced the ACh output, and

---

[2] Hanovia medium pressure 450 W mercury arc lamp with Kimax sleeve in a quartz
immersion well. Corex tubes (15 mm I.D., 1 mm wall) at 60 mm from lamp.

[3] In the electrically stimulated strip, naloxone itself is without effect.
Only when twitch tension is reduced by an opiate agonist does naloxone cause
an increase in twitch tension.

[4] Acetylcholine chloride (acetyl-1-^{14} C), Spec. act. 25mCi/mmole (Amersham).

TABLE 1

Effects of Opiates and Irradiation on Acetylcholine Release from
Myenteric Plexus–Longitudinal Muscle Strip

ACh Output

Per cent change from Period A

Drug	Drug Present (Period B)	After Washing (Period C)
Not irradiated		
1 None[a]	--	-8, -10
2 Lev 0.5 μM	-51, -66	-2, +6[b]
1.0 μM	-85, -90	-14, -12
3 Nal + Lev 1.0 μM[c]	-6. -8	-4, -13
4 Lev 1.0 μM + Nal[d]	-58 ± 5 (4)	+39 ± 13 (4)
5 MAPL 0.25 μM	-56 ± 8 (4)	-8 + 5[b] (4)
6 Nal + MAPL 0.25 μM[c]	-6, 13	-10, -12
7 MAPL 0.25 μM + Nal[d]	-39 ± 4 (4)	+1 ± 7 (4)
Irradiated		
1 None		-5, -6
2 MAPL 0.25 μM		-44 ± 3 (10)
3 Nal + MAPL 0.25 μM[c]		-1 ± 4 (4)
4 MAPL 0.25 μM + Nal[e]		-34, -36
0.50 μM + Nal[e]		-74 ± 3 (4)

Electrical stimulation was carried out in the presence of eserine (10 μM), and ACh release was measured as described in text. Collection period A represents ACh release in the absence of any drug; in 58 preparations the mean amount released was 92 (s.e.m.=4) ng per 100 mg tissue strip in 20 min. Between periods B and C the strip was washed repeatedly for 2 h. Experiments with MAPL were conducted in the dark except during the 20-min irradiation. For experiments with only two strips, individual results are shown; otherwise mean and s.e.m. are given, with number of strips in parentheses. Lev = levorphanol; Nal = naloxone 1.0 μM; MAPL = N-methyl quaternary derivative of N-β(p-azidophenyl)ethylnorlevorphanol.

(For Footnotes to TABLE 1, see next page).

(Footnotes to TABLE 1)

[a] Strips removed for 20 min from tissue bath and kept in Ringer solution at 18° C.

[b] Subsequent naloxone challenge did not alter the electrically induced twitch tension in this group of four strips.

[c] Naloxone concentration maintained until 1 h after starting the wash procedure.

[d] Opiate concentration maintained until the end of the experiment; naloxone added during collection period C.

[e] Naloxone added during collection period C.

---

this effect was reversed almost completely by washing. MAPL appeared to be approximately twice as potent as levorphanol. _6_: Naloxone largely prevented the action of MAPL. _7_: Naloxone reversed the effect of MAPL.

The effects of irradiation are shown in the second part of Table 1. _1_: In the absence of any drug, irradiation of the strips was virtually without effect. _2_: When strips were irradiated during incubation with MAPL, the inhibition of ACh release could not be reversed despite the extensive wash procedure. _3_: The presence of naloxone during irradiation with MAPL virtually blocked the MAPL effect, as evidenced by normal ACh release during period C. _4_: Naloxone could not reverse the effect of irradiation with MAPL.

Discussion

The data presented here confirm reports by others (5,10) that narcotic opiates inhibit the release of ACh from the myenteric plexus. We have found (data not presented here) that this effect is stereospecific for the D(-) isomer. When the opiates levorphanol and MAPL were tested in the dark, their inhibitory effect on ACh release could be reversed by washing, and naloxone blocked and reversed it. Irradiation of MAPL in contact with opiate receptors of the myenteric plexus resulted in an irreversible inhibition of ACh release, which could not be reversed by naloxone. However, preincubation of the strips with naloxone before and during irradiation in the presence of MAPL prevented these irreversible effects. These results indicate that MAPL competes with naloxone for occupancy of opiate receptor sites, and suggest that it may be attached there covalently upon exposure to ultraviolet radiation. It is possible, therefore, that MAPL will prove useful as an opiate receptor site labelling reagent.

Our results support the theory that occupancy of receptors by opiate agonists is a sufficient condition to bring about pharmacologic activity. They are inconsistent with Paton's "rate theory" (11), which correlates the rate of dissociation of an agonistic drug at equilibrium with its activity. It follows from this theory that agonists should be converted to antagonists after they become irreversibly attached to the receptor. Our results show, on the contrary, a persistent agonistic narcotic effect (i.e., persistent inhibition of ACh release). Thus, opiate action does not seem to require continuous stimulation such as would result from repetitive dissociation and combination of a drug with its receptor. Our results differ from those of Portoghese and his colleagues (12), who suggested that the long-lasting blockade of opiate analgesia observed in their experiments was due to alkylation of opiate receptors. Our findings are consistent with the interpretation that opiates may act by causing a specific alteration (e.g., a conformation change) of the receptor. Thus, they are compatible with the hypothesis that opiates allosterically inhibit an enzyme, such as a prostaglandin-stimulated adenylate cyclase (13).

We have shown that the persistent agonist effect caused by irradiation in the presence of MAPL is not reversed by an antagonist. On the other hand, exposure to the antagonist in the first place evidently prevents the binding of MAPL. These results strongly suggest the action of opiate agonists and antagonists on a common receptor site, as proposed by others (14-18). If the "dual receptor" hypothesis advanced by Martin (19) implies that narcotic agonists can combine only with agonistic receptor sites and antagonists only with antagonist receptor sites, our results are clearly incompatible with that hypothesis. However, our findings do not absolutely preclude separate sites for antagonists; the inefficacy of naloxone after photochemical attachment of MAPL could be explained if MAPL became attached to antagonist sites as well as to agonist sites.

A theory proposed by Goldstein (20) requires a conformation change of a dimeric receptor to bring about narcotic action. Narcotic antagonists are thought to prevent or reverse the conformation change even in the presence of a reversibly bound opiate. In the framework of this concept, our results would indicate that irreversible attachment of an opiate agonist prevents reversion of the receptor to its normal functional conformation.

Since naloxone prevents the irreversible photochemical effect observed here, it is evident that MAPL must occupy the opiate receptor sites during irradiation. It is conceivable, however, that the reactive azene generated by irradiation could alter receptors irreversibly by a "hit-and-run" mechanism, without any permanent attachment of the labelling reagent. This alternative explanation can be ruled out only by direct measurements of the stereospecific attachment of MAPL. Such experiments will be reported elsewhere.

Acknowledgements

We thank Dr. Kent Opheim for providing MAPL; Hoffman-La Roche, Inc., for levorphanol tartrate and dextrorphan tartrate; and Endo Laboratories for a gift of naloxone hydrochloride. Supported by NIDA Research Grant DA-972 and DA-249 as well as by the Drug Abuse Council.

References

1. B. A. WINTER and A. GOLDSTEIN, Mol. Pharmacol. 8, 601–611 (1972).

2. A. GOLDSTEIN, L. I. LOWNEY and B. K. PAL, Proc. Nat. Acad. Sci., U.S.A. 68, 1742–1747 (1971).

3. A. GOLDSTEIN, Life Sci., 14, 615–623 (1974).

4. K. OPHEIM and A. GOLDSTEIN, in preparation.

5. W. SCHAUMANN, Brit. J. Pharmacol. Chemother. 12, 115–118 (1957).

6. W. D. M. PATON, Brit. J. Pharmacol. 12, 119–127 (1957).

7. A. L. COWIE, H. W. KOSTERLITZ and A. J. WATT, Nature 220, 1040–1042 (1968).

8. H. W. KOSTERLITZ, R. J. LYDON and A. J. WATT, Brit. J. Pharmacol. 39, 398–413 (1970).

9. A. GOLDSTEIN and R. SCHULZ, Brit. J. Pharmacol. 48, 655–666 (1973).

10. B. M. COX and M. WEINSTOCK, Brit. J. Pharmacol. 27, 81–92 (1966).

11. W. D. M. PATON, Proc. Roy. Soc. Ser. B. 154, 21–69 (1961).

12. P. S. PORTOGHESE, V. G. TELANG, A. E. TAKEMORI and G. HAYASHI, J. Med. Chem. 14, 144–148 (1971).

13. H. O. J. COLLIER and A. C. ROY, Prostaglandins, 7, 361–376 (1974).

14. A. M. BECKETT, A. F. CASY and N. J. HARPER, J. Pharm. Pharmacol. 8, 874–884 (1956).

15. B. M. COX and M. WEINSTOCK, Brit. J. Pharmacol. 22, 289–300 (1964).

16. S. ARCHER and L. S. HARRIS, in Progress in Drug Research (E. Jucker, ed.) pp. 262–320, Birkhauser, Verlag, Basel und Stuttgart (1965).

17. A. E. TAKEMORI, H. J. KUPFERBERG and J. W. MILLER, J. Pharmacol. Exp. Ther. 169, 39–45 (1969).

18. P. S. PORTOGHESE, J. Pharm. Sci. 55, 865–887 (1966).

19. W. R. MARTIN, Pharmacol. Rev., 19, 463–521 (1967).

20. A. GOLDSTEIN, in Narcotic Antagonists (M. C. Braude, L. S. Harris, E. L. May, J. P. Smith and J. E. Villarreal, eds.) pp. 471–481, Raven Press, New York (1974).

AUTORADIOGRAPHIC LOCALIZATION OF THE OPIATE RECEPTOR IN RAT BRAIN

Candace B. Pert, Michael J. Kuhar and Solomon H. Snyder

Departments of Pharmacology and Experimental Therapeutics and Psychiatry and the Behavioral Sciences, Johns Hopkins University School of Medicine, Baltimore Maryland 21205

(Received in final form May 24, 1975)

One hour after injection of the potent opiate antagonist ^{3}H-diprenorphine (125 µCi, 13 Ci/mmole) 75-85% of the drug is associated with opiate receptor sites. Autoradiography of fresh frozen unfixed brain has been carried out to visualize receptor distribution. Dense clusters of autoradiographic grains are highly localized in the caudate-putamen, locus coeruleus, zona compacta of the substantia nigra and the substantia gelatinosa.

Recently, direct biochemical demonstration of the hypothetical receptor sites which mediate opiate action (1,2) has been accomplished (3-7). Using an in vitro rapid filtration procedure (3,4), it has been possible to study the subcellular (8), phylogenetic (9), neuroblastoma cell line (10) and monkey and human regional (11,12) distributions of opiate receptors.

In Rhesus monkey brain, opiate receptor distribution is strikingly heterogeneous (11,12) with a 30-fold difference in receptor content from the highest (amygdala) to the lowest (occipital pole) region examined, some regions (cerebellar cortex, white matter areas) containing no receptors. On one level, brain areas enriched in opiate receptor sites might be expected to mediate the pharmacological actions of opiates. In Rhesus monkeys, minute intracranial injections of morphine elicit analgesia only in the medial thalamus, periventricular and periaqueductal regions (13). These regions are indeed among the most receptor enriched examined (11). On another level, however, the physiological significance of the opiate receptor's uneven distribution is unclear. While no known neurochemical parallels this distribution (11), opiate receptors may normally interact with a previously undescribed endogenous substance (14).

We now report a procedure for light microscopic autoradiographic visualization of opiate receptor sites in rat brain. This procedure, which has been used previously to study the distribution of muscarinic receptors (15), is based upon autoradiographic techniques developed to visualize steroid hormone receptors in fresh, frozen unfixed brain tissue (16-18).

METHODS

Rats (170-200 g) were injected with saline containing 125 µCi of ^{3}H-diprenorphine (13 Ci/mmole) obtained from Amersham Corp (19) and sacrificed at various times following injection. Their brains were dissected into regions, and homogenized for 15 sec in 150 vol of ice-cold Tris-HCl buffer (.05M, pH=7.4 at 25°C) containing 100mM NaCl. Total ^{3}H-diprenorphine content was assessed by determining the radioactivity in one ml of the unfiltered homogenates by liquid scintillation spectrophotometry (4). For autoradiography, rats (170g) were injected with 125µCi of ^{3}H-diprenorphine (13Ci/mmole) and decapitated 1 hour later, the time at which maximal association of ^{3}H-diprenorphine with specific receptor sites occurs (Table 1). Brains were rapidly cut into 3-4mm coronal sections placed on microtome chucks and lowered slowly into liquid nitrogen "slush". Sections of 4 micron thickness were cut at -18°C in a Harris cryostat microtome. Sections were transferred by "thaw-mounting" in the dark to slides which had previously been coated with Kodak-NTB-3 emulsion (15). Slides were exposed for 5 weeks at low humidity (4°C) in a dark lead-lined cabinet and then developed at 17°C in Dektol for two minutes. Development was terminated by Kodak Liquid Hardener and slides were fixed in hypo (Kodak). After washing in running tap water, sections were stained with pyronine Y, dried, mounted with Permount and observed with a Zeiss Universal microscope. Control slides prepared for positive and negative chemography showed no evidence of significant fading of latent images or spurious generations of grains after 60-day exposures. The general autoradiographic procedure utilized in this study has been described previously (16-18).

RESULTS AND DISCUSSION

The autoradiographic localization of small diffusible molecules has traditionally been difficult and has required special techniques (16-18). Generally these frozen tissue methods, by avoiding all solvents, prevent the extraction and/or translocation of the radioactive ligand during tissue preparation and exposure. Before these methods could be successfully applied for visualization of opiate receptors, however, it was necessary to find conditions in which most ^{3}H-opiate was associated with specific receptor sites in vivo.

Unfortunately, the distribution of opiate in vivo is mostly governed by nonspecific influences such as blood flow, lipid solubility and drug ionization. Many workers (20-23) have examined the in vivo distribution of opiate agonists and antagonists without finding the marked brain regional differences or stereospecificity which would have indicated that specific opiate receptor interactions were affecting the distribution of a significant percentage of drug molecules. By using very low, subsaturating doses of ^{3}H-diprenorphine, an extremely potent opiate antagonist (24) it was possible to find conditions in which the majority of the drug was associated with opiate receptors in vivo (Table 1). The dissociation of opiate agonists from specific receptor sites is greatly accelerated by sodium (25). Therefore, ^{3}H-diprenorphine, rather than its agonist analogue etorphine, was chosen to attain maximal receptor labeling in the sodium-rich in vivo environment. Moreover, ^{3}H-diprenorphine has an extremely high affinity for the opiate receptor in vitro (1-2 x 10^{-10}M) and thus was expected to become selectively associated with receptors with time, as nonspecific, low affinity bound diprenorphine was cleared from brain.

TABLE 1
In Vivo Distribution of ^{3}H-Diprenorphine

Region	10 min	30 min	1 hr	2 hr	3 hr
		Time After Injection			
Cerebellum	170	110	80	75	80
Hindbrain	315	260	185	110	115
Midbrain	585	480	370	240	230
Ratio of Midbrain/Cerebellum					
Total cpm	3.4	4.3	4.6	3.2	2.8

^{3}H-Diprenorphine (125µCi) was injected into the tail vein, rats sacrificed at various times after injection and radioactivity content of three regions determined. Data are cpm/mg tissue and represent the means from 4-5 rats, whose values varied less than 20%.

One hour after injection of ^{3}H-diprenorphine (.008mg/kg, i.v., 125 µCi) the highest ratio of midbrain/hindbrain radioactivity content is attained (Table 1). The midbrain has 2 times as much binding in vivo as the hindbrain.

In _vitro_, the midbrain has 1.8 times as much stereospecific receptor binding as the hindbrain. The cerebellum, which is devoid of stereospecific binding _in vitro_ (3), has only 20% as much binding as the midbrain _in vivo_. Furthermore, after preinjection of rats with nonradioactive levallorphan (5mg/kg, i.v.) total brain content of ^{3}H-diprenorphine is reduced by 75% while preinjection with the same dose of the inactive (+) isomer of levallorphan is without effect. The strikingly heterogeneous regional distribution of injected ^{3}H-diprenorphine (which is consistent with that observed _in vitro_) as well as the marked stereo-specificity of ^{3}H-diprenorphine displacement suggests that 75-80% of the ^{3}H-diprenorphine is associated with opiate receptors under these conditions.

While not all ^{3}H-diprenorphine is specifically localized, there is suffi-cient labeling of receptor sites to obtain striking regional differences using autoradiography (Table 2). The rat striatum has previously been shown to con-tain the highest opiate-receptor content in rat brain (3). In the caudate-putamen, we observed a remarkable clustering of autoradiographic grains (Table 2, Figure 1). Grains are highly restricted to "patches" (Figure 1B) which are spaced irregularly over the corpus striatum (CS). In addition, a "streak" of autoradiographic grains of only a few hundred microns wide occurs all along the corpus striatum (CS) immediately adjacent and ventral to to the corpus callosum (CC) (Figure 1A). On either side of this narrow band of high density grains, the grain count is at background levels.

TABLE 2

Distribution of Autoradiographic Grains in Coronal Sections of Rat Brain

Region	$\bar{x}$ Grains/100^{2}microns
Nucleus caudatus putamen	
"streak" ventral to corpus callosum	11.5
"clusters"	10.5
low density areas	1.7
fibers	1.2
Substantia gelatinosa (spinal cord)	10.4
Locus coeruleus	10.0
Amygdala medialis	6.5
Amygdala centralis	5.8
Zona compacta of substantia nigra	6.5
Thalamus medialis	5.5
Periventricular substance	5.2
Habenula	5.1
Lateral habenula	5.0
Nucleus periventricularis (of hypothalamus)	3.8
Nucleus ventromedialis (of hypothalamus)	2.8
Dentate gyrus	2.1
Motor cortex	2.0
Zona reticulata of substantia nigra	1.9
Hippocampus	1.7
Corpus callosum	0.7
Fimbria	0.8
Ventricle III	1.3
Pyrifirm cortex	1.1
Cerebellum	0.8
Nucleus of cranial nerve V	0.8

Grain counts represent the means of 2400 square micron areas.

While grains in the medial thalamus are high and diffusely distributed, receptor sites are highly localized in the lateral edge of the medial habenu-lar nucleus. Figure 1C shows the medial habenular nucleus with an arrow point-ing toward the midline. Figure 1D shows an area slightly more lateral, with the lateral edge of the medial habenular nucleus in the upper right corner, the arrow again pointing toward the midline. The striking absence of grains in the lower left corner which shows the medial side of the medial habenular nucleus is noticeable.

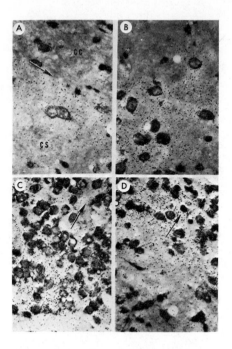

FIG. 1

Autoradiographs of corpus striatum (A,B) and habenular nucleus (C,D) of rats injected with ^{3}H-diprenorphine.

In general, we have observed patterns of high density grain localization with rather sharp distinct boundaries. For example, the areas surrounding the high density amygdaloid nuclei are only slightly above background. The locus coeruleus is highly labeled, while the nearby nucleus of cranial nerve V is not above background (Table 2). Interestingly, single units in the locus coeruleus are specifically inhibited by morphine (26). In agreement with in vitro studies (3,11,12) the cerebellum and white matter areas have grain counts of "background" levels. In all labeled regions grains appear at least 5 times more frequently in between cell bodies than over them. This suggests that receptor sites are primarily on dendritic processes, which is in good agreement with the synaptic localization of receptors by in vitro methods (8).

Selective labeling of certain cell types within a single area are potentially of great interest. Thus far, we have observed high density grain counts in parts of the zona compacta, but not the zona reticulata of the substantia nigra. The entire substantia gelatinosa of the dorsal horn is highly labeled in an extremely narrow band. This is consistent with the notion that morphine has an analgesic action at the spinal level (27).

We are currently preparing coronal sections of the complete rat central nervous system in order to obtain a detailed map on stereotoxic drawings of opiate receptor distribution. Presumably, brain neuronal groups with dense opiate receptor enrichment should be useful "target areas" for future electrophysiological and lesioning studies.

ACKNOWLEDGEMENT

We are grateful for the expert technical assistance of Mrs. Naomi Taylor

REFERENCES

1. V.P. Dole, Ann. Rev. Biochem. 39:821 (1970).

2. A. Goldstein, L. Aronow and S.M. Kalman,   Principles of Drug Action, Harper and Row, New York, p. 50 (1968).

3. C.B. Pert and S.H. Snyder, Science 179:1011 (1973).

4. C.B. Pert and S.H. Snyder, Proc. Nat. Acad. Sci., USA 70:2243 (1973).

5. E.J. Simon, J.M. Hiller and I. Edelman, Proc. Nat. Acad. Sci., USA 70:1947 (1973).

6. L. Terenius, Acta Pharmac. Toxic. 32:317 (1973).

7. A. Goldstein, Life Sci. 14:615 (1974).

8. C.B. Pert, A.M. Snowman and S.H. Snyder, Brain Res. 70:184 (1974).

9. C.B. Pert, D. Aposhian and S.H. Snyder, Brain Res. 75:356 (1974).

10. W.A. Klee and M. Nirenberg, Proc. Nat. Acad. Sci., USA 71:3474 (1974).

11. M.J. Kuhar, C.B. Pert and S.H. Snyder, Nature 245:5426 (1973).

12. J.M. Hiller , J. Pearson and E.J. Simon, Res. Comm. in Chem. Path. and Pharmac. 6:1052 (1973).

13. A. Pert and T. Yaksh, Brain Res. 80:135 (1974).

14. J. Hughes, Brain Res. 88:102 (1975).

15. M.J. Kuhar and H. Yamamura, Nature 253:560 (1975).

16. C.H. Anderson and G.S. Greenwald, Endocrinology 85:1160 (1969).

17. W.E. Stumpf and L.G. Roth, J. Histochem.Cytochem. 14:274 (1966).

18. J.L. Gerlach and B.S. McEwen, Science 175:1133 (1972).

19. J.W. Lewis, M.J. Rance and G. Raymond Young, J. Med. Chem. 17:465 (1974).

20. C.B. Pert and S.H. Snyder, Life Sci. (in press).

21. N.A. Ingoglia and V.P. Dole, J. Pharm. Exp. Ther. 175:84 (1970).

22. B.A. Berkowitz and E.L. Way, J. Pharm. Exp. Ther. 177:500 (1971).

23. D.H. Clouet and N. Williams, Biochem. Pharm. 22:1283 (1973).

24. K.W. Bentley, A.L.A. Boura, A.E. Fitzgerald, D.G. Hardy, A. McCoubrey, M.L. Aikman and R.E. Lister, Nature 206:102 (1965).

25. C.B. Pert and S.H. Snyder, Mol. Pharmac. 10:868 (1974).

26. J. Korf, B.S. Bunney and G.K. Aghajanian, Eur. J. Pharmacol. 25:165 (1974).

27. L.M. Kitahata, Y. Kosaka, A. Taub, K. Bonikos and M. Hoffert, Anaesthesiology 41:39 (1974).

AUTORADIOGRAPHIC EVALUATION OF THE INTRACEREBRAL DISTRIBUTION OF ^{3}H-ETORPHINE IN THE MOUSE BRAIN.

P. Schubert, V. Höllt and A. Herz

Department of Neuropathology and Department of Neuropharmacology, Max-Planck-Institut für Psychiatrie, Munich, Germany.

(Received in final form May 24, 1975)

To get more information on the intracerebral distribution of opiates, highly labeled etorphine, showing high affinity to opiate receptors, was applied and visualized by autoradiography. Five minutes after intravenous injection of ^{3}H-etorphine (2 µCi/g; spec. act. 41 Ci/mmole) the mice were killed by decapitation; the brains were quickly removed and frozen by CO_2. In the dark, 20 micron cryostat sections were cut at different levels of the brain and taken up on slides previously coated with a photographic emulsion. Following an exposure time of one to two weeks, the autoradiographs were developed, fixed, and counterstained. The distribution of the autoradiographic labeling was checked microscopically.

In general, the radioactivity applied was found sufficient to result in a distinct labeling of the tissue. Silver grains were seen nearly allover the tissue sections at the different levels. Comparing the individual structures obvious differences were evident. Although a complete mapping cannot be given here, this may be illustrated by two examples. The labeling of the cerebellum was considerably lower than that of the underlying brainstem. Here, radioactivity seemed to be accumulated in different brainstem nuclei (see Fig. left). A very differentiated and typical distribution pattern was found at the level of hippocampus (see Fig. right). Here, again labeling appeared to be concentrated in some nuclei, e.g. thalamic nuclei. Other nuclei, e.g. the nucleus habenulae showed only a very small radioactivity. Labeling of the cortex was considerably high and contrasted to the overall low-labeling of the hippocampal formation. Here, the labeling appeared to be particularly differentiated. Nearly no silver grains were found in the central part of the dentate gyrus and over the granule cell layer, whereas the molecular layer showed a distinct labeling. There was also general labeling over the remaining hippocampus with the pyramidal cells, except for a stripe-like layer just over the pyramidal cells of CA_4 which appeared free of labeling. This is the part where the mossy fiber-axons originating from the granule cells, pass through the basal dendritic layer of CA_4 neurons to terminate on the dendrites of the CA_{3-1} neurons.

Following the application of unlabeled inhibitors (naltrexone 1 mg/kg) together with the labeled opiate (^{3}H-etorphine), the overall labeling appeared to be reduced, compared to the labeling obtained after ^{3}H-opiate injection alone. Moreover, also the differences e.g. between labeling of the cerebellum and the brainstem appeared to be less obvious. The results show that autoradiography gives a more detailed information on the fine localization of the drugs within brain tissue than is possible by e.g. in vitro binding studies (2,3). But the statements which can be made are qualitative more than quantitative.

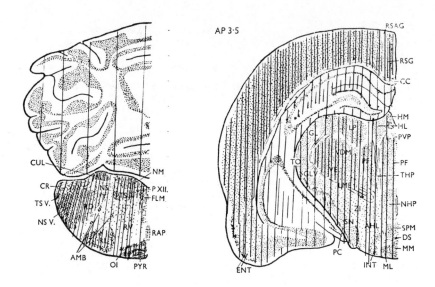

The distribution of ^{3}H-etorphine (2 μCi/g mouse) 5 minutes after i.v. injection at a frontal level (right, plane AP 3.5) and at the level of lower brainstem (left, plane AP 12) according to the stereotactic atlas (1).
The intensity of autoradiography labeling (grain density) is represented by the density of striation.

References

1) BUREŠ, J., M. PETRAN, J. ZACHAR, Electrophysiological Methods in Biological Research, Prag 1967.

2) KUHAR, M. J., C. B. PERT and S. H. SNYDER, Nature 245, 447-450 (1973).

3) HILLER, J. M., J. PEARSON and E. J. SIMON, Res. Comm. Chem. Pathol. Pharmacol. 6, 1052-1062 (1973).

PROSTAGLANDINS, CYCLIC AMP AND THE BIOCHEMICAL
MECHANISM OF OPIATE AGONIST ACTION

Ashim C. Roy   and   Harry O.J. Collier

Research Department, Miles Laboratories Limited,
Stoke Poges, Slough, SL2 4LY, England

(Received in final form May 24, 1975)

SUMMARY

The paper re-examines, in the light of recent evidence, the
original proposition that the ability of opiates to inhibit the
stimulation by E prostaglandins of cyclic AMP formation in rat
brain homogenate represents a biochemical mechanism that could
account for the analgesic and allied effects of these drugs.
It is concluded that subsequent evidence largely supports the
original proposition; but that this can now be made more definite. It is proposed that inhibition of an adenylate cyclase
of morphine-sensitive neurones is the decisive biochemical
consequence of the binding of an opiate agonist with its specific
receptor.

Early in 1974, we reported that opiates inhibit the stimulation by E prostaglandins of cyclic AMP formation in rat brain homogenate, presumably by
inhibiting the stimulation of a neuronal adenylate cyclase (1). On the basis
of its properties, we proposed that this inhibitory activity represents a
biochemical mechanism that could account for the analgesic and allied effects
of these drugs. The present paper re-examines the evidence relating to this
proposition that has since appeared (2-8), to assess how its validity now
stands. The original proposition carried the rider that opiate dependence
may arise through a biochemical hypertrophy that would compensate for the inhibition proposed. This rider will be discussed in other papers of this
symposium (9, 10).

CRITERIA AND PERFORMANCE

Our original hypothesis identified the inhibition of a biochemical process as
the cause of a group of pharmacological effects. The biochemical process is
the formation of cyclic AMP and the effects are the acute actions of opiates
that are specifically antagonized by naloxone. These agonist actions of
opiates, which are largely inhibitory, include analgesia and associated euphoria, respiratory depression, and the suppression of the response to electrical stimulation of guinea-pig ileum and mouse vas deferens (11, 12). They
are believed to arise from the interaction of opiates with what Kosterlitz
calls "morphine-sensitive neurones".

A test of our hypothesis would be to compare the observed properties of this
biochemical interaction with those of the pharmacological effects that it
intends to explain. These comparisons may be grouped under four heads: (a)
time of onset and site of action; (b) potency and effectiveness; (c) stereospecificity and specific antagonism; and (d) the appropriateness of this
biochemical interaction to the pharmacological effect.

a)   Time of onset and site of action. As regards time of onset, the incubation periods used in measuring the activity of opiates against PGE-activated cyclic AMP formation in vitro ranged between 5 and 20 min (1,4,5). That periods of 1-20 min were used by Kosterlitz and colleagues (11,12) to equilibrate a test opiate with isolated guinea-pig ileum or mouse vas deferens in determining agonist and antagonist potency suggests that the time-courses were roughly comparable of the effects of opiates on cyclic AMP formation and on evoked contraction of smooth muscles.

As regards site, the essential consideration concerns the morphine-sensitive neurone, which is one responding to low concentrations of morphine in a way that is competitively antagonised by naloxone. Any claim that a biochemical mechanism is the basis of opiate agonist action should ultimately be supported by evidence that the effect is more conspicuous or potent in cells or tissues richer in morphine-sensitive neurones. This requirement is best met by considering whether the response of a cell or tissue is related to the content of neurones with opiate receptors. Rat brain, in which most of our work has been done, is rich in such neurones (13,14). Moreover, there is a significant (P=0.01) correlation between the rank order of seven opiates in inhibiting E prostaglandin-activated cyclic AMP formation and in affinity for the opiate receptor (see below). More direct evidence could be obtained by separately testing the cerebellum, in which opiate receptors have not been found.

In cultured cells, the evidence is fuller. In glioma or glioma x fibroblast cells, morphine does not inhibit adenylate cyclase, whether or not it is stimulated with PGE_1 (3,5). In neuroblastoma or neuroblastoma x glioma cells, the effectiveness of morphine was much greater in cells rich in opiate receptors (5). Moreover, in a line of neuroblastoma x glioma cells rich in opiate receptors, Sharma et al (5) found an identical rank order of four opiate agonists for (i) affinity to the opiate receptor and (ii) potency in inhibiting basal adenylate cyclase.

So far, search has revealed only one possible exception to the restriction of the effect to morphine-sensitive neurones. This is the reversal by levorphanol and morphine of the inhibition by PGE_1 of platelet aggregation induced by adrenaline or ADP in human shed plasma (R.J. Gryglewski, A. Szczeklik, K. Bieron, personal communication). If this effect proves to be specific and stereospecific, it would not be the first time that blood platelets have biochemically simulated neurones.

b)   Potency and effectiveness. Only an interaction of a drug with a biochemical process in vitro that possesses appropriately high potency and a high, dose-related effectiveness is likely to apply in drug therapy in vivo, in which concentration of drug at the site of action is usually low. Moreover, of two interactions, the one with higher potency and effectiveness is likely to be the one operating at therapeutic doses of the drug. To compare the possible contribution to therapy of the inhibition of prostaglandin-activated and basal cyclic AMP formation in central neurones, we determined, in the same preparation of rat brain homogenate, the inhibitory effect of 4, 20, 100 and 500 μM morphine against these two types of cyclic AMP formation. Whereas, for PGE_1-activated formation, these concentrations of morphine yielded a smooth dose/response line, running from 32% to 95% inhibition, none of them had an appreciable effect on basal cyclic AMP formation.

It is reasonable to expect, too, that the potency of a drug's interaction with a biochemical mechanism in vitro should roughly match the
concentration of the drug at its site of pharmacological action in vivo.
In the main experiments so far reported, the dose/response line for inhibition by morphine of PGE-stimulated cyclic AMP formation runs from a
minimal to a maximal effect between about 10^{-7} to 10^{-4} Molar, or 29 ng
to 29 μg ml^{-1} (1-6). This range spans the concentrations of analgesic
doses of morphine in brain (0.1 to 0.5 μg per g).

In experiments on cyclic AMP formation in rat brain homogenate, the
absolute potencies of levorphanol, heroin and pethidine were close to
their potencies on mouse vas deferens (12). Etorphine, morphine and
methadone, however, were relatively weaker against cyclic AMP formation.
This discrepancy might be due to greater non-specific absorption on
materials in the brain homogenate or to some other experimental condition.

Not only absolute, but relative potencies in the biochemical interaction
should correspond with those in the pharmacological effect. In our
hands, the rank order of potency of seven opiates against prostaglandin-
activated cyclic AMP formation in rat brain homogenate was etorphine,
levorphanol, heroin, morphine, pethidine, methadone, dextrorphan. This
order was compared with those obtained for inhibition of evoked contraction of mouse vas deferens (12) and guinea pig ileum (11) and of
naloxone binding to the opiate receptor in rat brain homogenate (13).
The correlation coefficients for rank in the cyclic AMP test with those
in the other three tests were: mouse vas deferens, 1.0 ($\underline{P}$ <0.01); guinea
pig ileum, 0.786 ($\underline{P}$ <0.05); opiate receptor affinity 0.943 (P=0.01).

c) Stereospecificity and specific antagonism. When the potencies of levorphanol and dextrorphan were tested on prostaglandin-stimulated cyclic
AMP formation, levorphanol showed about 10-16 times the potency of
morphine, whereas dextrorphan was either inactive or of very low potency
(1, 2, 5, 7). In our hands, in a direct comparison, levorphanol was 326
(limits 264-403) times the potency of dextrorphan (2).

Four groups of investigators have now reported that naloxone antagonizes
the inhibition by morphine of PGE-activated cyclic AMP formation (1, 4,
5, 6). In three of these reports, the concentrations of naloxone used
were close to those of morphine; but, in one report (4), naloxone was
effective at one-tenth to one-hundredth the concentration of morphine.
In two reports (1, 4), naloxone alone somewhat depressed the reponse to
PGE$_1$.

d) Appropriateness of biochemical interaction to pharmacological effect.
Could a lowering of brain PGE or neuronal cyclic AMP account for the
agonist actions of opiates? The main evidence concerning E prostaglandins, cyclic AMP, pain and analgesia is as follows. E and F prostaglandins occur in the brain and, indeed, are liberated there in response
to noxious stimulation of the periphery (15). E prostaglandins stimulate
cyclic AMP formation in the brain (16, 17), although prostaglandin-
stimulated adenylate cyclase is a particularly labile enzyme (3, 8, 16).
In man, injection into the cerebrospinal fluid of bradykinin or blood
plasma, either of which is likely to liberate prostaglandin, causes
intense headache that is relieved by indomethacin (18), which potently
inhibits PG biosynthesis. Intravenous infusion of PGE$_1$ (19) or injection of pyrogen (18), which is known to liberate E prostaglandin in
the brain (20), also causes headache. In the rabbit, injection of
bradykinin into the cisterna magna elicits a violent flight response
that is prevented by indomethacin or by morphine (18). In this species

also, indomethacin potentiates the antiociceptive effect of morphine against tooth nerve stimulation (21). In the rat, theophylline or caffeine, which inhibits brain cyclic AMP phosphodiesterase in vitro (9, 22), lowers the nociceptive threshold (23). Also, intracerebroventricular PGE_1 (24) or cyclic AMP (25), in the rat or mouse, antagonises morphine analgesia. Intraperitoneal theophylline had a like effect (25). All this evidence supports the view that increase of PGE in the neighbourhood of appropriate central neurones and the stimulation of cyclic AMP formation within them would lead to pain, and that inhibition of this process would produce analgesia. Such an action might be expected if cyclic AMP either inactivated neurones that inhibit pain or activated neurones that excite pain. That acetylcholine, as well as opiates, antagonises PGE-activated cyclic AMP formation in neuroblastoma hybrid cells (7) would fit the seemingly paradoxical finding that centrally acting cholinergic drugs have a powerful antinociceptive effect that is antagonised by naloxone (26).

DISCUSSION AND CONCLUSIONS

Originally, we proposed that the biochemical interaction that we had observed might represent the biochemical mechanism of opiate analgesia because: (i) cyclic GMP rather than cyclic AMP might have been involved; (ii) opiates might have decreased cyclic AMP accumulation by affecting some other enzyme than adenylate cyclase; (iii) the stimulatory substance was not necessarily an E prostaglandin. The word "represents" allowed scope for such variation of the mechanism in detail, but it now seems needlesssly loose. That intraventricular injection of cyclic AMP, but not of cyclic GMP, intensified the opiate abstinence syndrome (27), fits the argument that cyclic AMP rather than GMP is involved in the agonist action of morphine. Inhibition of phosphodiesterase or activation of ATPase might offer alternative explanations for the lessening by morphine of cyclic AMP accumulation; but such effects have not been consistently observed (28-30). It therefore seems probable that inhibition of an adenylate cyclase is primarily in morphine agonist action. This probability is greatly strengthened by the experiments of Sharma et al (5) in cultured neuroblastoma hybrid cells.

The role of E prostaglandins remains unsettled. We did not conclude that morphine competes with E prostaglandin for a single receptor site, although we did not exclude this possibility, and we accept the evidence of Traber et al (3) that it does not. We consider that E prostaglandin was, rather, a means of picking out an adenylate cyclase that responded to morphine, because basal or fluoride-activated cyclic AMP formation showed little or no response (1, 2, 31). Sharma et al (5) have found that the basal adenylate cyclase activity of their hybrid strain of cells responded to about the same extent to 10^{-5} M morphine as did PGE_1-stimulated activity. Perhaps this means that the basal adenylate cyclase activity of a cell rich in opiate receptors is of a type represented by only a small fraction of the basal activity of a whole brain homogenate. In the meantime, it can be said that all investigators so far have found that E prostaglandin stimulates at least part of the adenylate cyclase that opiates inhibit (1-6).

Some observations should be mentioned that might seem contrary to the proposed mechanism of action. It has been observed that, in certain circumstances, morphine stimulates adenylate cyclase (30). It has also been observed that morphine stimulates prostaglandin biosynthesis (32, 33), although this effect is not antagonised by naloxone (10). Again, E prostaglandins and cyclic AMP simulate the effect of morphine on mouse vas deferens, but this effect is also not antagonised by naloxone (34). Taken in conjunction with the fore-going argument, however, these observations appear consistent with Claude Bernard's dictum that morphine exhibits a mixture or a succession of depressant and stimulant effects.

Another question arises: what is the relationship of this adenylate cyclase mechanism to the opiate receptor and the endogenous morphine-like peptide, enkephaline (34)? This question raises another: what happens _after_ the opiate molecule binds with its receptor? The foregoing analysis suggests that the inhibition of adenylate cyclase is the decisive biochemical con-sequence of this binding. The sequence of events might be that binding of opiate molecule to its receptor produces a conformational change in the catalytic site of adenylate cyclase that lessens the enzyme's ability to convert ATP to cyclic AMP, whereas binding of an E prostaglandin to a different but related site would enhance that ability. Alternatively, there might be a looser link between opiate receptor and catalytic site of adenylate cyclase, as may perhaps be implied by the formulation of Sharma et al (5) that the opiate receptor is a "regulator" of adenylate cyclase.

If the opiate receptor is a regulator of adenylate cyclase activity in morphine-sensitive neurones and opiate binding inhibits the enzyme, it follows that enkephaline would act as an endogenous inhibitor of adenylate cyclase by binding with the same site as does morphine. The nature of biochemical mechanisms is such that an endogenous activator may also be expected to exist. E prostaglandin might constitute this activator, but alternatively it may reinforce another, as yet unidentified one.

We thank Dr. W.A. Klee and Professor H.W. Kosterlitz for valuable discussions, Mr. L.C. Dinneen for statistical advice, Mr. N.M. Butt for technical help, Reckitt & Colman for etorphine, Roche Products Limited for dextrorphan and levorphanol and Sankyo Limited for naloxone.

REFERENCES

1. H.O.J. COLLIER, A.C. ROY, Nature, Lond. 248, 24-27 (1974).
2. H.O.J. Collier, A.C. ROY, Prostaglandins 7, 361-376 (1974).
3. J. TRABER, K. FISCHER, S. LATZIN, B. HAMPRECHT, FEBS Lett. 49, 260-263 (1974).
4. J. TRABER, K. FISCHER, S. LATZIN, B. HAMPRECHT, Nature, Lond. 253, 120-122 (1975).
5. S.K. SHARMA, M. NIRENBERG, W.A. KLEE, Proc. Nat. Acad. Sci. U.S.A. 72, 590-594 (1975).
6. J.C. BLOSSER, J.R. ABBOTT, W. SHAIN, Fedn. Proc. 34, 713 (1975).
7. J. TRABER, G. REISER, K. FISCHER, B. HAMPRECHT, FEBS Lett. 52, 327-332 (1975).
8. G.P. TELL, G.W. PASTERMAK, P. CUATRECASAS, FEBS Lett. 51, 242-245 (1975).
9. D.L. FRANCIS, A.C. ROY, H.O.J. COLLIER, this symposium.
10. H.O.J. COLLIER, D.L. FRANCIS, W.J. McDONALD-GIBSON A.C. ROY, S.A. SAEED, this symposium.
11. H.W. KOSTERLITZ, A.J. WATT, Br. J. Pharmac. 33, 266-276 (1968).
12. J. HUGHES, H.W. KOSTERLITZ, F.M. LESLIE, Br. J. Pharmac. 53, 371-381 (1975).
13. C.B. PERT, S.H. SNYDER, Proc.Nat.Acad.Sci.U.S.A., 70, 2243-2247 (1973).
14. E.J. SIMON, J.M. HILLER, I. EDELMAN, Proc.Nat.Acad.Sci.U.S.A. 70, 1947-1949 (1973).
15. P.W. RAMWELL, J.E. SHAW, Prostaglandins (eds. S. Bergström and B. Sam-uelsson) p. 283, Almqvist and Wiksell, Stockholm (1967).
16. F. BERTI, M. TRABUCCHI, V. BERNAREGGI, R. FUMAGILLI, Pharmac. Res. Comm. 4, 253-259 (1962).

17. W. WELLMANN, U. SCHWABE, Brain Research 59, 371-378 (1973).
18. F. SICUTERI, Bradykinin, Kallidin and Kallikrein (ed E.G. Erdös) p. 482, Springer, Heidelberg (1970).
19. S. BERGSTRÖM, L.A. CARLSON, L.G. EKELUND, L. ORÖ, Acta Physiol. Scand. 64, 332-339 (1965).
20. W. FELDBERG, K.P. GUPTA, A.S. MILTON, S. WENDLANDT, J. Physiol, Lond. 234, 279-303 (1973).
21. M.J. MATTILA, L. SAARNIVAARA, Ann. Med. exp. Fenn. 45, 360-363 (1967).
22. B. BEER, M. CHASIN, D.E. CLODY, J.R. VOGEL, Z.P. HOROVITZ, Science 176, 428-430 (1972).
23. G. PAALZOW, L. PAALZOW, Acta Pharm. Toxicol. 32, 22-32 (1973).
24. S. FERRI, A. SANTAGOSTINO, P.C. BRAGA, I. GALATULAS, Psychopharmacologia, Berl. 39, 231-235 (1974).
25. I.K. HO, H.H. LOH, E. LEONG WAY, J. Pharmac. exp. Ther. 185, 336-346 (1973).
26. L.S. HARRIS, W.L. DEWEY, Agonist and Antagonist Actions of Narcotic Analgesic Drugs (eds. H.W. Kosterlitz, H.O.J. Collier, J.E. Villarreal) p. 198, Macmillan, London (1972).
27. H.O.J. COLLIER, D.L. FRANCIS, Nature, Lond 255, 159-162 (1975).
28. H. KANETO, T. KAKU, M. KOIDA. International Soc. Neurochem. Meeting, Tokyo, 3, 479 (1973).
29. M.L. JAIN, B.M. CURTIS, E.V. BUKITIS, Res. Comm. Shem. Pathol. Pharmacol. 7, 229-232 (1974).
30. S.K. PURI, J. COCHIN, L. VOLICER, Life Sciences 16, 759-768 (1975).
31. R.L. SINGHAL, S. KACEW, R. LAFRENIERE, J. Pharm. Pharmac. 25, 1022-1024 (1973).
32. H.O.J. COLLIER, W.J. McDONALD-GIBSON, S.A. SAEED, Br.J.Pharmac. 52, 116P (1974).
33. H.O.J. COLLIER, W.J. McDONALD-GIBSON, S.A. SAEED, Nature, Lond. 252, 56-58 (1974).
34. J. HUGHES, Brain Research 88, 295-308 (1975).

INFLUENCE OF OPIATES ON THE LEVELS OF ADENOSINE 3':5'-CYCLIC MONOPHOSPHATE IN NEUROBLASTOMA X GLIOMA HYBRID CELLS.

Jörg Traber, Robert Gullis and Bernd Hamprecht

Max-Planck-Institut für Biochemie, 8033 Martinsried, Federal
Republic of Germany

(Received in final form May 24, 1975)

In neuroblastoma x glioma hybrid cells prostagland-
din E_1 (PGE_1) increases the level of adenosine 3':5'-
cyclic monophosphate. This response to PGE_1 is strongly
enhanced in cells that were incubated with morphine,
methadon, noradrenaline or carbamylcholine for several
hours. All these compounds increase the level of cyclic
GMP in the cells. As in untreated cells, the effect of
PGE_1 can be inhibited by morphine or noradrenaline. The
development of the increased response to PGE_1 is dependent on protein synthesis. The increased response to
PGE_1 is discussed in connection with morphine tolerance
and withdrawal.

Morphine is known to inhibit the contractions of intestinal
muscle evoked by prostaglandins E (PGE) (1). PGE_1, on the other
hand, stimulates neuroblastoma x glioma hybrid cells (2) to increase their intracellular levels of adenosine 3':5'-cyclic monophosphate (cyclic AMP). In many respects these hybrid cells be-
have like neurons. They extend long processes (3), contain vesicles comparable to those seen in cholingeric and adrenergic nerves (4), have high activity of choline acetyltransferase (3) and
fire action potentials on electrical or chemical stimulation
(3,5). In view of these facts and of the action of morphine on
the central nervous system we hypothesized that morphine might
also antagonize the action of PGE_1 in mouse neuroblastoma and
neuroblastoma x glioma hybrid cells. Experiments with these cells
showed that morphine inhibits the increase of the intracellular
level of cyclic AMP elicited by PGE_1 (6,7), that the action of
morphine is prevented in the presence of the morphine antagonist
naloxone (7), that the opiate action is stereospecific (5), that
PGE_1 and morphine must act through different receptors (8), and
that PGE_1 sensitive cell lines of nonneuronal character do not
respond to morphine (8). Similar results were obtained in other
laboratories by studying opiate binding or adenylate cyclase
activity in the same neuroblastoma x glioma hybrids or in brain
homogenates (9-11). Our finding that opiates elevate the levels
of intracellular guanosine 3':5'-cyclic monophosphate (cyclic
GMP) suggests that the inhibitory action of morphine on the elevation of cyclic AMP levels in the presence of PGE_1 may be
mediated by cyclic GMP (R.G., J.T. and B.H., submitted for publication).

Having seen acute effects of morphine in the hybrid cells,
we studied the longterm action of morphine in the hope to contri-

bute to the elucidation of phenomena like opiate tolerance, dependence and withdrawal.

Methods

The mouse neuroblastoma x rat glioma hybrid line 108CC15 (3) was cultured as described (2). For experimental incubation, the cells were kept for 10 min, 37°C, at the concentrations of PGE_1 and opiates specified, as described previously (7,12). After the incubation, the cells were assayed for content of cyclic AMP and the data referred to cellular protein (12). For longterm exposure to opiates (preincubation), the cells were maintained in the presence of a drug. Subsequently, the medium was removed, the cells were washed twice with incubation medium (12) and the experimental incubation was initiated.

Results

After preincubation of the hybrid cells with 10 μM morphine or methadon for 15 or 36 hours, PGE_1 elevated the levels of cyclic AMP to values up to 100 % higher than in the controls (Table 1).

Table 1

Effect of the Preincubation of the Hybrid Cells with Various Drugs on the Response to PGE_1 and Morphine

Pre-incubation with [a]	addition during main incubation							
	experiment 1				experiment 2			
	C	M	P[c]	P[c] + M[b]	C	M[b]	P[b]	P[c] + M[b]
	cyclic AMP (pmol per mg protein)							
C	19	14	910±8	436±25	38±5	38±8	1310±50	338±51
M	16	-	1280±55	874±92	57±5	45±5	2540±230	1220±20
D	12	23	818±49	269±25	50	28±3	1200±50	355±4
L	-	12	871±21	832±67	35±2	38±1	847±62	1010±120
Me	39	14	942±58	853±42	39±4	45±3	2440±140	2240±120
N	21	14	698±61	328±36	-	-	-	-
I	-	-	-	-	60	45±1	5620±100	2880±450
Ca	-	-	-	-	80	54±3	2560±60	990±86

[a] All concentrations 10 μmol 1^{-1}; [b] 0.1 mmol 1^{-1}; [c] 3 μmol 1^{-1}. C, control, no addition; M, morphine; P, PGE_1; D, dextrorphan; L, levorphanol; Me, L-methadon; N, Naloxone; I, D,L-isoproterenol; Ca, carbamylcholine. Experiment 1: preincubation 15 hours, 2.2×10^6 viable cells per plate, viability 98 %, passage number 10. Experiment 2: preincubation 36 hours, 4.4×10^6 viable cells per plate, viability 98,5 %, passage number 9.

Such treament with 10 μmol 1^{-1} levorphanol, a congener of morphine did not cause an increase in the response to PGE_1, but rather a slight depression. The same was observed if dextrorphan, the biologically inactive enantiomer of levorphanol, or naloxone, a morphine antagonist were used. The ß-adrenergic agonist isoproterenol, if employed at sufficiently high concentration, will act on the α-adrenergic receptors of the hybrid cells and prevent the increase of the level of cyclic AMP elicited by PGE_1 (5). Also cholinergic agonists like carbamylcholine were shown to interfere with the action of PGE_1 in the hybrid cells (13). Preincubation of the cells with isoproterenol or carbamylcholine elevated the response of the cells to PGE_1, by 400 and 100 %, respectively (Table 1). In cells pretreated with morphine, noradrenaline or carbamylcholine, morphine reduced the effect of PGE_1 to a smaller extent than in untreated cells, and the levels of cyclic AMP after incubation with PGE_1 and morphine were much higher than in untreated cells (Table 1). Preincubation with dextrorphan or naloxone had little effect on the response of the cells to morphine. However, no significant inhibition by morphine of the effect of PGE_1 could be found in cells pretreated with levorphanol or methadon (Table 1).

The increased response to PGE_1 of the hybrid cells develops within 6 to 15 hours after onset of the preincubation with morphine (Fig. 1). After each period of preincubation, the cells were incubated for 10 min with PGE_1 (curve a) or PGE_1 + morphine, (curve b). From curve b it can be seen that morphine cannot compensate the increased response to PGE_1 that developed during the preincubation with morphine. The increase in the response to PGE_1, that develops during prolonged treatment with morphine is prevented, if cycloheximide, an inhibitor of protein synthesis, is also present (J.T., and B.H., in preparation). Variation of the concentration of morphine present during a constant preincubation

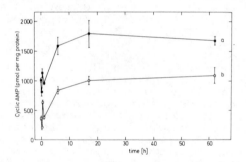

Fig. 1

Time course of the development of the increased response to PGE_1, during continuous pretreatment of the hybrid cells with 10 μmol l^{-1} morphine. 3.6×10^6 viable cells per plate, viability 95 %, passage number 8. Main incubation (10 min) in the presence of 3 μmol l^{-1} PGE_1 (curve a) or PGE_1 + 0.1 mmol l^{-1} morphine (curve b).

period demonstrates that a maximal effect was obtained in the range of 10 to 100 μmol l^{-1} (fig. 2). As concentrations of morphine during preincubation exceed 0.1 mmol l^{-1}, the levels of cyclic AMP obtained on stimulation by PGE_1 fall again (Fgi. 2, curve a). At this point morphine does not inhibit the action of PGE_1, although it does so if the morphine concentration during preincubation had been below 1 mmol 1^{-1}.

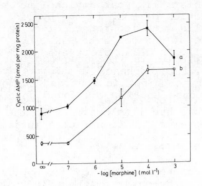

Fig. 2

Relationship between the response to PGE_1 and the concentration of morphine during the preincubation period of 15 hours. 3.0×10^6 viable cells per plate, viability 99 %, passage number 9. Main incubation (10 min) in the presence of 3 μmol 1^{-1} PGE_1 (curve a) or PGE_1 + 0.1 mmol 1^{-1} morphine (curve b).

Pretreatment of the cells with levorphanol, methadon or morphine hardly changes the sensitivity of the cells to PGE_1. The EC_{50} values are all in the range of 10 to 50 nmol 1^{-1}. Again, the maximal response to PGE_1 is enhanced after preincubation with methadone or morphine (J.T. and B.H., in preparation). As mentioned, morphine, acetylcholine and noradrenaline suppress the increase of the levels of cyclic AMP evoked by PGE_1 (5-7,13) and elevate the level of cyclic GMP (R.G., J.T. and B.H., submitted; R.G. and B.H., in preparation). In cells preincubated with 10 μmol 1^{-1} levorphanol or methadon, morphine does no longer inhibit the action of PGE_1. Since morphine still elevates the level of cyclic GMP in such cells (R.G. and B.H., in preparation), one could be tempted to conclude, that in these cells cyclic GMP can no longer obviate the action of PGE_1 on adenylate cyclase. This is not the case, however, since noradrenaline still strongly inhibits the action of PGE_1 (J.T. and B.H., in preparation). Although morphine alone does not affect the action of PGE_1, it enhances the effect of noradrenaline. Furtheron, noradrenaline also inhibits the action of PGE_1 in cells preincubated with morphine, isoproterenol, carbamylcholine or no addition (J.T. and B.H., in preparation). Also carbamylcholine blocks the effect of PGE_1 in normal cells (13) or in cells pretreated with isoproterenol or carbamylcholine (J.T. and B.H., in preparation).

The enhanced response to PGE_1 observed after pretreatment with morphine, is lost in the course of 3 hours after removal of morphine from the cultures.

Discussion.

The present investigation demonstrates that prolonged treatment of the hybrid cells with morphine, methadon, isoproterenol or carbamylcholine strongly enhances the response to PGE_1, expressed as the increase in the intracellular concentration of cyclic AMP. The common feature of these compounds is that at low concentrations they increase the intracellular level of cyclic GMP in the hybrid cells. Although this is also true for levorphanol, and although the effects of levorphanol in animals are practically identical to those of morphine, in contrast to morphine, no enhancement of the response to PGE_1 was found on pretreatment with levorphanol. This paradox is resolved, if one considers that the EC50 for stimulation of guanylate cyclase by levorphanol is one order of magnitude lower than that for morphine (R.G., J.T. and B.H., submitted) and that at elevated concentrations, levorphanol and morphine cause a second effect, i.e., they evoke an increase of cyclic AMP and a decrease of cyclic GMP and thereby, within a narrow range of opiate concentrations, an enormous fall of the ratio of concentrations of cyclic GMP and cyclic AMP. Thus, at 10 μmol 1^{-1} levorphanol during preincubation, the second effect of levorphanol may already be large enough to prevent the generation of the increased responsiveness to PGE_1. In addition, the elevation of the level of cyclic GMP in response to morphine is not sufficient to cause an inhibition of the response to PGE_1. If, however, noradrenaline is used, an agent more potent than morphine in elevating the level of cyclic GMP, the response to PGE_1 can be inhibited even in cells pretreated with levorphanol. The effects of pretreatment with methadon may be explained in the same way. In fact, even on pretreatment with morphine the responsiveness to morphine is lost, if the concentration of morphine during preincubation was high enough to cause the second effect mentioned (Fig. 2).

The above exemplifies the importance of the ratio of the concentrations of the 2 cyclic nucleotides in acute and longterm opiate action. The picture emerges that the effects observed at low opiate concentrations are those corresponding to the effects observed in an animal. The acute effects of opiates then are to increase the level of cyclic GMP and decrease the level of cyclic AMP. As has been shown (5), this event is accompanied by a depolarization of the cell membrane which, in a neuron, would mean activation. In contrast, PGE_1 increases the level of cyclic AMP and hyperpolarizes the membranes of the hybrid cells (5), which in a nerve cell would mean inhibition of neuronal activity. Since in an animal morphine causes analgesia, one may speculate that the neurons carrying opiate receptors are inhibitory neurons, which are activated by opiates or their physiological equivalent and inhibited by PGE_1 or other endogenous agents of comparable action. These "opiate neurons" should be linked to the neurons that, e.g. "register" pain. On prolonged treatment of the hybrid cells with opiates, PGE_1 causes an increased rise of the intracellular level of cyclic AMP. Now an increased concentration of opiate would be needed to compensate the effect of PGE_1. We like to suggest that this phenomenon is equivalent to what is known as opiate tolerance in animals and men. In terms of the "opiate neuron" this would mean that increased amounts of opiate are required to counteract the hyperpolarizing action of PGE_1 (or its physiological equivalent). In tolerant animals, therefore, the

"opiate neuron" has a tendency to fire less frequently, i.e. to have a reduced inhibitory effect (abstinence effect) unless sufficient opiate is provided. Such an abstinence effect can also be generated in the hybrid cells. If cells preincubated with morphine are challenged with PGE_1 or PGE_1 plus morphine, the levels of cyclic AMP are higher in the absence than in the presence of morphine (see Fig. 1). Thus, in cells pretreated with morphine the increased responsiveness to PGE_1 is more pronounced in the absence of morphine. Morphine abstinence was recently correlated with an increase in cyclic AMP levels in brain (14).
The development under the influence of morphine of an increased response to PGE_1 can be completely blocked by cycloheximide (J.T. and B.H., in preparation). Also in animals, the development of narcotic tolerance can be prevented by inhibition of protein synthesis (15). The material synthesized may or may not be closely related to the adenylate cyclase complex. Also the slow reversal of the tolerance phenomenon in the hybrid cells might be indicative that protein snythesis and degradation rather than short term regulatory processes might be involved in the tolerance phenomenon.

The fact, that neurohormones like noradrenaline and acetylcholine cause effects identical to that of morphine raises the possibility that compounds which stimulate the elevation of cyclic GMP in "opiate neurons" might exert a morphine-like action, if properly applied.

Acknowledgements

We thank Prof. A. Herz, the Farbwerke Hoechst A.G. and Hoffman-La Roche for drugs, Dr. J. Pike for prostaglandin E_1 and The Sonderforschungsbereich 51 of the Deutsche Forschungsgemeinschaft for financial support.

References

1. R. Jacques, Experientia, 25, 1059-1060 (1969).
2. B. Hamprecht and J. Schultz, Hoppe-Seyler's Z. physiol. Chem., 354, 1633-1641 (1973).
3. B. Hamprecht, Mosbacher Kolloquium, 25, 391-423 (1974).
4. M.P. Daniels and B. Hamprecht, J.Cell Biol., 63, 691-699 (1974).
5. J. Traber, G. Reiser, K. Fischer and B. Hamprecht, FEBS Lett., 52, 327-332 (1975).
6. J. Traber, Diplomarbeit, University of Munich (1973).
7. J. Traber, K. Fischer, S. Latzin and B. Hamprecht, Nature, 253 120-122 (1975).
8. J. Traber, K. Fischer, S. Latzin and B. Hamprecht, FEBS Lett., 49, 260-263 (1974).
9. H.O.J. Collier and A.C. Roy, Nature, 248, 24-27 (1974).
10. W.A. Klee and M. Nirenberg, Proc. Natl. Acad. Sci., U.S.A., 71, 3474-3477 (1974).
11. S.K. Sharma, M. Nirenberg and W.A. Klee, Proc. Natl. Acad. Sci. U.S.A., 72, 590-594 (1975).
12. J. Traber, K. Fischer, S. Latzin and B. Hamprecht, Proc 9th Int. Congr. Collegium Internat. Neuropsychopharmacologicum, i.p.
13. J. Traber, K. Fischer, C. Buchen and B. Hamprecht, Nature, in the press.
14. H.O.J. Collier and D.L. Francis, Nature, 255, 159-162 (1975).
15. A.A. Smith, M. Clarmin and J. Gavitt, J. Pharmacol. Exp. Ther., 156, 85-91 (1967).

OPIATE RECEPTORS AS REGULATORS OF ADENYLATE CYCLASE

Werner A. Klee, Shail K. Sharma* and Marshall Nirenberg

Laboratory of General and Comparative Biochemistry, NIMH,
and the Laboratory of Biochemical Genetics, NHLI, NIH,
Bethesda, Maryland   20014

(Received in final form May 24, 1975)

We have reported the presence of opiate receptors in some
neuroblastoma derived cell lines cultured in vitro and
that a neuroblastoma x glioma hybrid cell line, NG108-15, contains
a particularly large number of morphine receptors (1). Table 1
shows that whereas the hybrid cell line has opiate receptors

Table 1   RECEPTOR BINDING

	^{3}H-dihydromorphine	^{3}H naloxone	
	fmoles/mg protein		
HYBRIDS			
NG108-15	17	37	(19)
PARENTS			
N18TG-2	0	11	(6)
C6BU-1	1	1	(1)

The concentration of radioactive narcotic was 1 nM in
each case. In neither case is this close to a saturating amount,
naloxone one has twice the affinity of dihydromorphine and so to
be comparable the naloxone data should be divided by 2 (numbers in
parenthesis). NG108-15 (also called 108CC15) was obtained by B.
Hamprecht, T. Amano and M. Nirenberg (in preparation), N18TG-2
by Minna et al. (2), C6BU-1 by Amano et al. (3).

which are readily demonstrated by both radioactive ligands those
of N18TG2 were only detected with [3] H-naloxone binding whereas the
C6BU-1 line does not have a detectable number of opiate receptors
by either assay method. This group of cell lines with no, few
and an abundance of opiate receptors has provided us with
material with which to study the biochemical consequences of
the interaction of morphine with its receptor.

Collier and Roy reported that morphine and related drugs
inhibit the PGE$_1$ stimulated conversion of [3] H ATP into cAMP
by rat brain homogenates in a way that correlates with agonist
potency and receptor affinity (4,5). These experiments prompted us
to examine the effect of morphine on adenylate cyclase activity
and on the cAMP levels of NG108-15 hybrid cells and their parental
cell lines (6). We found that morphine inhibits the adenylate
cyclase activity of NG108-15 cells and lowers cellular cAMP levels
in the presence and in the absence of added PGE$_1$ (fig 1).

*Fogarty International Fellow, on leave from the Department of
Biochemistry, All India Institute of Medical Sciences, New Delhi,
India.

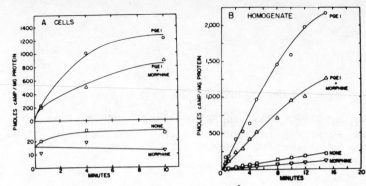

Figure 1. Inhibition by morphine (10^{-5} M) of the rate of cAMP accumulation in intact NG108-15 hybrid cells (part A) and of adenylate cyclase activity in homogenates (part B). Basal and PGE_1 (10^{-5} M) stimulated results are shown (6).

There is also a dramatic reduction in the adenosine stimulated rise in cellular cAMP levels in the presence of morphine (17). Thus, in this cell, morphine inhibits both stimulated and unstimulated adenylate cyclase.

Morphine inhibits the adenylate cyclase of the neuroblastoma parent somewhat, but does not affect the activity the enzyme found in the glioma parent (Table II). Thus, the de-

Table II Effect of morphine on adenylate cyclase activity of neuroblastoma and glioma parents

Addition*	N18TG-2	C6BU-1
	pmole/min/mg protein	
None	6	20
Morphine	4	19
Naloxone	5	20
Morphine + naloxone	5	20
PGE_1	75	24
PGE_1 + morphine	63	25
PGE_1 + naloxone	72	24
PGE_1 morphine + naloxone	70	23

*10 μm of each component

gree of inhibition of adenylate cyclase by morphine is correlated with the number of opiate receptors. There are a number of other properties of the enzyme of NG108-15 cells which show that the inhibition by opiates is mediated by their receptors. Thus, naloxone, an apparently pure antagonist of narcotic drugs reverses morphine inhibition of adenylate cyclase (6). Furthermore, the inhibition is sterospecific in that levorphanol, but not its inactive isomer, dextrorphan, inhibits adenylate cyclase (6). Traber et al. (7-9) have also reported that morphine reduces PGE elevation of cAMP levels and Blosser et al. (10) have reported that morphine inhibits the PGE_1 dependent activation of adenylate cylase in neuroblastoma or hybrid cell lines derived from neuroblastoma cells.

There is a good correlation between the concentrations at which opiate agonists displace ^{3}H-naloxone from the receptors and and those required for inhibition of adenylate cyclase. This agreement is readily apparent in the data presented in Table III.

Table III Comparison of narcotic affinity for the opiate
         receptor and ability to inhibit adenylate cyclase

Narcotic	Kd Narcotic receptor nM	Ki Adenylate cyclase nM
Etorphine	5	10
Levorphanol	200	200
Morphine	4,000	2,000
3-Allylprodine	10,000	50,000
Dextrorphan	10,000	--
Naloxone	20	--

However, we found that the opiate binding and enzyme inhibition
curves not superimposible (6). Enzyme inhibition takes place
over a much narrower range of drug concentrations than does displacement of ^{3}H-naloxone from the receptors. This behavior implies cooperativity among liganded receptors in their interaction
with the adenylate cyclase complex. Analysis of the data by means
of Hill plots shows that the slope for narcotic binding (reactionl
of scheme 1) is close to 1 indicating little or no cooperativity

$$(1) \quad M + receptor \underset{}{\overset{1}{\rightleftharpoons}} receptor \cdot M \underset{}{\overset{2}{\rightleftharpoons}} \left[enzyme \cdot receptor \cdot M \right]$$

in the formation of [narcotic·receptor] complex but that the
maximum slopes of the curves for adenylate cyclase inhibition by
narcotics (reaction 2) are between 2 and 3, indicating strong
positive cooperativity in the reactions that couple [narcotic-
receptor] complexes with adenylate cyclase.

     Coupling of opiate-receptor complexes to adenylate cyclase
may occur by any of 3 general mechanisms:
 1) Direct interaction of receptor and enzyme, by analogy with
enzyme systems composed of catalytic and regulatory subunits, or
linkage via a modulator (15).
 2) Opiate-receptor complexes may elicit the production of chemical messages, suggested as a rather unlikely possibility by H.O.J.
Collier (personal communication).
 3) Indirect coupling mediated by conformational transitions of
the membrane. The membrane conformation may reflect either the
proportions of receptors in states A and B or may change in reponse to the process of transition of the conformation of the
receptors between states A and B induced by the association and
dissociation of agonists (but not of antagonists, since Na$^+$ main-
tains receptors in the B state). The indirect coupling mechanisms,
which involve membrane changes, may allow opiate receptors to
express their interaction with narcotics in more than one way.
Thus, the inhibition of adenylate cyclase and the electro-
physiologocal effects of narcotics on NG108-15 cells found by
Traber et al. (9), Myers and Livengood (16) and in our own
laboratories can be different manifestations of the same
fundamental effects on membrane structure.

     An important property of many of the narcotic analgesics
is that of mixed agonist-antagonist behavior. Perhaps the best
studied example of such a compound is nalorphine which is a
potent antagonist of morphine, but also is a good analgesic in
its own right (11). How may this dualism of action be understood

in the context of opiate action as an inhibitor of adenylate
cyclase? Figure 2 shows the effects of nalorphine upon adenylate

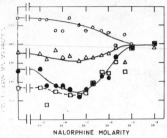

NALORPHINE MOLARITY

Figure 2. Effects of nalorphine on the adenylate cyclase activity
of homogenates of NG108-15 cells. The curves, reading from top
to bottom, represent experiments performed at the following
concentrations of morphine: none, 2×10 M, 10^{-4}M, and
2×10^{-5}M. The data have been normalized so that uninhibited
adenylate cyclase activity is constant.

cyclase activity at several concentrations of morphine. In the
absence of morphine, nalorphine inhibits the enzyme but only
partially when compared with the degree of inhibition produced
by morphine. In the presence of morphine, on the other hand,
the effect of nalorphine is to reverse the inhibition produced
by morphine. The reversal of morphine inhibition by nalorphine
is also not complete but only restores enzyme activity to the
level seen in the presence of nalorphine alone.

There is evidence that opiate receptors exist in two conformational states (12, 13) as shown below:

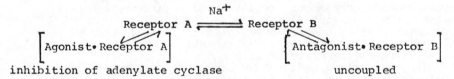

$$\text{Na}^+$$
$$\text{Receptor A} \rightleftharpoons \text{Receptor B}$$

$$\left[\text{Agonist} \cdot \text{Receptor A} \right] \qquad \left[\text{Antagonist} \cdot \text{Receptor B} \right]$$

inhibition of adenylate cyclase   uncoupled

Receptor form A has a high affinity for agonists and form B for
antagonists as shown. Binding of agonists to the receptor will
shift the equilibrium to the left and convert most receptors to
the [Agonist· Receptor A] complex which will result in inhibition of
adenylate cyclase. Conversely, when receptors are in the form of
the [Antagonist·Receptor B] complex, as the result of interaction
with a pure antagonist, adenylate cyclase is not inhibited. Mixed
agonist-antagonists, such as nalorphine, may have a comparable affinity for receptors in both states. The interaction of opiate
receptors with agonist-antagonist narcotics will then result in
the receptor complexes being partitioned between states A and B in
comparable amounts. Inhibition of adenylate cyclase will thus be
only partial as is observed.

When NG108-15 cells are cultured in the presence of morphine
for a number of days, the level of adenylate cyclase activity increases by approximately 50-100%. An experiment which demonstrates this phenomenon is shown in fig 3. The cells after 2 or
more days of exposure to morphine are tolerant in the sense that
adenylate cyclase activity is nearly normal when assayed in the

adenylate cyclase activity is nearly normal when assayed in the

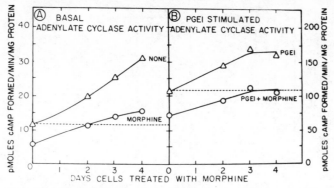

Figure 3. Basal and PGE$_2$ stimulated adenylate cyclase activity of homogenates of NG108-15 cells cultured in the presence of 10 M morphine for the times shown (17).

presence of morphine. They are dependent upon it in the sense that adenylate cyclase activity measured in its absence is abnormally high. The dependence phenomenon is dramatically seen when cAMP levels of cells cultured in the presence of morphine for 48 hours are measured after a brief exposure to naloxone.

Table IV cAMP levels of normal and addicted cells (17)

	CELLS		
Conditions of Assay	Normal	Addicted	% of Normal
	pmoles cAMP/mg protein		
basal	20	23	113
naloxone	21	37	175
PGE	264	81	31
PGE + naloxone	241	1183	491
adenosine	103	65	63
adenosine + naloxone	72	217	301
naloxone			

Addicted cells show as much as a 4 to 5 fold increase in cAMP levels over the control, in the presence but not in the absence of naloxone precipitated withdrawal. There is no change in the number of opiate receptors in tolerant cells (17).

Figure 4 summarizes the general conclusions which we have reached concerning tolerance and dependence on the basis of these and other (17), related, experiments. We find that morphine inhibits adenylate cyclase activity and thus decreases cAMP levels. On continued exposure to morphine the cells adapt by an increase in adenylate cyclase activity which results in tolerance and dependence. The fully tolerant cells have cAMP levels close to normal in the presence of morphine. When the opiate is withdrawn on addition of an antagonist, cAMP levels rise to abnormally high values. This abrupt increase in cAMP indicates that the cells are depen-

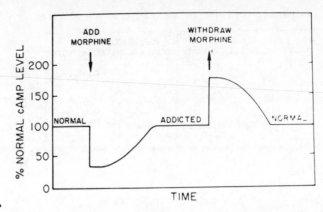

Figure 4.

dent upon morphine and is the biochemical counterpart of the
abstinence syndrome. Recovery of the cells from the addicted
state requires the return of adenylate cyclase activity to
its normal levels. These results support the suggestions of
Goldstein and Goldstein (14) and Shuster (19), made many
years ago, that drugs may act as enzyme inducers. Increases
in cAMP levels in the abstinence syndrome of animals
has recently been demonstrated by Collier and Francis (18).

REFERENCES

1. W.A. KLEE, M. NIRENBERG, Proc. Nat. Acad. Sci. U.S.A.,
   71, 3474-3477 (1974).
2. J. MINNA, D. GLAZER, M. NIRENBERG, Nature New Biol., 235
   225-231 (1972).
3. T. AMANO, B. HAMPRECHT, W. KEMPER, Exp. Cell Res., 85
   399-408 (1974).
4. H.O.J. COLLIER, A.C. ROY, Nature, Lond., 248 24-27 (1974).
5. H.O.J. COLLIER, A.C. ROY, Prostaglandins, 7 361-376 (1974).
6. S.K. SHARMA, M. NIRENBERG, W.A. KLEE, Proc. Nat. Acad. Sci.,
   U.S.A., 72 590-594 (1975).
7. J. TRABER, K. FISCHER, S. LATZIN, B. HAMPRECHT, FEBS Letts.,
   49 260-263 (1974).
8. J. TRABER, K. FISCHER, S. LATZIN, B. HAMPRECHT, Nature, Lond.,
   253 120-122 (1975).
9. J. TRABER, G. REISER, K. FISCHER, B. HAMPRECHT, FEBS Letts.,
   52 327-332 (1975).
10. J.C. BLOSSER, J.R. ABBOTT, W. SHAIN, Fed. Proc., 34 713 (1975).
11. R.I. TABER, D.D. GREENHOUSE, J.K. RENDELL, S. IRWIN,
    J. Pharmacol. Exp. Ther., 169 29-38 (1969).
12. C.B. PERT, G. PASTERNAK, S.H. SNYDER, Science, 182 1359-1361
    (1973).
13. E.J. SIMON, J.M. HILLER, J. GROTH, I. EDELMAN, J. Pharmacol.
    Exp. Ther., in press (1975).
14. D.B. GOLDSTEIN, A. GOLDSTEIN, Biochem. Pharmacol., 8 48 (1961).
15. M. RODBELL, M.C. LIN, Y. SALOMON, C. LONDOS, J.P. HARWOOD,
    D.R. MARTIN, M. RENDELL, M. BERMAN, Adv. in Cyclic Nucleotide
    Research, 5 3-29 (1975).
16. P. MYERS, D. LIVENGOOD, Fed. Proc., 43 359 (1975).
17. S.K. SHARMA, W.A. KLEE, M. NIRENBERG, in preparation.
18. H.O.J. COLLIER, D.L. FRANCIS, Nature, Lond., 255 159-162 (1975).
19. L. SHUSTER, Nature, Lond., 189 314-315 (1961).

EFFECTS OF PROSTAGLANDINS AND MORPHINE ON BRAIN ADENYLYL CYCLASE*

R.G. Van Inwegen, S.J. Strada, and G.A. Robison

Department of Pharmacology, The University of Texas Medical School at Houston, Houston, Texas 77025

(Received in final form May 24, 1975)

Data implicating involvement of cyclic nucleotides in the pharmacology of morphine is compromised by contradictory data in the literature. For example, *in vitro* morphine sulfate (MS) stimulated (1) and had no effect (2) on basal adenylyl cyclase (AC) in rat striatum, and inhibited AC of several brain areas (3). Acute MS injections increased AC of rat striatum (1) and mouse cerebral cortex (4), had no effect on AC of mouse and rat cerebral cortex, cerebellum and hypothalamus (4-6) and decreased AC of mouse brain stem (4). Dopamine (DA) and sodium fluoride (NaF) stimulated AC of rat striatum were unaffected by MS *in vitro* (1, 2, 7) or by acute injections (1, 6), but acute injections enhanced DA sensitive AC (7). Cyclic AMP levels increased in pituitary and striatum (8), decreased in hypothalamus (3) or did not change in cerebral cortex, cerebellum or hypothalamus (6) after acute MS injection. Chronic MS administration decreased (4) and increased (5) AC in mouse cerebral cortex, but did not affect AC in rat cerebral cortex, cerebellum and hypothalamus (5). Abstinence withdrawal of addicted mice decreased AC of cerebral cortex, cerebellum and hypothalamus (6). High K_m cAMP phosphodiesterase (PDE) of rat striatum was inhibited by MS both *in vitro* and by acute injection (1), but PDE in mouse cerebellum, hypothalamus, cerebral cortex, and brain stem were not affected by MS injections (4, 6). MS had no effect on high K_m PDE in striatum of addicted rats, but during abstinence the Vmax of high K_m PDE decreased (9). Our studies were designed to resolve some of these contradictions.

MATERIALS AND METHODS: Adenylyl cyclase (10), cAMP phosphodiesterases (11, 12), and protein (13) were assayed as described. Rats (150 gm, male Sprague-Dawley-Timco) were decapitated and tissues homogenized in 40 mM Tris - Cl pH 7.4; for AC assays the buffer contained 2 mM methyl-isobutyl-xanthine and 1 mM EGTA. Acutely injected and MS addicted rats (9) were killed one hour after final injection (i.p.). "Abstinence withdrawal" rats received final MS injections 1 hr and 20 mg/kg Naloxone 1/2 hr before sacrifice. Neuroblastoma-glioma hybrids (courtesy of Dr. M. Nirenberg) and BHK-21 c/13 cells (American Type Culture Collection) were cultured as described (14, 15). Confluent cells were trypsinized, washed, reseeded (3×10^6 cells per 100 x 20 mm dish in culture medium) and incubated 24 hrs prior to addition of MS (10μM) and/or PGE$_1$ (3μM). After 10 min incubation, the medium was discarded, PCA (0.4N) was added, and cells were scraped from the dishes for DNA (17) and cAMP purification and determination (16).

RESULTS: No consistent effects of MS were found *in vitro* or *in vivo* on basal, NaF stimulated-, or DA stimulated AC of striata of naive, addicted, or addicted rats in withdrawal (Table I). The dose response curves for DA stimulation of AC of striatum were the same for naive, acutely injected (10 mg/kg), addicted, and addicted rats in abstinence or precipitated withdrawal. PDE in striata from all these treatments showed similar kinetics (total Vmax = 135 nM/min/mg and associated K_m = 0.3 - 0.4 mM; Vmax extrapolated from low concentrations of cAMP = 5.0 pm/min/mg, and associated K_m = 2μM).

Prostaglandin stimulation of AC was relatively small (10-25%) ± GTP in control or indomethacin treated rats (Table II). PGE$_1$, PGE$_2$, and 16,16-dimethyl PGE$_2$ gave similar results, but PGF$_{1\alpha}$ and PGF$_{2\alpha}$ and PGA$_1$ were ineffective. Morphine did not antagonize the stimulatory effect of prostaglandins and/or GTP or DA or NaF. In one experiment, PGE$_1$ (10μM) stimulated pituitary AC approximately twofold (Y.C. Clement-Cormier, J. J. Heindel, and G. A. Robison, *personal communication*), but MS (100 μM) had no effect on this or on basal activity.

In agreement with reported data (18), PGE$_1$ (3μM) increased 10-fold the cAMP accumulation in neuroblastoma-glioma hybrid cells, and MS (10μM) markedly inhibited (70%) this stimulation. PGE$_1$ increased 5-fold the cAMP accumulation in BHK cells, but MS had little or no effect on this stimulation.

---

*Supported by a grant (DA-00744) from the U.S. Public Health Service.

TABLE I: ADENYLYL CYCLASE OF STRIATUM. Basal = pm/min/mg; others are % basal. *In vitro* = 100 μM Morphine Sulfate (MS) in assay; A-# = Acute injection of # mg MS/kg; ADD. = addicted; ABST. = abstinence withdrawal; PW = precipatated withdrawal; DA = 100 μM Dopamine, NaF = 5 mM sodium fluoride, Nal = 100 μM Naloxone, MS = 100 μM.

	CONTROL	IN VITRO	A-10	A-20	A-50	ADD.	ABST.	PW.
BASAL	110	100	99	120	115	85	110	94
NaF	190	200	190	210	205	197	180	180
DA	190	200	180	200	215	160	160	170
MS	109	-	-	-	-	95	102	102
Nal	105	102	110	-	-	95	105	100

TABLE II: *IN VITRO* EFFECTS OF MS ON CEREBRAL CORTEX ADENYLYL CYCLASE. Exp. rats had 20 mg/kg indomethacin i.p. 24 and 2 hours before sacrifice. Basal activity = pm/min/mg; others =% basal. Data = average of 3 experiments. MS, DA, and NaF as in Table I; norepinephrine (NE), epinephrine (EPI), and isoproterenol (ISO) = 50 μM; PGE_1 = 100 μM (same results with 10 μM); GTP = 20 μM guanosine triphosphate.

	BASAL	NE	EPI	DA	ISO	NaF	PGE_1	GTP	$GTP+PGE_1$
NAIVE	99	204	205	192	185	412	113	146	162
NAIVE + MS+	99	-	-	190	200	-	112	145	158
EXP.	103	155	-	160	135	313	125	119	140
EXP. + MS+	101	-	-	162	-	-	124	120	134

DISCUSSION: We were able to confirm the previously reported finding that morphine inhibits the prostaglandin-induced rise in cAMP levels in cultured neuroblastoma-glioma hybrid cells (18, 19). This effect of morphine does not occur in the parental cell lines, which lack morphine receptors, and neither does it occur in BHK cells, which presumably also lack these receptors. To this extent our data support the hypothesis of Collier and Roy (20) that cAMP may be involved in the action of morphine. Unfortunately we were not able to resolve the contradictory data from noncultured brain cells, for we were unable to see any consistent effect of morphine on AC or PDE from any brain area, either in response to morphine injected *in vivo* or added *in vitro*. This may reflect nothing more than the complexity of the brain and our inability to control the many factors which are known to affect AC and PDE in this tissue, such as ions, nucleotides, neurotransmitters, and other potential modulators. Continued studies of the mechanism by which morphine affects AC activity in cultured cells seem warranted and may eventually contribute to a better understanding of how morphine affects brain function *in vivo*.

REFERENCES: 1) Puri, S.K., J. Cochin and L. Volicer, Life Sciences 16: 759-768 (1975); 2) Tell, G.P., G.W. Pasternak and P. Cuatrecasas, FEBS Letters 51: 242-245 (1975); 3) Iwatsubo, K. and D.H. Clouet, Fed. Proc. 32: 536 Abs. (1973); 4) Chou, W.S., A.K.S. Ho and H.H. Loh, Proc. West. Pharmacol. Soc. 14: 42-46 (1971); 5) Naito, K. and K. Kuriyama, Japan J. Pharmacol. 23: 274-276 (1973); 6) Singhal, R.L., S. Kacew, and R. Lafreniere, J. Pharm. Pharmacol. 25: 1022-1024 (1973); 7) Iwatsubo, K., G.J. Gold and D.H. Clouet, The Pharmacologist 16: 270 abs. (1974); 8) Costa, E., A. Carenzi, A. Guidotti and A. Revuelta, Frontiers in Catecholamine Research pp. 1003-1010. Pergamon Press, London. (1973); 9) Volicer, L., S.K. Puri and J. Cochin, Adv. Cyclic Nuc. Res. 5: 814 Abs. (1975); 10) Thompson, W.J., S.A. Little and R.H. Williams, Biochemistry 12: 1889-1894 (1973); 11) Thompson, W.J. and M.M. Appleman, Biochemistry 10: 311-316 (1971); 12) Weiss, B., R. Lehne and S.J. Strada, Anal. Biochem. 45: 222-235 (1972); 13) Schacterle, G.R. and R.L. Pollack, Anal. Biochem. 51: 654-655 (1973); 14) Klee, W.A. and M. Nirenberg, Proc. Nat. Acad. Sci. 71: 3474-3477 (1974); 15) Pledger, W.J., W.J. Thompson and S.J. Strada, J. Cyclic Nuc. Res. In Press (1975); 16) Heindel, J., R. Rothenberg, G.A. Robison and A. Steinberger, J. Cyclic Nuc. Res. 1: 69-79 (1975); 17) Burton, K. Biochem. J. 62: 315-323 (1956); 18) Traber, J., K. Fischer, S. Latzin and B. Hamprecht, Nature 253: 120-122 (1975); 19) Sharma, S.K., M. Nirenberg, and W.A. Klee, Proc. Nat. Acad. Sci., 72: 590-594 (1975); 20) Collier, H.O.J., and A.C. Roy, Nature 248: 24-27 (1974).

REGIONAL ALTERATIONS IN CYCLIC NUCLEOTIDE LEVELS
WITH ACUTE AND CHRONIC MORPHINE TREATMENT

Kenneth A. Bonnet

Department of Psychiatry, New York University School of Medicine
New York, New York 10016[1]

(Received in final form May 24, 1975)

Systemic morphine briefly elevated the caudate cyclic AMP level
and subsequently depressed those levels in the substantia nigra
and hypothalamus. Thalamic cAMP was unaffected within sixty minutes of the injection. Cyclic GMP was reduced in all four structures by thirty minutes. Tolerant animals evidenced increased
cAMP levels in all but the hypothalamus and reduced cGMP in all
four structures. A challenge injection of morphine elevated the
two nucleotides briefly in the substantia nigra, depressed only
cAMP in the hypothalamus and did not alter levels in the other
structures.

The acute analgesic effects of morphine and the phenomena of tolerance
and dependence have been reported to involve the brain cyclic AMP system.
Pharmacological administration of agents that increase or mimic cAMP antagonize
morphine-induced analgesia and accelerate tolerance and dependence development
(1). Chronic morphine produces alterations in cerebral cortex adenyl cyclase
activity and withdrawl reduces the NaF-stimulated adenyl cyclase in most regions
in a manner that is prevented by methadone maintenance(2-4).

Many of the effects of narcotics may result from interactions with neurotransmitters or their receptors in the central nervous system(5). Norepinepherine and dopamine sensitive adenyl cyclases have been described in the
mammalian brain, and stimulation of muscarinic cholinergic receptors has been
shown to increase cyclic GMP levels (6-8). Moreover, norepinepherine and cAMP
have recently been shown to have effects on pyramidal tract neurons that are
reciprocal and antagonistic to those of acetylcholine and cGMP (9). Morphine
has recently been reported to inhibit prostaglandin-stimulated cAMP formation
in brain homogenates, and the possibility has been raised that adenyl cyclase
may act as an opiate receptor (10,11). However, no reports have appeared to
date concerning an involvement of cGMP in opiate action.

The rapid pharmacologic action of morphine, and the rapid rise and fall
of intracellular cyclic AMP following hormonal stimulation would seem to
dictate procedures permitting rapid fixation of tissue and the measurement of
cyclic nucleotide levels directly. Studies in this laboratory with repeated
intracerebral injections of morphine into specific structures showed initial
analgesic responses mediated through the thalamus, posterior hypothalamus and
substantia nigra, with subsequent tolerance development evident only in the
medial thalamus and particularly in the substantia nigra (Bonnet and Rogers, in
preparation). Thus, the present studies were designed to follow region-specific

[1]Supported by Grant DA-01113 from the U.S. Public Health Service. I thank
Seraphim Rimarenko for excellent technical assistance.

alterations of cAMP and cGMP by simultaneous determinations in caudate, hypo-thalamus, substantia nigra and thalamus of drug-naive and morphine-tolerant rats at various times following a challenge injection of morphine.

Materials and Methods

Male Fisher rats (Microbiological Associates, F344 strain) were received at 55 days of age and maintained in suspended wire cages, three per cage, at least five days before use. Acute animals were injected with 1 ml/kg saline or 10 mg/ml morphine sulfate subcutaneously and sacrificed at various post-injection times. Chronic animals were implanted with a subcutaneous pellet containing 37 mg morphine base and twenty-four hours later with a 75 mg pellet. They were then sacrificed at various times following subcutaneous saline or morphine injection forty-eight hours after the last pellet implant. Naloxone was injected at 2 mg/kg i.p. in isotonic saline.

Animals were sacrificed by rapid submersion in liquid nitrogen, then quick withdrawl to immersion of only the head and upper thorax for three minutes. Full cerebral circulation was evident for more than five seconds at which time the medial epithalamus area had reached +10 C. Cooling reached −4 C by ten seconds and −43 C by thirty seconds. This appeared to avoid the ischemic and anoxic effects which may contribute to rapid postmortem changes in cerebral cyclic nucleotides (12,13). Heads were stored at −100 C, or in liquid nitrogen for less than two weeks. Brains were removed from frozen heads in a cold room, bisected along the longitudinal fissure and placed, medial surface down, on a freezing microtome stage at −35 C. Hemispheres were sectioned to predetermined levels using a stereotaxic atlas as a guide (14), and structures of interest were extracted by visual guidance using precooled punches made for each struc-ture. The extracted structure was immediately weighed at −24 C and homogenized in ice-cold 6% trichloroacetic acid.

The supernatant of the acid extract was extracted exhaustively with ether, taken to dryness in a stream of nitrogen and resuspended in 0.05M sodium acetate buffer (pH 6.2) containing 4 mM EDTA. Cyclic AMP was assayed in triplicate by the protein binding assay of Gilman (15). Cyclic GMP was assayed by the radioimmunoassay of Steiner, et al.(16).

Results and Discussion

Cyclic nucleotides in various brain regions compared well to determinations reported from tissues fixed by microwave irradiation (17,18).

The acute effects of a 10 mg/kg injection of morphine on brain region levels of cAMP are shown in Table 1. At one minute postinjection there is a brief increase in the caudate level, accompanied by a rapid and long-lasting decrease in the levels in the hypothalamus. The subsequent decrease in cAMP in the substantia nigra parallels the time course for the development of behaviorally assessed analgesia. No significant alteration in thalamic levels were apparent at the times studied. The depletion in the hypothalamus and substantia nigra is probably related to the recently reported in vitro inhibition of prostaglandin stimulated cAMP formation in brain homogenate, and corresponds in magnitude to the effect of morphine in a whole-cell, opiate receptor competent neuroblastoma-gliaoma cell culture (10,11). An alternate possibility may involve the depletion of catecholamines from these structures (19) and possibly the early release of calcium that may result in a rapid activation of phosphodiesterase activity (20).

The acute effects of morphine on brain region cGMP levels are given in Table 2. The decrease in cGMP in all four structures is remarkably similar in

TABLE 1.

Effects of Acute and Chronic Morphine Sulfate on Levels
of Cyclic AMP in Four Rat Brain Structures

Structure	Minutes Following Morphine Injection (10 mg/kg)					
	0	1	5	10	30	60
DRUG NAIVE						
Caudate	.76(.001)	1.12(.158)*	1.26(.365)	1.01(.190)	.92(.107)	.93(.121)
Subs. Nigra	.49(.046)	.39(.077)	.44(.113)	.28(.098)*	.33(.042)*	.42(.128)
Hypothalamus	1.13(.339)	.69(.096)*	.75(.239)	.60(.125)*	.67(.095)*	.65(.082)*
Thalamus	.56(.071)	.79(.101)	.75(.161)	.68(.071)	.70(.077)	.59(.030)
MORPHINE PELLETED						
Caudate	1.23(.217)**	1.48(.156)	1.14(.260)	.86(.157)	1.05(.121)	1.10(.063)
Subs. Nigra	.78(.097)**	1.19(.159)*	.83(.207)	.61(.036)	.69(.078)	.60(.033)
Hypothalamus	1.15(.180)	1.36(.307)	1.17(.246)	.74(.095)*	.78(.099)	.75(.005)*
Thalamus	.97(.120)**	1.16(.070)	1.06(.033)	.84(.013)	.76(.067)	.84(.071)

Figures are expressed as mean (S.E.M.) picomoles of nucleotide per milligram of frozen tissue. Each mean represents four experiments done in triplicate. Differences from the preinjection level significant at the p<.05 level by the t test are designated (*), and differences between drug-naive and preinjection morphine pelleted levels significant at the p<.01 level designated (**).

TABLE 2.

Effects of Acute and Chronic Morphine Sulfate on Levels of Cyclic GMP in Four Rat Brain Structures

Structure	Minutes Following Morphine Injection (10 mg/kg)					
	0	1	5	10	30	60
DRUG NAIVE						
Caudate	47.8(1.1)	47.5(2.8)	43.1(2.5)	18.7(6.1)*	17.7(3.4)*	36.6(5.5)*
Subs. Nigra	38.1(6.9)	32.8(3.5)	25.6(6.5)	11.9(3.2)*	10.4(3.3)*	19.4(4.9)*
Hypothalamus	53.2(5.6)	45.9(3.9)	44.5(4.8)	32.8(7.3)*	19.0(3.4)*	32.6(3.9)*
Thalamus	52.5(3.8)	63.6(7.5)	48.8(3.8)	22.5(2.9)*	29.8(10.8)*	33.8(4.8)*
MORPHINE PELLETED						
Caudate	24.0(7.4)**	36.6(14.9)	29.5(5.6)	24.3(4.2)	25.8(4.3)	32.9(1.2)
Subs. Nigra	22.3(6.1)**	44.5(9.8)*	27.3(10.8)	27.0(8.4)	18.3(2.9)	12.1(1.2)
Hypothalamus	21.3(11.2)**	22.2(11.1)	37.2(8.9)	26.7(10.4)	26.8(9.2)	20.9(0.5)
Thalamus	33.3(12.8)**	23.4(12.7)	49.7(3.5)	36.8(4.3)	31.1(1.5)	25.9(1.8)

Figures are expressed as mean (S.E.M.) femtomoles of nucleotide per milligram of frozen tissue. Each mean represents three or four experiments done in triplicate. Significant differences are designated as in Table 1.

time and magnitude and has a time course similar to behaviorally observed analgesia as well. The role of muscarinic receptors are usually associated with increases in nervous system cGMP, and the decrease in cGMP may reflect decreased acetylcholine release at such sites (21). However, the uniformity of the effect across all four structures is reminiscent of the morphine-induced decrease in brain region calcium levels which decrease quickly and in all regions with an acute morphine injection (22). Goldberg, et al., have indicated that optimal tissue calcium ion levels are necessary for the maintenance of steady state levels of cGMP (23). Though both cyclic nucleotides decline, the relative concentration of cAMP increases 2-3 fold, and it is possible that the increase in cAMP relative to cGMP is important in effecting an analgesic response.

Naloxone injected twenty minutes prior to morphine (2 mg/kg, i.p.) prevented the morphine-induced depletion in both nucleotides in all structures with the possible exception of cAMP in the hypothalamus.

Morphine pelleted animals evidenced increased steady state levels of cAMP in caudate, substantia nigra and thalamus, but not in the hypothalamus. In contrast to the time course of effects of the acute morphine injection, the challenge injection in tolerant animals produced an early elevation in cAMP of the substantia nigra which dissipated by five minutes, and a subsequent decrease in cAMP in the hypothalamus. Caudate levels were not altered significantly from the tolerant pre-injection level and remained elevated above the drug-naive level throughout, as did thalamic levels. These elevations in cAMP contrast with the reduction in cerebral cortex adenyl cyclase activity reported for 72 hour morphine pelleted mice (2) but agree more with the increased adenyl cyclase activity reported by Naito, et al., with 14-28 days of chronic morphine treatment (3).

In contrast to the elevations in cAMP with morphine pelleting, the cGMP levels were depressed by about 40% in all four structures (Table 2). The challenge injection of morphine produced parallel elevations in cGMP and cAMP in the substantia nigra at one minute only, and showed a similar (not significant) trend in the thalamus at five minutes. The new steady state levels of cGMP resemble the peak effect of acute morphine and may reflect a reduced release of acetylcholine or sustained calcium depletion. These and other possibilities are being explored.

In the tolerant state the ratio of cAMP to cGMP is very high, but the ratio does not change appreciably with the challenge injection except in the hypothalamus were the cAMP decreases relative to the stable and depressed cGMP level. It is interesting to note that tolerance does not develop to the analgesic effects of up to ten repeated injections of 10 micrograms of morphine into the posterior hypothalamus, but animals so treated evidence subsequent tolerance to the analgesic effects of a systemic injection of morphine.

It must be pointed out that the effects reported here are seen only in the first hour following acute morphine, and in acutely tolerant animals. Long-term chronic narcotic administration often produces neurochemical effects that are dissimilar or opposite to those seen in acute tolerance or dependence (24). Studies in progress indicate substantially lowered cAMP levels in caudates of animals treated with morphine pellets for at least three weeks. Nonetheless, the alterations in cyclic nucleotides under the conditions reported here may represent a locus in which adaptive alterations underly the predisposition to the signs of physical dependence, and may alter local proteosynthesis in the acute state in a manner which initiates the probable altered state underlying the phenomenon of tolerance.

References

1. I.K. HO, H.H. LOH, and E. L. WAY, J. Pharmac. exp. Ther., 185, 336 (1973).

2. W.S. CHOU, A.K.S. HO, and H.H. LOH, Proc. West. Pharmac. Soc., 14, 42 (1971).

3. K. NAITO and K. KURIYAMA, Japan. J. Pharmac., 23,274-276 (1973).

4. R.L. SINGHAL, S. KACEW, R. LAFRENIERE, J. Pharm. Pharmac.,23, 274-276 (1973).

5. K. NAKAMURA, R. KUNTZMAN, A. MAGGIO and A. CONNEY, J. Pharm. Pharmac., 25, 584-587 (1973).

6. E. GARELIS abd N.H. NEFF, Science, 183, 532 (1974).

7. J.W. KEBABIAN and P. GREENGARD, Science, 174, 1346-1348 (1971).

8. F.W. WEIGHT, G. PETZOLD and P. GREENGARD, Science, 186, 942-944 (1974).

9. T.W. STONE, D.A. TAYLOR and F.E. BLOOM, Science, 187,284-287 (1974).

10. H.O.J. COLLIER and A.C. ROY, Nature,248, 24-27 (1974).

11. S.K. SHARMA, M. NIRENBERG and W.A. KLEE, Proc. Nat. Acad. Sci.(Wash.) 72,590-594 (1975).

12. J.A. FERENDELLI, M.H. GAY, W.C. SEDGEWICK and M.M. CHANG, J. Neurochem. 19,979-987 (1972).

13. W.D. LUST, J.V. PASSONNEAU and R.L. VEECH, Science, 181, 280-282 (1973).

14. J. KOENIG and R. KLIPPEL, The Rat Brain: A Stereotaxic Atlas, Krieger, New York (1963).

15. A.G. GILMAN, Proc. Nat. Acad. Sci., 67,305 (1970).

16. A.L. STEINER, C.W. PARKER and D.M. KIPNIS, J. Biol. Chem.,247, 1106 (1972).

17. M.J. SCHMIDT, D.E. SCHMIDT, G.A. ROBISON, Science, 173, 1142-1143 (1971).

18. A. GUIDOTTI, D.L. CHENEY, M. TRABUCCHI, M. DOTEUCHI and C. WANG, Neuropharmac., 13, 1115-1122 (1974).

19. K. NAKAMURA, R. KUNTZMAN, A. MAGGIO and A. CONNEY, J. Pharm. Pharmac., 25, 584-587 (1973).

20. J. SCHULTZ, J. Neurochem., 24, 495(1975).

21. E.F. DOMINO and A.E. WILSON, Biochem. Pharmacol., 24, 927-928 (1975).

22. H.L. CARDENAS and D.H.ROSS, J. Neurochem., 24, 487 (1975).

23. N.D. GOLDBERG, R.F. O'DEA, M.K. HADDOX, in P. GREENGARD and G.A. ROBISON (eds.) Advances in Cyclic Nucleotide Research 3, Raven Press, New York (1973).

24. E.F. DOMINO and A.E.WILSON, Psycholpharmacol., 41, 19-22 (1975).

POSSIBLE ROLE OF CYCLIC AMP AND DOPAMINE IN MORPHINE TOLERANCE AND PHYSICAL DEPENDENCE

Chander S. Mehta[1] and Willam E. Johnson

College of Pharmacy, Washington State University, Pullman,Wash. 99163.

(Received in final form May 24, 1975)

In chronically morphinized rats undergoing naloxone induced withdrawal the cerebellar Cyclic 3',5' adenosine monophosphate (Cyclic AMP) was significantly higher than the controls. The cerebellar dopamine (DA) and norepinephrine (NE) were decreased, elevated or unchanged depending on the duration of morphine treatment. The corpus striatal DA levels during withdrawal were markedly elevated and the striatal cyclic AMP levels were unchanged. The NE levels in the striatal tissue were either elevated or unchanged depending upon the duration of morphine administration. In sharp contrast to the chronically morphinized rats undergoing naloxone induced withdrawal, the rats made morphine dependent over a period of eight weeks showed quite moderate changes in the striatal and cerebellar cyclic AMP and DA levels. Thus alterations in the DA and the cyclic AMP levels in the central nervous system (CNS) may play an important role in the naloxone induced stereotyped morphine withdrawal behavior.

Cyclic AMP has been strongly implicated as a second messenger which mediates the pharmacological actions of numerous hormones in many tissues (1,2,3,4). However, no strong evidence exists for the assignment of a definitive role for cyclic AMP in brain function. Nevertheless, psychopharmacological agents are known to influence the cyclic AMP content of the rat brain and activity of the phosphodiesterase, an enzyme which hydrolyzes the cyclic nucleotide. These include a number of phenothiazine tranquilizers (5,6), tricyclic antidepressants (7,8,9) and hypnosedatives (submitted for publication). In addition to various psychopharmacological drugs, many aspects of the adenyl cyclase-cyclic AMP system in the CNS have been extensively studied. Gessa and co-workers (10) reported that this enzyme system was possibly involved in causing profound behavioral changes in rats and cats. Their studies demonstrated that dibutyryl cyclic AMP (a lipophillic analog of cyclic AMP which readily crosses cell membranes) when injected into rat lateral ventricles and other areas of the CNS produced marked behavioral changes, such as increased locomotor activity, catatonia, and convulsions.

Antagonism of the analgetic effect to morphine has been observed when exogenous cyclic AMP was administered to morphine tolerant and nontolerant mice (11). Cyclic AMP has also been found to accelerate the development of morphine tolerance and physical dependence in morphine pellet implanted mice (12). Thus the involvement of brain adenyl cyclase-cyclic AMP system in affecting behavioral pattern in animals and its possible role in the alteration of the phenomenon of tolerance to and physical dependence on morphine,

---

[1]Present address: School of Pharmacy, Texas Southern University, 3201 Wheeler Avenue, Houston, Texas 77004.

would suggest a central role for the cyclic nucleotide in the biochemical mechanisms of narcotic dependence.

The studies relating the effects of morphine and other narcotic agents on the biogenic amines of the CNS have employed decapitation as method of sacrifice. The excitation and long time required to remove brain would affect the endogenous levels of these biochemicals. Likewise, the alteration of endogenous cyclic AMP in the CNS of the morphine dependent animal has not been examined. It therefore seemed of interest to study using microwave irradiation as the method of sacrifice, the effects of chronic morphine treatment on the endogenous cyclic AMP and biogenic amines such as DA and NE in rat brain.

Methods

Male Sprague-Dawley rats (Hilltop laboratory) with an initial weight of 130 to 150 g were used throughout this study. The animals were housed at an automatically controlled temperature of $25^{\circ}C$ and a lighting schedule of 12 hours light alternated with 12 hours darkness. Standard Purina Chow and water were available ad libitum to all rats. The animals were sacrificed between 1.30 and 3.30 p.m. A styrofoam tube closed at both ends was used to confine the rat before sacrifice in the microwave oven (Model Toshiba, 1250 watts, 2450 mc). The closed dark environment calmed the animal and helped minimize apparent excitment. The period of 30 seconds was used to irradiate all animals since this interval completely denatures adenyl cyclase and phosphodiesterase enzymes (13). After microwave irradiation, the rat heads were excised and cooled in ice for easy handling. The brains were removed from skulls and cerebellar and striatal tissues were separated, weighed, quickly frozen in liquid nitrogen and stored at $-20^{\circ}C$ until assayed for cyclic AMP, DA, NE and protein content. Brain levels of cyclic AMP were assayed by the modified method of Brown et al.(14), as described by Rabinowitz and Katz (15). Results were expressed as pico moles (pm) of cyclic AMP per mg protein (16). Endogenous biogenic amines were assayed by the fluorometry method (17). The statistical evaluations of the data were determined with a two tailed Students' "t" test and a P value of less than 0.05 was considered significant.

Morphine Treatment

Morphine sulfate (calculated as morphine base) was dissolved in normal saline and given IP in doses of 5, 10, 20 and 40 mg morphine base per kg every 12 hours on the first, second, third and fourth days, respectively. Thereafter the dose was maintained at 40 mg/kg every 12 hours for the remainder of the period until sacrifice. Each rat was injected with 1 ml/kg saline before being sacrificed with 30 second microwave irradiation.

Those morphine dependent rats which underwent naloxone induced withdrawal were treated as above, except 4 mg/kg naloxone HCl was injected IP instead of normal saline. Control rats were injected twice daily with 1 ml/kg normal saline instead of the drug. The control group for naloxone induced withdrawal rats were administered 4 mg/kg naloxone HCl.

Results

Effect of Chronic Morphine Treatment

The time course of the morphine induced alteration in cyclic AMP, DA and NE in rat cerebellum and corpus striatum is shown in Fig. 1.

Cyclic AMP level of cerebellum of the chronically morphinized rat was significantly lower (P<0.001) on the first week of morphine treatment. But on fourth week the cyclic AMP concentration was significantly higher than saline controls (P<0.01). However, on the eighth week cerebellar cyclic AMP level had returned to control levels. No significant change in the cyclic AMP content of corpus striatum was observed during the entire eight weeks of morphine treatment.

DA content of the cerebellar tissue was essentially unchanged for the eight weeks of the drug treatment. Also the striatal DA level on the first week

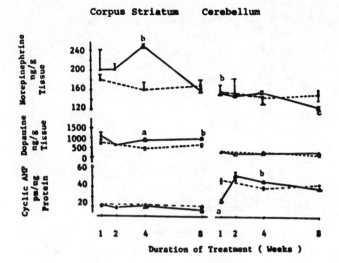

Corpus Striatum   Cerebellum

Duration of Treatment (Weeks)

FIG. 1

Effect of chronic morphine treatment on the endogenous levels of cyclic AMP, DA and NE in the rat cerebellum and corpus striatum. Morphine treatment▲———▲; control●- - - -●. Mean ± SE of 6 animals / point.

was not significantly different from the control group. However, significantly higher levels of striatal DA over that of control rats were observed in the fourth and eighth weeks of chronic morphine administration.

With respect to NE content, no significant difference was observed in the cerebellar or corpus striatal levels of NE except on the fourth week of morphine treatment where a significant elevation (P<0.01) of striatal NE was observed.

Effect of Naloxone Induced Morphine Withdrawal

Rats treated for up to eight weeks with morphine and subjected to naloxone induced withdrawal gave the following results as graphically shown in Figs. 2 and 3.

Striatal levels of cyclic AMP were not significantly different from controls. However, a significant elevation (P<0.001) in cerebellar cyclic AMP was observed on the fourth and eighth weeks when compared to respective saline controls.

The cerebellar DA level was significantly higher than control on the fourth week. Also the fourth week DA level was significantly greater (P<0.001) than the second week DA level of morphine treated rats. Marked increase in striatal DA levels were observed on the fourth and eighth weeks in morphine dependent rats undergoing naloxone induced withdrawal.

The cerebellar NE level was significantly higher (P<0.001) than the control on the first week. However, in the eighth week the test animals showed a significant (P<0.05) decline in cerebellar DA when compared to saline controls. The striatal NE level was significantly higher than the control

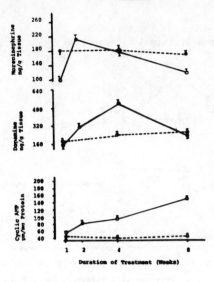

FIG. 2

Effect of naloxone induced withdrawal on the endogenous levels of cyclic AMP, dopamine and norepinephrine in the morphine dependent rat cerebellum. Each value represents the mean ± SE of 6 rats. Morphine treatment○——○, Saline control●----●.

($P<0.001$), on the fourth week of morphine treatment when followed by naloxone induced withdrawal.

Discussion

Morphine induced stereotyped behavior of continuous sniffing, licking and biting without normal behavior such as grooming, eating or locomotion, has been observed in rats undergoing chronic morphine treatment (18,19,20). Ahyan and Randrop (20) reported that reserpine and α-methyl tyrosine supressed these morphine induced stereotyped behaviors. They also noted that FLA-63, an agent which specifically depletes NE without affecting levels of DA through the blockage of DA β-hydroxylase, was found to inhibit this characteristic behavior. The intraventricular administration of NE reversed this blocking action of FLA-63 upon the stereotyped behavior. Our data shows that the levels of striatal DA and NE were higher than controls on the fourth week of morphine treatment. This suggested that at least for the first four weeks, elevations in the levels of NE and DA could both be involved in stereotyped behavior. The striatal DA level was significantly higher than the control even on the eighth week of morphine treatment, without any decrease in the stereotyped behavior. The importance of the central stores of both NE and DA in the manifestation of abstinence syndrome in morphine dependent animals as speculated by others (21) was confirmed by our data.

Naloxone induced abstinence withdrawal in morphine dependent rats caused a great increase over the controls in the cerebellar cyclic AMP levels. This data was in agreement with the elevations in cyclic AMP observed in the whole brains of rats that were implanted with morphine pellets (22). However, no such increase in cyclic AMP was observed in the striatal tissue of rats chronically treated with morphine.

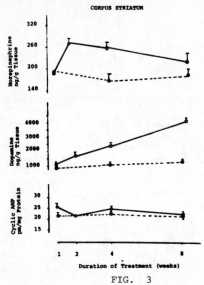

CORPUS STRIATUM

FIG. 3

Effects of naloxone induced withdrawal on the endogenous levels of cyclic AMP, DA and NE in morphine dependent rat corpus striatum. Each value represents the mean ± SE of 6 rats. Morphine treatment o——o, Saline control •----•.

According to other published reports the morphine analgesia in tolerant and nontolerant mice was antagonized by the administration of cyclic AMP, dibutyryl cyclic AMP, or theophylline, an inhibitor of phosphodiesterase (11, 12). The development of tolerance to morphine and physical dependence on the drug was also considerably facilitated by the increase in cyclic AMP levels (12). Our data showing marked increase in cerebellar cyclic AMP after naloxone administration would suggest that cyclic AMP acts as a morphine antagonist through some unknown mechanism; at least with respect to analgesia and tolerance. Naloxone HCl perhaps manifested its pharmacological response as a morphine antagonist, by increasing the levels of endogenous brain cyclic AMP. However, naloxone per se showed no elevations in brain cyclic AMP in rats that were never exposed to morphine (submitted for publication).

For the first four weeks during morphine withdrawal, a significant linear increase in the cerebellar DA level was observed. However, the cerebellar NE showed no such increase. This might suggest that DA was more than a mere precurssor to NE in the rat cerebellum.

Marked elevation of striatal DA level during morphine withdrawal suggested that an increase in neostriatal dopaminergic activity could cause the stereotyped behavior such as the wet dog shakes during morphine withdrawal in rats. In sharp contrast to the chronically morphinized rats undergoing naloxone induced withdrawal, the rats made morphine dependent over a period of eight weeks showed quite moderate changes in striatal and cerebellar cyclic AMP and DA levels. Thus alterations in the DA and the cyclic AMP levels in the CNS may play an important role in the stereotyped morphine withdrawal behavior.

135

References

1. G.A. ROBISON, R.W. BUTCHER, and E.W. SUTHERLAND, Annu. Rev. Biochem. 37 149-174 (1968).
2. E.W. SUTHERLAND, G.A. ROBISON and R.W. BUTCHER, Circulation 37 279-306 (1968).
3. B. McL. BRECKENRIDGE, Annu. Rev. Pharmacol. 10 19-34 (1970).
4. G.A.ROBISON, R.W. BUTCHER, E.W. SUTHERLAND, Fundamental Concepts in Drug Receptor Interactions, p 59-91 Acad. Press, London (1969).
5. P. UZUNOV and B. WEISS, Neuropharmacology 10 697-708 (1971).
6. M.I. PAUL, G.L. PAUK and B. R. DITZION, Pharmacol. (Basel) 3 148-154 (1970).
7. B. BEER, M. CHASIN, D. CLODY, J. R. VOGEL and Z. P. HOROVITZ, Science 176 428-430 (1972).
8. J. H. McNEILL and L. D. MUSCHEK, Fed. Proc. 30 330 (1971).
9. G.C. PALMER, Life Sci. 12 345-355 (1973).
10. G.L. GESSA, G. KRISHNA, J. FORN, A. TAGLIMONTE and B.B. BRODIE, Role of Cyclic AMP in Cell Function, p.371-381 Raven Press, N.Y. (1970).
11. I.K. HO, H. LOH and E.L. WAY, J. Pharmacol. Exp. Ther. 185 336-346 (1973).
12. I.K. HO, H. LOH and E.L. WAY, J. Pharmacol. Exp. Ther. 185 347-357 (1973).
13. M.J. SCHMIDT, D. SCHMIDT, and G.A. ROBISON, Advance in Cyclic Nucleotide Research, p. 425-434 (1972).
14. B.L. BROWN, J. ALBANO, R.P. EKINS, A.M. SGHERZI and E. TAMION, Biochem. J. 121 561-562 (1971).
15. B. RABINOWITZ and J.KATZ, Clin. Chem. 19 312-314 (1973).
16. O.H. LOWRY, N.J. ROSEBROUGH, A.L. FARR and R.J. RANDALL, J. Biol. Chem. 193 265-275 (1951).
17. M.K. SCHELLENBERGER and J.H. GORDON, Anal. Biochem. 49 356-372 (1971).
18. R. FOG, Psychopharmacologia (Berl.) 16 305-312 (1970).
19. V.P. VENDERNIKOU, Psychopharmacologia (Berl.) 17 283-288 (1970).
20. I.H. AHYAN and A. RANDROP, Psychopharmacologia (Berl.) 27 203-212 (1972).
21. Y. MARUYAMA and A.E. TAKEMORI, J. Pharmacol. Exp. Ther. 178 20-29 (1971).
22. C.S. MEHTA and W.E. JOHNSON, Fed. Proc.33 493 (1974).

CHANGES IN BRAIN CYCLIC AMP METABOLISM AND ACETYLCHOLINE AND DOPAMINE DURING NARCOTIC DEPENDENCE AND WITHDRAWAL

Z. Merali, R.L. Singhal, P.D. Hrdina and G.M. Ling

Department of Pharmacology, University of Ottawa
Ottawa, Canada K1N 9A9

(Received in final form May 24, 1975

Effects of morphine administration were studied on cyclic AMP metabolism in several regions of rat brain. In the cortex, cerebellum and thalamus-hypothalamus, morphine dependence did not alter the activity of either adenylate cyclase or phosphodiesterase. However, during withdrawal from the opiate treatment, adenylate cyclase activity declined in all three regions studied. In contrast, the striatal cyclic AMP metabolism was enhanced during morphine treatment as reflected by elevated endogenous cyclic AMP and increased adenylate cyclase. Furthermore, narcotic dependence produced significant increases in acetylcholinesterase activity of rat striatum. Whereas morphine withdrawal reversed the changes in striatal acetylcholine levels and acetylcholinesterase activity, the enhanced striatal dopamine remained unaltered. Although the activity of striatal adenylate cyclase was significantly reduced when compared to the morphine-dependent rats, the drop in cyclic AMP levels was not significant. Methadone replacement did not affect the changes in striatal dopamine seen in morphine-withdrawn rats. Whereas dopamine stimulated equally well the striatal adenylate cyclase from control or morphine-dependent animals, it failed to stimulate the striatal enzyme from rats undergoing withdrawal. The crude synaptosomal fraction of the whole brain from morphine-dependent rats exhibited an increase in cyclic AMP which was accompanied by elevated adenylate cyclase and protein kinase activity. Naloxone administration suppressed this rise in cyclic AMP and reversed the morphine-stimulated increases in the activities of adenylate cyclase and protein kinase. Following the withdrawal of morphine treatment, alterations in cyclic AMP metabolism were similar to those noted in morphine-naloxone group. Furthermore, substitution of morphine with methadone antagonized the observed alterations in cyclic nucleotide metabolism during withdrawal.

There is evidence to suggest that several of the actions of opiate analgesics are related to alterations in the metabolism of cyclic AMP and biogenic amines in the central nervous system. Administration of cyclic AMP has been reported to antagonize analgesic effects of morphine and to accelerate the development of tolerance to and physical dependence on this narcotic agent (1). Conversely, opiate treatment has been found to alter cyclic AMP turnover in mouse brain (2,3). Similarly, some of the effects of narcotics including the development of physical dependence can be modified by manipulations of brain amine levels (4-6). In addition, administration of opiates has been shown to alter the metabolism of brain biogenic amines (7-9). Recently, dopamine-sensitive adenylate cyclase was identified in mammalian brain (10) and was presumed to represent the "dopamine-receptor." Since chronic morphine treatment alters both dopamine and cyclic AMP metabolism, it is conceivable that cyclic AMP acts in the dopamine-mediated transmission as a "second messenger." As is the case for certain antipsychotic drugs (11,12), it seems possible that narcotic analgesics may exert their pharmacological effects, at least in part, by modulating a specific dopamine-sensitive adenylate cyclase in brain tissue. We were therefore prompted to examine the influence of morphine dependence and withdrawal on the metabolism of cyclic AMP, acetylcholine and dopamine in rat brain. In addition, the effect of morphine dependence on the interrelationship of dopamine and cyclic AMP was investigated in the most prominent dopaminergically innervated area of the brain, the striatum. Our results demonstrate that development of morphine dependence is accompanied by enhanced cyclic AMP metabolism in the striatum as well as in crude synaptosomal fraction of the whole brain and that during withdrawal, the activity of dopamine-sensitive adenylate cyclase is virtually blocked.

Experiments were conducted on male Sprague-Dawley rats weighing approximately 100 g and having free access to food and water. In acute studies, morphine sulphate (15 mg/kg) was injected s.c. and the animals were killed 1 hr later. Rats were made dependent to morphine either by (a) modification of the method described by Takemori (13) where animals were injected twice daily with a 15 mg/kg dose of morphine sulphate i.p. for the first week, 30 mg/kg during the second week and 45 mg/kg in the third week of treatment ("slow schedule") or (b) by the method of Pinsky (personal communication) in which rats were given morphine sulphate by i.p. injection twice daily in doses increasing from 10 mg/kg to 270 mg/kg/injection over a period of 6 days ("rapid schedule"). Upon completion of narcotic treatment, one group (morphine-dependent) was killed 6-8 hr after the last injection, while rats in another group (morphine-withdrawn) were maintained without any additional treatment for 48 (after "slow schedule") or 24 hr (after "rapid schedule"). The third group of morphine-dependent rats received methadone (15 mg/kg; i.p.) twice daily for 48 (after "slow schedule") or 24 hr (after "rapid schedule") and constituted the "methadone-replaced" groups. In certain experiments, another group was included (morphine-naloxone) in which withdrawal was precipitated with a single dose of naloxone (2.7 mg/kg) and the animals killed 5 min later. Rats were decapitated and brains rapidly excised in cold room (4°) for the measurement of various neurochemical parameters as described in previous publications (9,19).

One hour after the injection of morphine (15 mg/kg), no significant change was detected in the activity of either basal or fluoride-stimulated form of adenylate cyclase in cerebral cortex, cerebellum and thalamus-hypothalamus. The activity of the cyclic AMP degrading enzyme, phosphodiesterase also remained unaltered in these brain regions of rats treated acutely with morphine. Similarly, morphine dependence ("slow schedule") did not alter significantly the activity of adenylate cyclase or phosphodiesterase in either of the regions examined. However, whereas withdrawal (48 hr) from morphine treatment significantly decreased both the basal and the fluoride-stimulated forms of adenylate cyclase, the activity of phosphodiesterase remained virtually unaltered. It is of interest that methadone replacement in morphine-dependent rats generally prevented these neurochemical alterations in animals undergoing withdrawal. From the same group of dependent rats, the striatal regions were utilized for the determination of acetylcholine, dopamine and the activity of acetylcholinesterase. Data in Fig. 1 show that the development of narcotic dependence was accompanied by an accumulation of striatal acetylcholine. This may be due either to the simultaneous suppression of acetylcholinesterase activity observed in present experiments and/or to the inhibitory effect of morphine upon the release of brain acetylcholine (14).

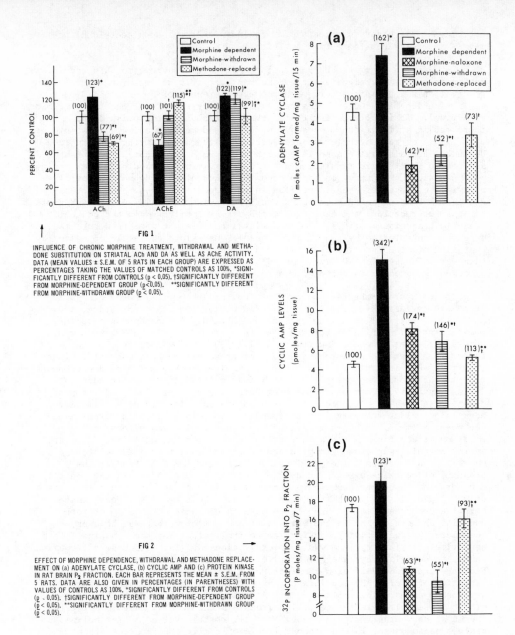

FIG 1

INFLUENCE OF CHRONIC MORPHINE TREATMENT, WITHDRAWAL AND METHA-
DONE SUBSTITUTION ON STRIATAL ACh AND DA AS WELL AS AChE ACTIVITY.
DATA (MEAN VALUES ± S.E.M. OF 5 RATS IN EACH GROUP) ARE EXPRESSED AS
PERCENTAGES TAKING THE VALUES OF MATCHED CONTROLS AS 100%. *SIGNI-
FICANTLY DIFFERENT FROM CONTROLS (p < 0.05). †SIGNIFICANTLY DIFFERENT
FROM MORPHINE-DEPENDENT GROUP (p<0.05).   **SIGNIFICANTLY DIFFERENT
FROM MORPHINE-WITHDRAWN GROUP (p < 0.05).

FIG 2

EFFECT OF MORPHINE DEPENDENCE, WITHDRAWAL AND METHADONE REPLACE-
MENT ON (a) ADENYLATE CYCLASE, (b) CYCLIC AMP AND (c) PROTEIN KINASE
IN RAT BRAIN P_2 FRACTION. EACH BAR REPRESENTS THE MEAN ± S.E.M. FROM
5 RATS. DATA ARE ALSO GIVEN IN PERCENTAGES (IN PARENTHESES) WITH
VALUES OF CONTROLS AS 100%. *SIGNIFICANTLY DIFFERENT FROM CONTROLS
(p - 0.05). †SIGNIFICANTLY DIFFERENT FROM MORPHINE-DEPENDENT GROUP
(p < 0.05). **SIGNIFICANTLY DIFFERENT FROM MORPHINE-WITHDRAWN GROUP
(p < 0.05).

Withdrawal of morphine treatment resulted in a significant reduction of
striatal acetylcholine levels well below those found in control animals. Our
data on acetylcholine depletion in morphine-withdrawn rats are in agreement
with those reported by Domino and Wilson (14) and are compatible with the work
of Crossland (15) who demonstrated that morphine withdrawal resulted in an
"explosive release" of brain acetylcholine. It has been suggested that this
phenomenon may be partly responsible for the hyperactive state seen upon acute
withdrawal of morphine in both animals and man. Replacement with methadone did

not prevent the observed effects of morphine-withdrawal upon acetylcholine levels and acetylcholinesterase activity.

In addition to these changes in the cholinergic system, morphine administration resulted in a significant enhancement of striatal dopamine (Fig. 1), an observation which is in accord with the recent report of Johnson and Clouet (16). The dopamine content remained significantly elevated even after morphine withdrawal. It is of interest that methadone replacement abolished the increases in striatal dopamine seen in morphine-dependent animals. Iwamoto et al. (17) reported that naloxone-precipitated withdrawal jumping in morphine-dependent animals may be associated with elevated brain dopamine and might be subject to cholinergic regulation since physostigmine blocked both the jumping response and the increase in brain dopamine. Recently, a dopamine-sensitive adenylate cyclase has been identified in the caudate nucleus. Considerable evidence has accumulated to support the hypothesis that this enzyme represents a "dopamine-receptor" and that cyclic AMP may be implicated in the central synaptic transmission (10,18). The striatal regions obtained from rats made dependent on morphine by the "rapid schedule" had elevated levels of homo-vanillic acid and tyrosine hydroxylase activity, indicating increased dopamine turnover. The cyclic AMP levels of this region were also significantly enhanced as compared to those of control animals (Table 1).

In contrast to the cerebrocortical, cerebellar or thalamo-hypothalamic adenylate cyclase which remained unaltered during the dependent state, the activity of striatal adenylate cyclase was markedly enhanced upon morphine administration. During withdrawal, the reduction in cyclic AMP levels was not significant; however, the enzyme activity dropped significantly when compared to that of the morphine-dependent group although it was still higher than that seen in controls. In order to examine whether morphine dependence affects the "dopamine-receptor", dopamine-stimulated increases in adenylate cyclase activity in striatal tissue preparations were studied. Addition of dopamine (40 µM) in vitro to striatal homogenates, significantly stimulated adenylate cyclase activity in non-dependent rats (Table 1). In morphine-dependent animals, in which adenylate cyclase activity was already enhanced, addition of dopamine caused a further increase in enzyme activity. However, in the morphine-withdrawn group, dopamine failed to activate adenylate cyclase over its basal values. The net increase in cyclic AMP formation in the presence of dopamine was 12.7 and 13.3 pmol/mg tissue/2.5 min in the control and morphine-dependent groups, respectively. In contrast, the increment was only 0.3 pmol in the morphine-withdrawn rats. These results suggest that morphine dependence may be associated with an enhanced metabolism of both dopamine and cyclic AMP in the rat striatum. During withdrawal however, adenylate cyclase activity declined to control values and the dopamine-sensitive adenylate cyclase was completely blocked. This blockade of dopamine sensitive adenylate cyclase may be related to withdrawal symptoms. Our findings are concordant with those of Ho et al. (1) who reported that administration of cyclic AMP accelerated the development of tolerance to and dependence on morphine. Since cyclic AMP has been implicated in the transmission of impulses in the central nervous system, we also have investigated the question whether morphine dependence alters the cyclic AMP metabolism in brain synaptosomes. The endogenous levels of cyclic AMP in crude synaptosomal fraction of the whole brain of rats rendered dependent to morphine ("rapid schedule") exhibited a 3-fold increase over those of non-treated controls (Fig. 2b). This elevation was accompanied by significant stimulation of both adenylate cyclase and protein kinase activity (Fig. 2a,c).

Administration of naloxone to morphinized rats precipitated withdrawal symptoms that included loss in body weight, teeth chattering and "wet-dog shakes." Moreover, naloxone significantly suppressed the morphine-induced

TABLE 1

Effect of Morphine Dependence and Withdrawal on Basal and Dopamine-
Stimulated Adenylate Cyclase and Cyclic AMP Levels
of Rat Striatum

Each value represents the mean ± S.E.M. from 4 to 6 rats in the group.
Rats were made morphine-dependent by the "rapid schedule" as described in the
text. Rats in "morphine withdrawn" group were deprived of morphine injections
for 24 hr. For determination of the dopamine-sensitive adenylate cyclase,
striatal homogenates were incubated with 40 µM dopamine for 2.5 min at 30° and
measured the amount of cyclic AMP formed. Data are also given in percentages
(in parentheses) taking the value of control rats as 100%.

Treatment	cAMP (pmol/mg)	Adenylate Cyclase (pmol cAMP formed/mg)		pmol cAMP formed in presence of DA over its respective basal value
		-DA	+DA (40 µM)	
Control	0.63±0.06 (100)	36.6±1.10 (100)	49.3±2.61 (100)	12.7 (100)
Morphine-Dependent	0.87±0.07 (138)*	59.8±1.41 (163)*	73.1±4.58 (148)*	13.3 (105)
Morphine-Withdrawn	0.79±0.04 (126)*	49.2±3.29 (134)*†	49.5±2.40 (100)*†	0.3 (2.4)*†

*Significantly different when compared with control values (p <0.05).

†Significantly different when compared with the morphine-dependent group
(p <0.05).

increases in cyclic AMP levels and reversed the morphine-induced stimulation
in adenylate cyclase and protein kinase (Fig. 2a,b,c). It is also of interest
that 24 hr following morphine withdrawal, the alterations in cyclic AMP levels
as well as in adenylate cyclase and protein kinase activities were similar to
those noted in the morphine-naloxone group. Furthermore, replacement of
morphine with methadone in morphine-dependent animals not only antagonized the
alterations seen during withdrawal, but also abolished the morphine-induced
changes in the cyclic AMP levels and protein kinase activity.

In conclusion, the present study indicates that brains of rats rendered
dependent to morphine display region-specific alterations in cyclic AMP metabolism. Of the several regions examined, the most pronounced changes in cyclic
AMP and adenylate cyclase activity were observed in the striatum. In this
brain region, elevated acetylcholine levels as well as enhanced dopamine
turnover (as reflected by increased homovanillic acid levels and tyrosine
hydroxylase activity) also were noted in opiate-dependent rats. It is conceivable that altered cyclic AMP metabolism might be involved in the development of opiate dependence and that the blockade of dopamine-sensitive adenylate cyclase might play a role in the phenomena of abstinence syndrome.

Acknowledgements

This investigation was supported by the Non-Medical Use of Drugs Directorate of Health and Welfare Canada under its program of Research on Drug Abuse (RODA) and by grants from the Ontario Mental Health Foundation. The authors are grateful to Mr. S. Klosevych, Director of Medical Communications and his staff for their skilled assistance in the preparation of the illustration.

References

1. I.K. HO, H.H. LOH, and E. LEONG WAY, J. Pharmacol. Exp. Ther. 185, 347-357 (1973).
2. W.S. CHOU, A.K.S. HO, and H.H. LOH, Proc. West. Pharmacol. Soc. 14, 42-46 (1971).
3. K. NAITO, and K. KURIYAMA, Japan. J. Pharmacol. 23, 274-276 (1973).
4. D.M. BUXBAUM, G.G. YARBROUGH, and M.E. CARTER, J. Pharmacol. Exp. Ther. 185, 317-327 (1973).
5. Y. MARUYAMA, and A.E. TAKEMORI, J. Pharmacol. Exp. Ther. 185, 602-608 (1973).
6. E. EIDELBERG, and R. ERSPAMER, J. Pharmacol. Exp. Ther. 192, 50-57 (1975).
7. C. GAUCHY, Y. AGID, J. GLOWINSKI, and A. CHERAMY, Europ. J. Pharmacol. 22, 311-319 (1973).
8. D.G. CLOUET, and M. RATNER, Science 168, 854-856 (1970).
9. Z. MERALI, P.K. GHOSH, P.D. HRDINA, R.L. SINGHAL, and G.M. LING, Europ. J. Pharmacol. 26, 375-378 (1974).
10. J.W. KEBABIAN, G.L. PETZOLD, and P. GREENGARD, Proc. Nat. Acad. Sci. U.S.A. 69, 2145-2149 (1972).
11. M. KAROBATH, and H. LEITICH, Proc. Nat. Acad. Sci. U.S.A. 71, 2915-2917 (1974).
12. P. GREENGARD, J. Psychiat. Res. 11, 87-90 (1974).
13. A.E. TAKEMORI, J. Pharmacol. Exp. Ther. 130, 370-374 (1960).
14. E.F. DOMINO, and A. WILSON, J. Pharmacol. Exp. Ther. 184, 18-32 (1973).
15. J. CROSSLAND, Drugs and Cholinergic Mechanisms in the Central Nervous System, p. 355, Forvarest Forskninganstalt, Stockholm (1970).
16. J.C. JOHNSON, and D.C. CLOUET, Fed. Proc. 32, 757 (1973).
17. E.T. IWAMOTO, I.K. HO, and E. LEONG WAY, J. Pharmacol. Exp. Ther. 187, 558-567 (1973).
18. Y.C. CLEMENT-CORMIER, R.G. PARRISH, G.L. PETZOLD, J.W. KEBABIAN, and P. GREENGARD, J. Neurochem. (1975) In press.
19. R.L. SINGHAL, S. KACEW, and R. LAFRENIERE, J. Pharm. Pharmacol. 25, 1022-1024 (1973).

EFFECT OF CYCLIC NUCLEOTIDES AND PHOSPHODIESTERASE INHIBITION ON MORPHINE TOLERANCE AND PHYSICAL DEPENDENCE

I. K. Ho, H. H. Loh, H. N. Bhargava and E. Leong Way

Department of Pharmacology and Langley Porter Neuropsychiatric Institute, University of California, San Francisco, California 94143.

(Received in final form May 24, 1975)

Summary

The effects of cyclic nucleotides and theophylline were assessed in mice rendered tolerant to and physically dependent on morphine by the pellet implantation procedure. Tolerance was quantified by the increase in amount of morphine to produce analgesia and dependence by the decrease in amount of naloxone to precipitate withdrawal jumping. By these criteria, pretreatment with a single intravenous injection of cyclic 3',5'-adenosine monophosphate (cAMP) was found to enhance markedly tolerance and dependence development. Repeated injections of theophylline were also effective. Cycloheximide and beta-adrenergic blockers prevented the accelerating effect of cAMP and with more frequent administration also decreased the development of tolerance and dependence. It is concluded that cAMP may have a role in morphine tolerance and dependence development.

In recent years, considerable evidence has been obtained on the biochemical processes that may be concerned in the development of tolerance to and physical dependence on morphine. In our laboratory, we have found that the development of morphine tolerance and physical dependence can be altered by pharmacologic manipulations. Either syndrome may be inhibited or accelerated by selection of compounds which act by different mechanisms. These changes can be achieved with a dose of an agent that may or may not change morphine responses acutely. These studies have been summarized in a review (1). In brief, evidence has been obtained suggesting that serotonin gamma-amino-butyric acid, and adenosine 3', 5'-cyclic monophosphate (cAMP) may play some associated role in morphine tolerance and dependence development.

The possibility that cAMP might interact with morphine is suggested by numerous reports indicating that morphine can alter the functional state of the biogenic amines which have been repeatedly demonstrated to have the ability to modify morphine action (2). Moreover, morphine was found to activate cerebral adenyl cyclase (3). We should like to summarize our previous findings (4, 5, 6) on the effects of cAMP on morphine tolerance and dependence and also present some more recent data.

Supported by grants DA-0037 and DA-00563 from the National Institute of Drug Abuse. I. K. Ho is the recipient of a Faculty Development Award from the Pharmaceutical Manufacturer Association Foundation in Basic Pharmacology. Contribution number 75-4.

Experimental Procedures

The methods for assessment of tolerance and physical dependence were similar to those previously reported (7). Mice were rendered tolerant to and physically dependent on morphine by the s.c. implantation of a specially formulated morphine pellet for 3 days. On the 4th day, the pellet was removed and 6 hours later the degree of tolerance and physical dependence development was assessed. Tolerance was quantified by determining the increase in the median analgetic dose of morphine (AD50) using the tail-flick procedure. Physical dependence was measured by determining the amount of naloxone (ED50) to precipitate withdrawal jumping. An inverse relationship exists between the two parameters; a decrease in the naloxone ED50 is indicative of increased physical dependence.

Various cAMP agonists and antagonists were tested for their effects on tolerance and physical dependence development. Usually, a single injection of a drug was made prior to implantation of a morphine or a placebo pellet and the effect of this maneuver on the morphine AD50 and the naloxone ED50 was made on the 4th day 6 hours after pellet removal. Thus, the assessment of the effect of the agent was made 80 hours after its administration. With shorter acting compounds, it was sometimes necessary to repeat with an additional dose at daily intervals for two additional days. Under these conditions, the assessment for the drug effect was made 30 hours after its last administration. The specific conditions for each chemical agent will be described in Results.

Results

Effect of cAMP on the development of tolerance.

Under conditions where pretreatment with cAMP did not alter the acute response to morphine, cAMP markedly accelerated tolerance development (6). In mice receiving one single injection of cAMP 10 mg/kg i.v., two hours prior to morphine pellet implantation, the AD50 of morphine was found to be considerably higher than that of controls. In saline-treated animals, morphine pellet implantation effected a 10-fold increase in the AD50 (from 7.5 to 76 mg/kg). In the cAMP group, the AD50 was increased more than 3-fold (from 8 to 270 mg/kg). Based on the relative increase in their respective AD50 values, the cAMP group was more than 3 times as tolerant as the control group. Similar experiments with a 2.5 mg/kg dose of cAMP resulted in a doubling of the morphine AD50 over that of saline-treated mice.

Cycloheximide prevented the accelerating effect of cAMP on morphine tolerance development. As shown on the right in Figure 1, in mice rendered tolerant to morphine by pellet implantation, a single injection of cAMP two hours before implanting a morphine pellet resulted in a morphine AD50 3 times that of a similarly implanted group receiving saline instead of cAMP. In a third group of mice receiving cycloheximide daily in addition to cAMP, the cAMP effect was prevented; the increase in the morphine AD50 noted after pellet implantation in the cAMP group was no greater than that in the animals given the vehicle. Likewise, the group receiving cycloheximide alone exhibited an AD50 nearly identical with the group given the vehicle. Thus, cycloheximide, under conditions which did not affect the morphine AD50 or mortality, blocked the accelerating effect of cAMP on tolerance development. With high doses and more frequent administrations, cycloheximide will also block the development of tolerance to morphine (8) but it is difficult to prevent deaths under such conditions.

Figure 1

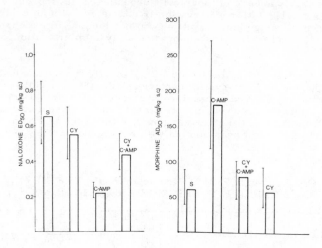

Effect of cycloheximide on cAMP enhancement of morphine dependence and tolerance development. The naloxone ED50 and morphine
AD50 plus 95% confidence limits were determined 6 hours after
removal of a morphine pellet implanted for 72 hours.   S denotes
saline;   CY, cycloheximide.   The doses were CY 20 mg/kg i. p. ;
cAMP 10 mg/kg i.v. From Ho et al., (6)

Effect of cAMP on the development of morphine physical dependence

The injection of cAMP prior to morphine pellet implantation also
accelerated the development of physical dependence (6). Enhancement of
dependence development by cAMP was indicated by a decrease in the amount
of naloxone needed to induce precipitated withdrawal jumping.   In mice
previously rendered dependent by pellet implantation, the administration
of cAMP immediately after pellet removal did not alter the naloxone ED50
significantly.   In contrast, in implanted mice pretreated with cAMP, a
higher degree of physical dependence was evidenced by a decrease in the
naloxone ED50 to one-fourth that of the group receiving the vehicle.   Enhancement of morphine physical dependence development by cAMP also was
shown after abrupt withdrawal; the body weight loss, which occurred after
removal of the morphine pellet, was greater with cAMP pretreatment.

Cycloheximide prevented the accelerating effect of cAMP on the development of physical dependent on morphine.   As shown on the left in Fig. 1, in
mice pretreated with a single injection of cAMP two hours before morphine
pellet implantation, the naloxone ED50 was one-third that of morphine
pellet-implanted animals treated with saline.   The administration of cycloheximide once daily at a dose which did not significantly alter the naloxone
precipitated withdrawal response reduced the enhancing effect of cAMP.
The naloxone ED50 of the cAMP-plus-cycloheximide-treated group was
about twice that of the cAMP-treated group and not significantly different
from morphine implanted animal treated with saline.

More frequent administration of cycloheximide not only blocked the accelerating effect of cAMP on morphine dependence development but also reduced the development of physical dependence in morphine pellet-implanted mice. The latter observation is consistent with an earlier study that dependence development, resulting from repeated injections of morphine for three weeks, is blocked by the daily administration of cycloheximide (8).

Two other nucleotides, adenosine-2',3'-cyclic monophosphate (2',3' cAMP) and guanosine-3',5'-cyclic monophosphate (3',5'-cGMP) were also assessed for their effect on morphine tolerance and physical dependence. As shown in Table 1, following pretreatment with a dose similar to that for cAMP (10 mg/kg i.v.) neither compound altered the morphine AD50 or naloxone ED50 of animals of implanted with a morphine pellet.

Table 1

EFFECT OF 2',3'-cAMP AND 3',5'-cGMP ON THE DEVELOPMENT OF MORPHINE TOLERANCE AND DEPENDENCE.

Compound	Morphine AD50*	Naloxone ED50*
Vehicle	60 (46 - 78)	0.53 (0.46-0.62)
2',3'-cAMP	90 (63 -128)	0.48 (0.28-0.83)
3',5'-cGMP	84 (14 -171)	0.45 (0.32-0.63)
3',5'-cAMP +	270 (200-360)	0.08 (0.05-0.12)

*determined after subcutaneous administration (mg/kg) 6 hours after removal of a morphine pellet implanted for 3 days; parentheses include the 95% confidence limits. +From Ho et al., (6)

Effect of theophylline on tolerance and dependence

The phosphodiesterase inhibitor, theophylline, enhanced tolerance and physical dependence development. The compound was administered at dose of 100 mg/kg intraperitoneally commencing 2 hours before morphine pellet implantation and repeated every 24 hours for 2 additional days. A control group received the vehicle instead of theophylline. The morphine AD50 and naloxone ED50 were determined in the usual manner 6 hours after pellet removal.

As shown on the left of Figure 2, theophylline treated animals were about 3 times more tolerant than the control group. The morphine AD50 of the theophylline pretreated group was 235 mg/kg whereas it was 78 mg/kg for the control group receiving the vehicle.

The development of a higher degree of physical dependence after theophylline pretreatment is shown by the data summarized on the right of Figure 2. The naloxone ED50 of the theophylline group (0.29 mg/kg) was one-third that of the control group (0.76 mg/kg).

Effect of beta adrenergic blockers

The enhancing effect of cAMP on tolerance and physical dependence development was blocked by pretreatment with the beta-adrenergic blockers. A single injection of dichloroisoproterenol (DCI, 40μg) pronethalol (70 μg), and propanolol (70 μg) intracerebrally 20 minutes prior to cAMP, prevented the accelerating effect of cAMP on tolerance and physical dependence development. Under these conditions and physical dependence development was not significantly altered by the individual beta blockers. In time course studies conducted with propanolol, the compound was found to be largely ineffective when given 24 and 48 hours after cAMP. When given 20 minutes or 4 hours after cAMP its action was greatly reduced (Loh et al., unpublished).

Figure 2

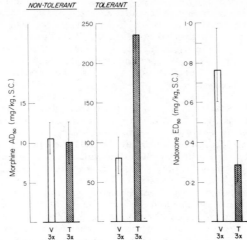

Effect of theophylline on the development of tolerance and physical dependence. V denotes the vehicle and T, theophylline 100 mg/kg i.p., administered at daily intervals for 3 days.

Administration of DCI for three days intracerebrally, resulted in a decrease in tolerance development. As shown in Table 2, an 11-fold tolerance developed in morphine implanted animals treated with saline whereas with DCI treatment, only a 4-fold tolerance developed. The three daily injections of DCI in the placebo pellet implanted animals did not alter the response to morphine (9). Similar results were obtained with experiments on propanolol.

Repeated administration of DCI also inhibited the development of physical dependence. When DCI was given prior to and during the development of dependence, the naloxone ED50 increased 8-fold as shown in Table 2. The acute administration of DCI to the dependent animals did not alter withdrawal response as evidenced by the fact that the naloxone ED50 of saline and DCI treated were nearly identical. Also, acute or chronic treatment with saline in morphine implanted animals did not alter the naloxone ED50.

Table 2

EFFECT OF SINGLE AND REPEATED INJECTIONS OF DCI ON
MORPHINE AD 50 AND NALOXONE ED50

| | Morphine AD50 * | | Naloxone ED50* |
	P	M	M
Saline	4.5 + 0.9	50.0 + 9.0	0.15 + 0.03
DCI 3X	5.0 + 1.0	22.0 + 4.5	1.20 + 0.20

*mg/kg + S.E.M. P denotes a placebo pellet implant;
M a morphine pellet. From Bhargava et al., (9).

Discussion

The results confirm our previous findings that cAMP may be involved with processes concerned with morphine tolerance and dependence development (6). Although cAMP was administered intravenously, it is also effective at much lower doses after intracerebral administration. The striking finding is that a single injection of the cAMP produces a marked effect that is measurable 80 hours after its administration. Some degree of selectivity in action must exist, since two other nucleotides tested were inactive. The inhibition of tolerance and dependence by the beta adrenergic blockers, DCI and propanolol are also compatible with an action that may be mediated by cAMP.

The effects noted with theophylline were less dramatic but consistent with the above findings. Although enhancement of tolerance and dependence developed was observed, it was necessary to repeat the theophylline administration. We can only presume that the degree of phosphodiesterase inhibition was insufficient or that theophylline possesses other pharmacologic effects that may be opposite to those elicited by cAMP.

Since the accelerating effect of cAMP on morphine tolerance and dependence development is blocked by cycloheximide, it appears that cAMP is participating in processes that may be initiating or accelerating selective synthesis of a protein or other macromolecule. Furthermore, the mechanism can be turned off as evidenced by the fact that the beta blockers completely prevented the accelerating effect of cAMP when they were administered before cAMP. This effect was obtained under conditions where the beta blocker per se did not affect tolerance and physical dependence. The mechanism by which blockade of cAMP action is elicited is not clear since the site of action of cAMP should be distal to the site of blockade, if one considers the beta-receptor to be a subunit of adenyl cyclase in the cellular membrane (10). However, since the enhancing effect of cAMP on tolerance and dependence was obtained with cAMP administered exogenously, an action at other sites can not be excluded and only further studies can provide an answer.

References

1. WAY, E.L., Proc. 5th Int. Congr. Pharmacology, San Francisco 1972, vol. 1, p.77-94 Karger, Basel (1973).
2. WAY, E.L. and F.H. SHEN, in Narcotic Drugs, Biochemical Pharmacology (D.H. Clouet, ed). p.229-253, Plenum Press, New York, (1971).
3. CHOU, W.S., A.K.S. HO, and H.H. LOH, Proc. West. Pharmacol. Soc. 14, 42-45 (1971).
4. HO, I.K., S.E. LU, H.H. LOH, and E.L. WAY. Nature (London) 328, 397-8 (1972).
5. HO, I.K., H.H. LOH, and E.L. WAY. J. Pharmacol. exp. Ther. 185, 336-346 (1973).
6. HO, I.K., H.H. LOH, and E.L. WAY. J. Pharmacol. exp. Ther. 185, 347-357 (1973).
7. WAY, E.L., H.H. LOH and F.H. SHEN. J. Pharmacol. exp. Ther. 167, 1-8 (1968).
8. LOH, H.H., F. SHEN and E.L. WAY. Biochem. Pharmacol. 18, 2711-2721 (1969).
9. BHARGAVA, H.N., S.L. CHAN and E.L. WAY. Proc. West. Pharmacol. Soc. 15, 4-7 (1972).
10. ROBISON, G.A., R.W. BUTCHER and E.W. SUTHERLAND. Ann N.Y. Acad. Sci. 139, 703-723 (1967).

MORPHINE ABSTINENCE AND QUASI-ABSTINENCE EFFECTS AFTER
PHOSPHODIESTERASE INHIBITORS AND NALOXONE

David L. Francis, Ashim C. Roy and Harry O.J. Collier

Research Department, Miles Laboratories Limited,
Stoke Poges, Slough, SL2 4LY, England

(Received in final form May 24, 1975)

SUMMARY

Naive or morphine-dependent rats received a single subcutaneous
injection of a phosphodiesterase inhibitor; their behavioural
responses were then recorded after a small subcutaneous dose of
naloxone. In naive rats, the potent phosphodiesterase inhibitor,
3-isobutyl-1-methylxanthine (IBMX) produced acutely a state in
which a small dose of naloxone (0.03 to 1.0 mg/kg subcutaneously)
precipitated a quasi-morphine abstinence syndrome that was
difficult to distinguish from the true abstinence syndrome,
precipitated by the same dose of naloxone in rats made dependent
on morphine. IBMX also intensified the true morphine abstinence
syndrome. The potency with which IBMX, theophylline, caffeine
and RO 20-1724 exerted these effects corresponded with their
potency as inhibitors of cyclic-3',5'-AMP phosphodiesterase in
rat brain homogenate. These and previous findings indicate that:
(i) morphine-abstinence effects express increased activity of a
central cyclic AMP mechanism; and (ii) naloxone can potently
stimulate behaviour in animals not treated with any opiate drug.

A "quasi-abstinence" effect has been defined as "an effect resembling one
elicited by withdrawal of a drug on which an animal has been made dependent,
but produced by another treatment in a naive animal never exposed to drug nor
to a like-acting congener that induces such dependence" (1). It has been
argued that the study of such effects could increase understanding of dependence mechanisms. Pursuing this possibility, it was found (2) that theophylline, an inhibitor of rat brain phosphodiesterase (3,4,5), when given to
naive rats, produced a number of behavioural signs resembling those of drug
withdrawal in morphine or heroin dependent rats (2). Like the true morphine
abstinence syndrome (TMAS), this quasi-morphine abstinence syndrome (QMAS)
could be intensified by naloxone. The syndrome was attenuated by heroin, and
the effect of heroin was in turn antagonised by naloxone. That the effects of
theophylline thus resembled those of morphine withdrawal suggested that increased activity of a brain cyclic nucleotide mechanism may be associated with
the expression of abstinence.

The relationship of this QMAS to the TMAS and the involvement of cyclic nucleotides in both phenomena have recently been further investigated (6).
Theophylline and other inhibitors of phosphodiesterase in rat brain, caffeine
(3) and 3-isobutyl-1-methylxanthine (IBMX) (7), when given shortly before
challenge to morphine-dependent rats greatly potentiated naloxone-precipitated
jumping and other abstinence signs (6). Imidazole, a phosphodiesterase
stimulant (8) reduced jumping precipitated by naloxone in morphine-dependent
rats and overcame the ability of theophylline to increase jumping (6). Intracerebroventricular injection of cyclic AMP and, to a lesser extent, dibutyryl

149

cyclic AMP significantly increased withdrawal jumping. By this route, cyclic AMP increased the severity of the abstinence syndrome as a whole but cyclic GMP or dibutyryl cyclic GMP did not significantly intensify naloxone-precipitated abstinence effects (6). These results suggested that the morphine-abstinence syndrome is associated with heightened activity of a brain cyclic AMP mechanism. In the investigation described below induction of the QMAS by phosphodiesterase inhibitors, its relationship to the TMAS and the part played by naloxone have been further studied.

METHODS

Studies in vivo. Male albino Wistar rats (125-175g) were housed six per cage in a room illuminated from 08.30h to 16.00h. Observations of the QMAS and TMAS were made between 13.00h and 16.30h in a separate room. Room temperature was 22 ± 2°C. Morphine alkaloid (150 mg/kg) was given subcutaneously (s.c.) in a sustained-release preparation (9). IBMX, theophylline and caffeine citrate were given s.c. in saline; RO 20-1724 (4-(3-butoxy-4-methoxybenzyl)-2-imidazolidinone) was given s.c. in $20\%^{w}/v$ gum acacia in saline. Naloxone hydrochloride and naltrexone hydrochloride were given s.c. in saline. The doses stated refer to the active bases. The procedure used for inducing dependence and precipitating the abstinence syndrome has been described elsewhere (9). Phosphodiesterase inhibitors were given s.c. 1h before saline or naloxone challenge. Methods of observation of abstinence signs and of statistical analysis of the data were as previously described (6,9,10).

Studies in vitro. Homogenates of rat brain were prepared in Tris-HCl buffer (50mM, pH7.5) containing 250mM sucrose, 2mM MgCl$_2$, 0.5mM EGTA and 5mM 2-mercaptoethanol at 0-4°. The cyclic 3',5'-AMP phosphodiesterase assays were carried out by the method of Brooker et al (11) with slight modifications, using 5μM substrate. This assay is based upon the production of tritiated nucleoside from tritiated cyclic AMP by the action of phosphodiesterase and Crotalus atrox venom 5'-nucleosidase.

RESULTS

The relationship of the QMAS to the TMAS. Table 1 shows the close resemblance between the effects of naloxone challenge in naive rats treated with IBMX 1h beforehand and in morphine-dependent rats. Naloxone alone (1.0mg/kg) had little effect on the behaviour of naive rats except to cause restlessness. IBMX alone (10mg/kg) significantly increased the incidence of six quasi-abstinence signs and the total quasi-abstinence score (P <0.001). When IBMX-treated rats were challenged with naloxone, the incidence of eleven of the observed signs was significantly greater than in the group treated with naloxone alone (Table I). The total score for the group treated with IBMX plus naloxone was significantly greater than for the groups treated either with naloxone or with IBMX alone (P <0.001). Jumping, which very rarely occurs in rats treated with saline, naloxone or IBMX alone, occurred with high frequency in rats treated with IBMX and challenged with naloxone. There was no significant differences in the incidence of any individual signs nor in the total score after naloxone challenge between rats pretreated 1h before challenge with IBMX alone and rats made dependent upon morphine.

In another experiment, in a total of 30 rats, naltrexone was tested for its ability to elicit the QMAS after pretreatment with IBMX. IBMX, 10mg/kg, significantly increased the median total quasi-abstinence score elicited by 0.3mg/kg of naltrexone from 2.5 to 7.5 (P <0.05); and by 3.0mg/kg of naltrexone to 10 (P <0.001).

TABLE I

Production of Quasi Morphine-Abstinence Signs in
Rats by Pretreatment with IBMX

| | % Incidence of sign after treatment | | | | |
Sign	(a) V+V	(b) V+N	(c) IBMX+V	(d) IBMX+N	(e) M+V+N
Jumping	0	0	0	$50^{a,b,c}$	$67^{a,b,c}$
Chattering	0	0	17	$58^{a,b,c}$	$92^{a,b,c}$
Squeak on touch	0	0	17	$50^{a,b}$	$75^{a,b,c}$
Squeak on handling	8	15	42	$100^{a,b,c}$	$100^{a,b,c}$
Diarrhoea	0	0	33^{a}	$92^{a,b,c}$	$92^{a,b,c}$
Chewing	17	0	33	$83^{a,b,c}$	$92^{a,b,c}$
Ptosis	8	0	50^{a}	$100^{a,b,c}$	$92^{a,b,c}$
Body shakes	8	0	67^{a}	$50^{a,b}$	$50^{a,b}$
Head shakes	0	15	33^{a}	33^{a}	8
Paw tremor	17	0	33	50^{b}	33^{b}
Rearing	67	62	$100^{a,b}$	$100^{a,b}$	$100^{a,b}$
Restlessness	0	38^{a}	42^{a}	$83^{a,c}$	58^{a}
Salivation	0	0	0	$33^{a,b,c}$	$33^{a,b,c}$
Licking penis	0	50	33	67^{a}	42
Median total score	1.5	2	5^{a}	$9^{a,b,c}$	$10^{a,b,c}$
Interquartile range	0-2	0.5-2	4-6	8-11	8-12
No. of rats	12	13	12	12	12

V, Vehicle; N, naloxone, 1mg/kg subcutaneously (s.c.); IBMX, 3-isobutyl-
1-methylxanthine, 10mg/kg s.c. 1h before saline or naloxone challenge; M,
morphine, 150mg/kg s.c. in a sustained-release preparation given 24h
before naloxone challenge. Signs were recorded during 15 min after
challenge. Letters a-e in the body of the table indicate comparisons
between columns where a significantly greater effect was found; where the
letter is not underlined, P <0.05; where it is underlined once, P <0.01;
where it is underlined twice, P <0.001.

Time-course of QMAS induced by IBMX. The median total quasi-abstinence score
elicited by naloxone (1.0mg/kg) was determined in rats pretreated with IBMX
(10mg/kg) or saline at either 20, 60 or 180 min before challenge. The highest
score occurred in rats tested 20 min after treatment with IBMX, although this
score was not significantly greater than that occurring when rats were challenged at 60 min. The score at 20 min was, however, very significantly
greater than the score for rats challenged at 180 min (P <0.001). These
results indicate that the induction of the QMAS by IBMX is an acute effect of
fairly short duration.

Naloxone and the QMAS - Dose/response effects. The dose-related effects of
naloxone (0.001-10mg/kg) on the incidence of quasi- and true abstinence
effects can be seen in Fig. 1. Naloxone alone had very little effect on naive
rats, other than to induce a slight increase in the incidence of squeak on
handling and of restlessness. At 3.0mg/kg naloxone, however, the total score
was also just significantly greater than for the group of saline-treated rats
(P <0.05). When groups of 8-12 rats were pretreated with IBMX (10mg/kg) 1h
before challenge with naloxone, the naloxone dose/response curve for several
abstinence signs was shifted to the left. Statistical analysis indicated
that, after IBMX, the lowest dose of naloxone given (0.03mg/kg) elicited a
significant increase in chewing and chattering (P <0.025). At 0.3mg/kg the

incidence of several signs was significantly greater, as was the total quasi-abstinence score (P <0.003). However, rats treated 24h before challenge with sustained-release morphine (150mg/kg s.c.) responded by jumping at rather lower doses of naloxone than did rats pretreated only with IBMX. For morphine-dependent rats the lowest dose of naloxone to elicit a significant increase in any individual signs was 0.06mg/kg which increased the incidence of diarrhoea, ptosis, licking the penis and jumping (P <0.05) and of chewing and chattering (P <0.01).

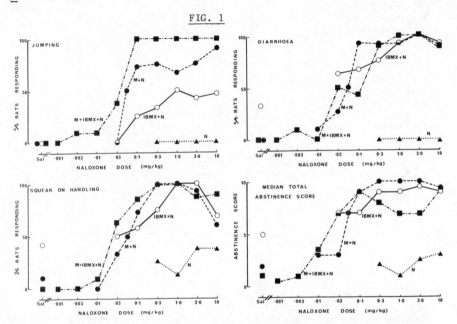

FIG. 1

The effects of dose on quasi- or true abstinence signs elicited by na-loxone given subcutaneously (s.c.) to rats after various pretreatments; ▲ naive rats; ○ rats pretreated 1h before naloxone with IBMX (10 mg/kg s.c.); ● rats pretreated 24h before naloxone with sustained-release morphine (150mg/kg s.c.), and ■ rats pretreated 24h before naloxone with sustained-release morphine (150mg/kg s.c.) and 1h before naloxone with IBMX (10mg/kg s.c.); Sal, saline challenge.

When groups of morphine-dependent rats were treated with IBMX (10mg/kg) 1h before challenge, the naloxone dose/response curve was shifted still further to the left. The lowest dose of naloxone required to elicit a significant increase in any abstinence sign was then 0.01mg/kg, which caused an increase in the incidence of chewing and restlessness (P <0.03) and in the total abstinence score (P <0.0007).

QMAS, TMAS and phosphodiesterase inhibition. The potency of the various drugs in inducing the QMAS or potentiating the TMAS was compared with their ability to inhibit 3',5'-cyclic AMP phosphodiesterase of rat brain homogenate and to stimulate PG biosynthesis. The results (Table II) show that the ability to increase the QMAS and TMAS relates to potency in inhibiting phosphodiesterase rather than in stimulating PG biosynthesis.

TABLE II

Comparison of relative potencies of four phosphodiesterase (PDE) inhibitors in inducing the QMAS, potentiating the TMAS, inhibiting rat brain PDE and stimulating prostaglandin (PG) biosynthesis. IC 25, concentration to inhibit by 25% cyclic AMP breakdown; SC 50 concentration to increase by 50% total PG production by bull seminal vesicle homogenate (12); NT, not tested.

Drug	Induction of QMAS (Median total abstinence score)	Potentiation of TMAS (% increase in jumping)	Inhibition of rat brain PDE (IC 25)	Stimulation of PG biosynthesis (SC 50)
IBMX	10	10	10	1.3
Theophylline	1	1	1	1
Caffeine	0.8	0.5	0.8	0.9
RO 20-1724	<0.8	NT	<0.8	NT

DISCUSSION

These experiments show how closely the quasi-morphine abstinence syndrome, elicited by naloxone in naive rats treated with IBMX, resembles the true abstinence syndrome, precipitated by naloxone in morphine-dependent rats. At 1.0mg/kg naloxone, neither the median total scores, nor the incidence of any single abstinence sign differed significantly between the QMAS and TMAS (Table I). At 0.1mg/kg naloxone, the resemblance was almost as close, but jumping was less in the quasi-abstinent group (P <0.005). The closeness of resemblance between quasi and true abstinence in these experiments suggests that IBMX modifies a mechanism that is a prerequisite of the expression of the morphine-abstinence syndrome. That IBMX also intensifies the TMAS (Fig. 1) further supports this suggestion.

An interesting difference between the quasi and true syndromes is their time-course of induction. Whereas the QMAS was highest at 20 min after injection of IBMX and had declined by 180 min, the TMAS required about 24h exposure to sustained-release morphine to reach as high a degree of intensity. This indicates that the quasi-abstinent state is a direct effect of IBMX, whereas a true state of morphine dependence requires an endogenous induction process. Indeed, acutely, heroin suppresses both the quasi- and true morphine abstinence syndromes (2,9).

The question therefore arises: what action of IBMX on a biochemical process produces, acutely and directly, a state so closely resembling the true morphine abstinence syndrome? Table II suggests that this action is mainly the inhibition of phosphodiesterase. This accords with the finding that heroin, which potently and specifically inhibits prostaglandin-stimulated cyclic AMP formation in rat brain homogenate (13), also specifically suppresses the QMAS (2). Another property of IBMX that could contribute to the effects described is its moderate ability to stimulate prostaglandin biosynthesis. If the state of quasi-morphine abstinence is due to inhibition of a brain phosphodiesterase, then increased cyclic nucleotide participates in the mechanism of the QMAS. This raises the question: which of the two cyclic nucleotides known to occur in brain - cyclic AMP and cyclic GMP - is primarily involved? The evidence that this is cyclic AMP is indirect, but strong. In experiments reported elsewhere, we have shown that intracerebroventricular cyclic AMP, but not cyclic GMP, intensifies the true morphine-abstinence syndrome (6). Furthermore, RO 20-1724, which is reported selectively to inhibit cyclic AMP phosphodiesterase (14), produces the QMAS.

Our results argue that the true abstinence syndrome is due to increased activity of a neuronal cyclic AMP mechanism, without necessarily implying that inhibition of phosphodiesterase is the cause of this increase. This mechanism of the morphine-abstinence syndrome accords with the finding of Mehta and Johnson (15) that the intensity of the syndrome in precipitated morphine abstinence in the rat can be associated with the level of brain cyclic AMP. It also accords with the finding of Clark et al (16) that the activity of microsomal protein kinase in rat brain increases in morphine abstinence.

Naloxone is generally believed to act as a "pure" opiate antagonist and to have no other specific pharmacological effects. There have, however, been occasional reports that naloxone has some effects in naive preparations or animals, at doses comparable with those used in antagonising opiates (17-20). In our hands, naloxone at 1.0mg/kg increased restlessness (Table I) and, at 3.0mg/kg, also increased total abstinence score (P <0.05) (Fig. 1). Its potency in these effects was enhanced by 10-100 fold by pretreatment with 10 mg/kg of IBMX. After IBMX also, naloxone at the lowest dose used (0.03 mg/kg) significantly stimulated two behavioural signs and produced a recognisable quasi-abstinence syndrome. The cause of this will be considered in another paper at this symposium (12).

We thank M.A. Collins, N.J. Cuthbert and J.F. de C. Sutherland for help in observing animals, N.M. Butt for biochemical assistance and L.C. Dinneen for statistical advice; Sankyo Limited for naloxone, Hoffman La Roche Inc. for RO 20-1724 and Endo Limited for naltrexone.

REFERENCES

1. H.O.J. COLLIER, Pharmacology 2, 58-61 (1974).
2. H.O.J. COLLIER, D.L. FRANCIS, G. HENDERSON, and C. SCHNEIDER, Nature. Lond. 249, 471-473 (1974).
3. B. BEER, M. CHASIN, D.E. CLODY, J.R. VOGEL, and Z.P. HOROVITZ, Science 176, 428-430 (1972).
4. W.Y. CHEUNG, Biochemistry 6, 1079-1087 (1967).
5. S. KATZ, and A. TENENHOUSE, Br.J.Pharmac. 48, 505-515 (1973).
6. H.O.J. COLLIER, and D.L. FRANCIS, Nature.Lond. 255, 159-162 (1975).
7. J. SCHULTZ, and J.W. DALY, J.Biol.Chem. 248, 853-859 (1973).
8. R.W. BUTCHER, and E.W. SUTHERLAND, J.Biol.Chem. 237, 1244-1250 (1962).
9. H.O.J. COLLIER, D.L. FRANCIS, and C. SCHNEIDER, Nature.Lond. 237, 220-223 (1972).
10. D.L. FRANCIS, and C. SCHNEIDER, Brit.J.Pharmacol. 41, 424P (1971).
11. G. BROOKER, L.J. THOMAS, and M.M. APPLEMAN, Biochemistry 7, 4177-4181 (1968).
12. H.O.J. COLLIER, D.L. FRANCIS, W.J. McDONALD-GIBSON, A.C. ROY, and S.A. SAEED, this symposium.
13. H.O.J. COLLIER, and A.C. ROY, Prostaglandins 7, 361-376 (1974).
14. T. POSTERNAK, Ann.Review.Pharmacol. 14, 23-33 (1974).
15. C.S. MEHTA, and W. JOHNSON, Fedn.Proc. 33, 493 (1974).
16. A.G. CLARK, R. JOVIC, M.R. ORNELLAS, and M. WELLER, Biochem. Pharmac. 21, 1989-1990 (1972).
17. J.E. VILLARREAL, and G.E. DUMMER, Fedn.Proc. 32, 688 (1973).
18. J.J. JACOB, E.C. TREMBLAY, and M-C. COLOMBEL, Psychopharmacologia (Berl.) 37, 217-223 (1974).
19. L.A. DYKSTRA, D.E. McMILLAN, and L.S. HARRIS, Psychopharmacologia (Berl.) 39, 151-162 (1974).
20. S.G. HOLTZMAN, J.Pharmacol.exp.Ther. 189, 51-60 (1974).

AN ANALYSIS AT SYNAPTIC LEVEL OF THE MORPHINE ACTION IN STRIATUM AND N. ACCUMBENS: DOPAMINE AND ACETYLCHOLINE INTERACTIONS.

E. Costa, D. L. Cheney, G. Racagni and G. Zsilla

Laboratory of Preclinical Pharmacology, NIMH, Saint Elizabeths Hospital, Washington, D. C. 20032

(Received in final form May 24, 1975)

Pharmacologically effective concentrations of opiates reduce the acetylcholine (ACh) released from peripheral (1) and central synapses (2). Jhamandas and Dickinson (3) have provided evidence that during precipitated withdrawal cholinergic mechanisms are activated. Although this and other evidence (4, 5) indicates that brain ACh may participate in the action of opiates, the molecular mechanisms that mediate this action remain obscure. A current research trend (6) proposes that in brain the interaction of drugs with specific neuronal systems can be studied by measuring the changes in transmitter turnover rate (7). This rationale has been applied also to the brain cholinergic system (8). By using steady-state (9) and non steady-state (10) methods to measure ACh turnover the action of morphine on ACh turnover rate has been studied in the whole brain of mice (8). These studies have shown that single doses of morphine (up to 350 μmoles/kg i. p.) change neither the steady state nor the turnover rate of ACh in whole brain (8). While this finding gives no definitive information as to the possibility that the action of morphine is preferentially located in a discrete cholinergic neuronal pathway it suggests that the running stereotypy elicited by 350 μmoles/kg i.p. fails to change the turnover rate of ACh in whole brain (8). However, the turnover rate of ACh in the whole brain of mice was increased during tolerance to and dependence on morphine (8). This change is promptly reversed by naloxone which does not influence the turnover rate of brain ACh per se (8). To answer the question as to whether a specific cholinergic neuronal pathway is preferentially affected by ACh we turned our attention to the rat because in this species by using infusion of radioactive phosphorylcholine it is possible to measure the turnover rate of ACh in discrete brain structures (11). These experiments showed that in rats catatonic with high doses of morphine the turnover rate of striatal ACh is normal (12). In contrast the turnover rate of ACh in cortex was decreased by morphine in a dose related manner (12). In rats that had developed tolerance and physical dependence to morphine, the striatal ACh turnover rate had decreased significantly, but the cortical ACh turnover rate was not different from controls (8, 12). In these rats the decreased turnover rate of striatal ACh was promptly reversed by Naloxone (8, 12).

It was difficult to explain these results with a model where cholinergic neurons were to be depicted as the primary target of morphine action. Moreover these results indicated that the factors involved in the regulation of ACh turnover rate are different in acute and chronic administration of morphine. In view of

this consideration we examined whether other neuronal systems influenced by morphine were involved in the control of cholinergic
function in striatum but not in cortex. Stimulation of postsynaptic dopamine (DA) receptors by (+) amphetamine, (3,4-dihydroxy-
phenylalanine) (DOPA) and apomorphine elicits a decrease of ACh
turnover rate in striatum but not in cortex (13). In rat the
value of striatal DA turnover rate is increased by morphine
doses that are ED_{80} for analgesia (14) but this increase of DA
turnover rate is suppressed by the development of morphine tolerance (14).

In order to bring about a clearer understanding of the possibility that the action of morphine on brain cholinergic pathways
is modulated via a modification of the DA system we performed the
experiments reported in the present paper.

Taking advantage of the technique developed in this laboratory
to assay ACh content in stereomicroscopically isolated brain nuclei (15) and of the constant rate infusion of deuteriated phosphorylcholine we measured the turnover rate of ACh in stereomicroscopically dissected nuclei of rat brain. This development includes the constant rate intravenous infusion of deuteriated phosphorylcholine (PCh-D4) for a prolonged time period to achieve a
high degree of labelling of the ACh stores, but at a sufficiently
low rate in order not to increase the Ch concentration in plasma
or in brain nuclei. Thus we report on the action of morphine on
the turnover rate of ACh in two nuclei receiving dopaminergic
afferents: N. caudatus and N. accumbens. In these nuclei and in
the hypothalamus we have measured the turnover rate of DA and
norepinephrine (NE) in rats treated with morphine. Since extra-
neuronally released DA activates adenylyl cyclase (16) and
elicits an increase of striatal cAMP content (14) we have
measured whether morphine, while it increases the turnover rate of
striatal DA also causes an activation or a blockade of DA receptors.

The results obtained indicate that the action of acute morphine on cholinergic neurons is indirect through an action other
than the morphine effects on dopaminergic neurons.

Methods

The assay of ACh content in stereomicroscopically dissected
nuclei of the rat brain was performed as previously described(17).
Choline acetyl-transferase (CAT) was measured according to Schrier
and Schuster (18). The turnover rate of ACh in various brain
nuclei was measured by killing the rats with a microwave radiation
(19) at various times after a constant rate infusion of deuteriated phosphorylcholine (D4) (21) and measuring the enrichment of
the isotopic variant in choline (Ch) and ACh extracted from stereomicroscopically isolated brain nuclei.

In figure 1 we report the relative enrichment of ^{2}H in the Ch
on ACh extracted from N accumbens and N. interpeduncularis at
various times after the infusion of 20 μmoles/kg/min. and 15
μmoles/kg/min of PCh-D4. These results illustrate that the increment in the enrichment differs with each of the two perfusion
rates of the deuteriated precursor. Since with the infusion of
20 μmoles/kg/min after 14 and 16 minutes the steady state of Ch

156

FIGURE 1

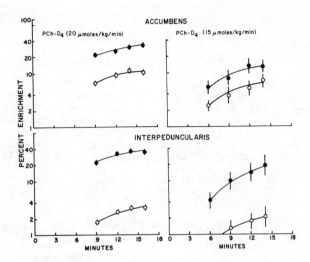

Fig 1 changes with time in the per cent enrichment of ^{2}H (measured as ratio of m/e 60/58) at the retention time of ACh (3.5 min)
and Ch (8 min.) in Nuclei accumbens and interpeduncularis. Mass
fragmentographic conditions and in instrumentation as described before (20).Open circles ACh, closed circles Ch. At time 0 the in
fusion with D$_4$ phosphorylcholine was initiated. D9 Ch and ACh
were used as internal standards.

had changed, these data could not be used to calculate ACh turnover rate by the finite difference method (11). In fact this
method assumes maintenance of steady state conditions in the precursor and product pools.

The DA and NE turnover rate was measured as previously described (22) using a pulse injection of 500 μc/kg i.v. of ^{3}H
tyrosine (30 ci/mM). The concentration of cAMP in striatum and
N. accumbens was measured according to Guidotti et al. (23).

Results

The data presented in table 1 show that morphine increases
the turnover rate of DA in striatum and N. accumbens of rats. It
appears that this drug preferentially affects DA turnover in
striatum but this selectivity can be abolished by increasing the
doses of morphine. With 52 μmoles/kg of morphine one can observe
a preferential effect of morphine on DA neurons, because this
dose still fails to increase the turnover rate of NE in the hypothalamus.

Since an increase of DA turnover rate in N. accumbens and

TABLE 1

TURNOVER RATE OF DOPAMINE IN STRIATUM AND NUCLEUS ACCUMBENS AND
OF NE IN HYPOTHALAMUS OF RATS INJECTED WITH MORPHINE.

DRUG	μmoles/kg i.p.	NE Turnover Rate nmoles/g/hr	DA Turnover Rate** nmoles/g/hr	
		Hypothalamus	N. Accumbens	Striatum
Saline	--	3.6 ± 0.32	26 ± 4	23 ± 6.5
Morphine	30	4.3 ± 0.76	32 ± 4.5	39 ± 2.8*
	52	4.7 ± 0.92	40 ± 5.6*	42 ± 3.6*

Each value represents the mean of at least four experiments. DA
concentrations in nucleus accumbens (nmoles/g) 56±1.2 S.E.M. (N=
20) DA concentrations in striatum (nmoles/g) 61±1.6 S.E.M. (n=20);
NE concentrations in hypothalamus (nmoles/g) 5.9 ± 0.62 S.E.M.
(N=16).
** Values are Mean ± SEM, *P<0.05

TABLE 2

STRIATAL AND N. ACCUMBENS CONTENT OF cAMP IN RATS RECEIVING MOR-
MORPHINE, (+)-AMPHETAMINE AND APOMORPHINE

Drug (μmoles/kg i.p.)	cAMP (pmoles/mg protein ± S.E.M.)	
	Striatum	N. Accumbens
Saline	5.8 ± 0.4	8.6 ± 0.2
Apomorphine (3.6)	9.9 ± 1.1 *	14 ± 1.1*
(+) Amphetamine (6.4)	9.7 ± 0.5 *	16 ± 1.6*
Morphine (52)	6.2 ± 0.31*	9.3 ± 0.5

Rats were killed in 2 sec. with a microwave beam (19) focussed to
the head (75 W/cm^2) at 15 minutes after the injection.   Each
mean refers to at least five rats.
*P<0.05

striatum of rats is elicited by antipsychotics (24) which block
DA receptors and by (+)-amphetamine (14) which stimulates DA receptors we have investigated the action of morphine on the cAMP
content of striatum and N. accumbens. The data reported in Table
2 show that morphine in doses that increase the turnover rate of
DA in striatum and N. accumbens fails to increase the concentration of cAMP in these two structures. In contrast a dose of (+)-
amphetamine that increases the turnover rate of DA in striatum
and N. accumbens (25) increases the cAMP content in both structures. Since the same change in cAMP content is elicited by apomorphine that directly stimulates the postsynaptic DA receptors,
it can be surmised that morphine in doses that increase the turnover rate of DA fails to activate DA receptors.

The action of morphine on striatal cAMP content was then compared to that of haloperidol. Both drugs were devoid of a direct
action on the cAMP content of striatum (Table 3). However the
action of haloperidol differs from that of morphine: the former
blocks the increase of cAMP elicited by (+)-amphetamine and apo-

FIGURE 2

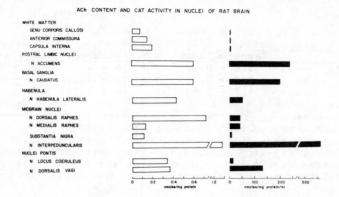

ACh CONTENT AND CAT ACTIVITY IN NUCLEI OF RAT BRAIN

morphine whereas morphine is devoid of such an effect. The
data presented in figure 2 show the ACh content and CAT activity
of various brain structures isolated stereomicroscopically. In
various brain nuclei both parameters do not follow the same pattern of distribution. In white matter where the ACh present is
stored cholinergic axons the ratio between ACh and CAT content is
much greater than that in N. dorsalis Vagi where ACh is stored
in cholinergic cell bodies. In N. caudatus and N. accumbens the
ratio between CAT/ACh resembles that of N. dorsalis Vagi and
differs from that of locus coeruleus. Since in the latter the
ACh is perhaps present in nerve terminals (17) we have surmised
that the ratio of CAT/ACh in Nuclei caudatus and Accumbens indicates that both structures contain small cholinergic interneurons.
In N. caudatus this suggestion is directly supported by histochemical evidence (26).

Since nuclei caudatus and accumbens. contain small cholinergic
axons which appear to be innervated by DA axons we have studied
the action of morphine on the turnover rate of ACh in N. caudatus,
N. accumbens and cortex parietalis (100 μg tissue protein) was
compared to that of rats receiving saline. The data reported in
Table 4 show that morphine fails to change steady state of ACh or
Ch in these three brain structures. However it decreases the
turnover rate of ACh in cortex parietalis and N. accumbens but
not in N. caudatus. Thus with regard to cortex and N. caudatus
these results obtained with stable isotope labelling are identical to those previously reported where labelling was performed
with ^{14}C phosphorylcholine (8).

Discussion

The experiments presented establish:

1) Morphine action on brain DA neurons can be differentiated

TABLE 3

EFFECT OF MORPHINE AND HALOPERIDOL ON THE INCREASE OF STRIATAL
cAMP CONTENT ELICITED BY APOMORPHINE AND (+)-AMPHETAMINE

Pretreatment (μmol/kg)	(cAMP (pmoles/mg protein) in rats receiving		
	Saline	Apomorphine	(+)-Amphetamine
None	6.1 + 0.41	9.8 + 0.78*	10 + 0.31*
Haloperidol (1.3 i.p.)	6.1 + 0.52	5.8 + 0.74	6.4+ 0.33
Morphine (52 s.c.)	6.2 + 0.31	9.2 + 0.53*	8.7+ 0.23*

*$P < 0.05$ when compared with saline treated rats.
Haloperidol and morphine were injected 10 minutes before saline
apomorphine or (+)-amphetamine; the rats were killed with microwave radiation (see table 2) 10 minutes after either apomorphine
(1.8 μmoles/kg s.c.) or (+)-amphetamine (16.4 μmoles/kg i.p.)

from that of antipsychotics and (+) amphetamine despite the
apparent similarity indicated by the measurement of DA turnover
rate (25).

2) Morphine action on brain cholinergic mechanisms does not
stemm from a direct modification by this drug of the dynamic
equilibrium of ACh in cholinergic neurons.

3) This indirect action can not be explained as related to
the action that morphine exerts on DA neurons because this hypothesis could not be reconciled with the different action of morphine on the turnover of ACh in N. accumbens and N. caudatus
(Table 4).
In addition our results suggest two considerations of more general significance: a) The study of morphine action at the molecular level can be initiated in various simplified model systems,
however the final verdict on the biological significance must be
inferred only from in vivo studies with brain structures. Brain
function is expressed by interaction of various regulatory
systems which operate at synaptic level, here regulation of
neuronal excitability is expressed by regulation of first and
second messenger production and action, b) Our results imply that
morphine interacts with another neuronal system that in nucleus
caudatus and N. accumbens regulates dopaminergic and cholinergic
systems. Among the known factors involved in the control of cholinergic and dopaminergic neurons in striatum and pars compacta
of substantia nigra GABA emerges as a possible transmitter that
may participate in morphine action. There is indication that
GABA mechanisms can be affected by morphine (27). Also this
action may be indirect through an unknown endogenous substrate
mobilized by morphine. These indications and the results presented in this paper have stimulated our interest in the study
of a possible GABA mediation of morphine action. These studies
are now in progress. Theoretically the action of morphine on DA
and ACh mechanisms in N. caudatus could be explained by assuming
that morphine prevents the release of GABA at two possible sites
of action: at presynaptic sites in DA nerve terminals and in the

TABLE 4

TURNOVER RATE OF ACh IN STEREOMICROSCOPICALLY ISOLATED BRAIN NUCLEI, AFTER A SINGLE INJECTION OF MORPHINE

	Treatment	ACh (nmoles/mg protein)	Ch (nmoles/mg protein)	k_B hr^{-1}	$TRACh_a$ (nmoles/mg prot/hr)
N. Accumbens	Saline	0.50 ± 0.001	0.40 ± 0.024	6.2 ± 0.76	3.1
N. Accumbens	Morphine	0.54 ± 0.044	0.42 ± 0.0010	2.9 ± 0.27*	1.6*
N. Caudatus	Saline	0.57 ± 0.044	0.30 ± 0.043	8.0 ± 0.13	4.6
N. Caudatus	Morphine	0.52 ± 0.031	0.35 ± 0.035	8.3 ± 0.75	4.3
Cortex parietalis	Saline	0.23 ± 0.001	0.44 ± 0.001	3.2 ± 0.15	0.74
Cortex parietalis	Morphine	0.25 ± 0.044	0.44 ± 0.050	2.3 ± 0.14*	0.58*

*$P < 0.05$

Rats were infused for various times with phosphorylcholine-D4 (15 µmoles/kg/min i.v.) and the enrichment of deuterium measured mass fragmentographically according to Hanin et al.(21) at various times (6, 9, 12 and 14 minutes) of infusion. Saline or morphine (70 µmoles/kg i.p.) were injected 10 minutes before the infusion. Rats were killed by microwave radiation (see Table 2).

and in the neuronal loop that controls excitability of DA cell bodies by feedback inhibition.

REFERENCES

1. Schaumann, W. Brit. J. Pharmacol. 12: 115 (1957)
2. Beleslin, D. and Polak, R. L. J. Physiol., Lond. 117: 411 (1965)
3. Jhamandas, K., and Dickinson, G. Nature New Biology 245: 219 (1973)
4. Collier, H. O. J. and Francis, D. L. Nature 237: 220 (1972)
5. Dole, V. P. Biochemistry of addiction. Ann. Rev. Bioch. 39: 821 (1970)
6. Costa, E. and Neff, N. H. Handbook of Neurochem., Vol. 4, Plenum Publ. Co., New York, p. 45 (1970)
7. Montanari, R., Costa, E., Beaven, M. A., and Brodie, B. B. Life Science 2: 232 (1963)
8. Cheney, D. L., Costa, E., Hanin, I., Racagni, G. and Trabucchi, M. Cholinergic Mechanisms Ed. by P. G. Waser, Raven Press, New York P. 217, 1975.
9. Cheney, D. L., Costa, E., Hanin, I., Trabucchi, M. and Wang, C. T. J. Pharmacol. Exp. Ther. 192: 288 (1975)
10. Domino, E. F., and Wilson, A. E. J. Pharmacol. Exp. Ther. 184: 18 (1973)
11. Racagni, G., Cheney, D. L., Trabucchi, M., Wang, C. and Costa, E. Life Sciences 15: 1961 (1974)
12. Cheney, D. L., Trabucchi, M., Racagni, G., Wang, C. and Costa, E. Life Sciences 15: 1977 (1974)
13. Trabucchi, M., Cheney, D. L., Racagni, G. and Costa, E. Brain Research 85: 130 (1975)
14. Costa, E., Carenzi, A., Guidotti, A. and Revuelta, A. In: Usdin, E. and Snyder, S. (eds): Frontiers in Catecholamine Research, London, England, Pergamon Press pp 1003   (1973)
15. Koslow, S. H., Racagni, G., and Costa, E. Neuropharmacology 13; 1123 (1974)
16. Clement-Cormier, Y. C., Kebabian, J. W., Petzold, G. L. and Greengard, P. Proc. Nat. Acad. Sci. USA 71: 1113 (1974)
17. Cheney, D. L., LeFevre, H. F. and Racagni, G. Neuropharmacology, Vol. 14, 1975 in press
18. Schrier, B. K., and Schuster, L. J. Neurochem. 14: 977 (1967)
19. Guidotti, A., Cheney, D. L., Trabucchi, M., Doteuchi, M., Wang, C. and Hawkins, R. A. Neuropharmacology 13: 1115 (1974).
20. Racagni, G., Trabucchi, M. and Cheney, D. L. Naunyn-Schmiedeberg's Arch. Pharmacol. (1975) in press.
21. Hanin, I. and Schuberth, J. J. Neurochem. 23: 819 (1974)
22. Neff, N. H., Spano, P. F., Groppetti, A., Wang, C. T. and Costa, E. J. Pharmacol. Exp. Ther. 176: 701 (1971)
23. Guidotti, A., Weiss, B. and Costa, E. Mol. Pharmacol. 8: 521 (1972)
24. Zivkovic, B., Guidotti, A., Revuelta, A., and Costa, E. J. Pharmacol. Exp. Ther. (1975) in press.
25. Carenzi, A., Guidotti, A., Revuelta, A. and Costa, E. JPET (1975) in press.
26. Butcher, S. G., and Butcher, L. L. Brain Research 71: 167 (1974)
27. Dostrovsky, J. and Pomeranz, G. Nature New Biology 246: 222 (1973)

STEREOSPECIFICITY OF INTRAVENTRICULARLY
ADMINISTERED ACETYLMETHYLCHOLINE ANTINOCICEPTION[1]

William L. Dewey, George Cocolas[2], Ellen Daves and Louis S. Harris

Department of Pharmacology
Medical College of Virginia
Richmond, Virginia 23298

(Received in final form May 24, 1975)

We have previously reported that the intraventricular injection of acetylcholine increases latency in the mouse tail-flick test, the ED50 being 7.3 ug (1). This effect was reversed by five narcotic-antagonist analgesics in the same order of potency in which they antagonized morphine, and was found to be due to muscarinic receptor stimulation. It was also pointed out at that time that the intraventricular injection of acetylcholine would block the writhing response to intraperitoneally administered p-phenylquinone. In this preliminary communication, we present our results of the effect of the intraventricular injection of acetylcholine on writhing induced by intraperitoneally administered acetylcholine. In addition, we present results of our studies in which we demonstrated stereospecificity of intraventricularly administered acetylmethylcholines in causing antinociception.

Mice were anesthetized with carbon dioxide and injected in either lateral ventricle with 0.05 ml solution containing the proper concentration of acetylcholine or acetylmethylcholine to give the desired dose. Ten minutes later, the p-phenylquinone or acetylcholine was injected intraperitoneally to produce the writhing responses which either were counted for one minute periods at 5 and 10 minutes following the intraperitoneal injection of p-phenylquinone or during the first six minutes after acetylcholine. Other mice were exposed to the tail-flick apparatus prior to and 10 minutes after the intraventricular injection of the acetylmethylcholines. The effects of intraventricularly administered acetylcholine on intraperitoneally administered acetylcholine induced writhing are presented in Table 1.

Table 1

The Effect of Intraventricularly Administered Cholines on Writhing in Mice

Drug	Dose (ug)	Writhing Agent	Percent Inhibition
Acetylcholine	2	Acetylcholine	12
Acetylcholine	4	Acetylcholine	25
Acetylcholine	8	Acetylcholine	50
Acetylcholine	16	Acetylcholine	75

ED50 = 8 (4.2 - 15.2) ug

1. Supported by USPHS grants DA00326 and NS09088
2. School of Pharmacy, University of North Carolina, Chapel Hill, N.C. 27514

Drug	Dose (ug)	Writhing Agent	Percent Inhibition
α-CH$_3$ acetylcholines			
R-	32	p-phenylquinone	0
RS	32	p-phenylquinone	0
S+	32	p-phenylquinone	3
β-CH$_3$ acetylcholines			
R-	32	p-phenylquinone	0
RS	32	p-phenylquinone	79
S+	32	p-phenylquinone	98

The percent inhibition expressed in the table was calculated using the number of mice that writhed as an index and not taking into account the number of times each mouse reacted. The ED50 and the 95% confidence when the total number of writhes was used as the index of activity was found to be 4.8 (2.8 - 8.2) ug.

The results presented in the table show that the intraventricular injection of alpha substituted acetylcholines were inactive in inhibiting the writhing response in mice. The alpha substituted cholines have been shown to have specific activity for nicotinic receptors. These findings agree with our previous report in which we showed that the nicotinic blocking drug, mecamylamine, did not block the antinociceptive action of intraventricularly administered acetylcholine.

The racemate and the S(+) isomer in the beta methyl substituted acetylcholines were active in inhibiting the writhing response. A more complete study showed that the S(+) isomer had an ED50 and 95% confidence limits of 13.5 (9.5 - 19.2) ug and the racemate was 15.5 (8.4 - 28.7) ug. The R(-) isomer was completely inactive. The intraventricular injection of the R(-) isomer did increase tail-flick latency in mice comparable to the racemate, but both were less active than the S(+) isomer (57% inhibition for the R(-) and the racemate and 74.5 percent for the S(+) isomer at 32 ug). It is the S(+) conformation of the beta methyl substituted acetylcholines which resembles the preferred conformation of acetylcholine as reported by Canepa et al. (2,3). We have reported previously that the S(+) isomer of beta substituted acetylcholine is more potent than the racemate or the R(-) isomer at peripheral muscarinic sites (4). The present results indicate that there is also stereospecificity for muscarinic receptors in the brain.

References

1. Pedigo, N., Dewey, W.L. and Harris, L.S.: J. Pharmacol. Exptl. Therap. (in press).

2. Chothia, C. and Pauling, P.: Chem. Comm. 626 (1969).

3. Canepa, F.G., Pauling, P. and Sorum, H.: Nature 210, 907 (1966).

4. Cocolas, G.H., Robinson, E.L., Dewey, W.L. and Spaulding, T.C.: J. Pharm. Sci. 60, 1749-1752 (1971).

A PHARMACOKINETIC APPROACH TO MORPHINE ANALGESIA AND ITS RELATION TO REGIONAL TURNOVER OF RAT BRAIN CATECHOLAMINES

Bengt Dahlström, Gudrun Paalzow and Lennart Paalzow

Department of Pharmacology, Pharmaceutical Faculty, University of Uppsala, Biomedicum, Box 573, S-751 23 Uppsala, Sweden

(Received in final form May 24, 1975)

Morphine concentrations in plasma and four discrete areas of the rat brain following intravenous administration, can be described by a three-compartment open model. The pharmacokinetic behavior of morphine was the same in each of the different parts of the brain. When relating this behavior to the effects of morphine on the threshold for vocalisation and vocalisation-after-discharge, it was possible to develop a pharmacokinetic model which suggests that morphine induces its analgesic effect by a change of activities in at least two neurophysiological systems.

As a result of investigations of morphine-induced changes of catecholamine turnover in different parts of the brain and of the consequences of modulating central monoaminergic activity prior to morphine administration, it was suggested that one of the two neurophysiological systems could be dopaminergic. In this system morphine increases the turnover of dopamine, most probably by releasing this transmitter from limbic structures that initiate the effect of morphine on the threshold for vocalisation-afterdischarge (the emotional component of pain reactions).

Our investigations into the mechanism of analgesic action of morphine and related compounds have aimed at combining two important relationships:
(1) The relation between morphine analgesia and the kinetic behavior of this drug;
(2) The relation between morphine analgesia and the activity of certain neuronal brain systems producing this effect.
When these relationships can be established and described on a strictly kinetic bases, we will have reached a point when a given effect of morphine can be followed in a chain of pharmacologic and physiologic events.

Male Sprague-Dawley rats were used throughout the studies. The influence of morphine on different pain reactions was studied by a technique previously described (1,2), based principally on the work by Carroll and Lim (3) and Hoffmeister and Kroneberg (4). By a standardized electrical stimulation of the tails of the animals, three responses to nociceptive stimulation can be qualitatively and quantitatively followed in each rat. In untreated animals, these responses appear in the following order: Firstly, a motor response (spinal reflex), secondly, a vocalisation response (mediated from structures of medulla oblongata), and finally a vocalisation afterdischarge (vocalisation after withdrawal of stimulus). The latter response is considered to be a response mediated by a system involved in the emotional component of the pain reactions and includes brain structures such as the thalamus-hypothalamus and rhinencephalon (3,4). This technique opens the possibility of studying different pain responses integrated at different levels of the central nervous system.

165

1. Pharmacokinetics of Morphine in Plasma and Discrete Areas of the Brain

Recently, we have described a specific and sensitive gas liquid chromatographic procedure for determination of morphine concentrations in the pico-nanogram range (5). Utilizing this method we followed the concentration of morphine in plasma, in the whole brain, the hypothalamus, the diencephalon-striatum and the medulla oblongata-pons-midbrain regions of the brain after intravenous administration of 2.5 mg/kg morphine.

As can be seen in Fig. 1, maximal brain levels were obtained 15-20 min after administration and the time course of morphine showed the same kinetic behavior in all the different parts of the brain. Furthermore, morphine exhibited a fairly even distribution with the highest concentration in the telencephalic cortex and the lowest in the diencephalon-striatum brain portion.

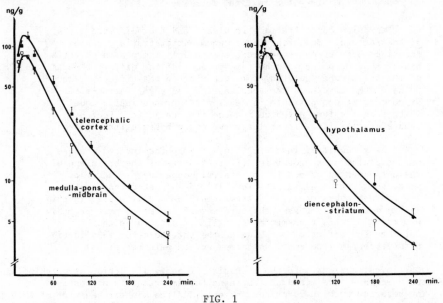

FIG. 1

Regional brain concentrations of morphine after i.v. administration of 2.5 mg/kg. Each point represents the mean $\pm$ S.E. from 5-10 rats. (Obtained from Dahlström, B. and Paalzow, L. Submitted for publication in J. Pharmacokinetics and Biopharmaceutics.)

The plasma curve as well as the brain curves all appeared to be composed of three exponential terms, and by using the digital computer program SAAM-25, all morphine concentration data were simultaneously fitted to five separate sets of three-compartment open models. These calculations showed that the kinetic behavior of morphine in the rat can be described by a three-compartment open model and the computed transfer constants of this model can be seen in Fig. 2.

2. Morphine Analgesia and Kinetic Behavior

To test the current concept that a direct and reversible pharmacological effect is associated with a particular drug concentration at the site of action, we have investigated the relation between morphine analgesia and the kinetic behavior of this drug. In such a study one should expect that a given tissue level of morphine at the site of action should always yield the same intensity of pharmacological response during phases of distribution (rising tissue levels), as well as when the tissue levels are on the decline. Assuming that in the case of analgesia, the site of action of morphine is restricted to the central nervous system, we adapted the three-compartment model to the effects of morphine on nociceptive stimulation.

The time course of morphine activity on the threshold for vocalisation and vocalisation-afterdischarge has been investigated in 4 doses from 1.7 to 5.0 mg/kg i.v. and the effects after 2.5 mg/kg are illustrated in Fig. 2. As is apparent from this figure, the time course of the two effects are different from that of morphine concentrations in the brain (Fig. 1). By using the SAAM-25 program (6) it was, however, possible to develop a pharmacokinetic model (Fig. 2) which can describe both the time course of morphine in the brain as well as the time course of the two effects studied. (Data obtained from Dahlström, B., Paalzow, L., Segre, G. and Ågren, A: In preparation for publication).

In this model, the solution of the three-compartment open model described above serves as a function generator sending its signal (S) to two added sub-units, 4 and 7, symbolizing two physiological events in the brain. It should be observed that S and -S are signals and not a transfer of material and that the added units do not affect the kinetics of morphine in the brain (compartment 2). When the effects of morphine on the threshold for vocalisation and vocalisation afterdischarge are obtained by summing up signals from units 4 and 7 good fits were obtained between computed effect data and experimentally registered data (Fig. 2). However, computing effect data from a more simple model omitting units 5 to 7 did not show a good fit (Fig. 2). To be able to obtain the satisfactory fits the computer uses different amounts of signals from units 4 and 7. In physiological terms this could mean that the two effects of morphine can be described by the sum of activities in at least two physiological systems. Furthermore, for each of the two effects one system is of greater importance than the other. Moreover, this model suggests that morphine induces a changed activity in some physiological systems, which develops and declines with a time course different from the mass movement of morphine. As a consequence of these kinetic studies we have taken into consideration some neurophysiological systems which might initiate morphine analgesia.

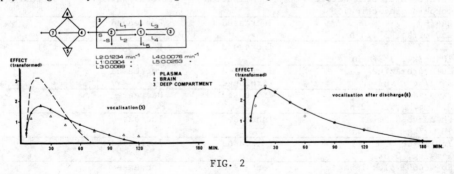

FIG. 2

The effect of morphine (2.5 mg/kg i.v.) on the threshold for vocalisation (unit 5) and vocalisation-afterdischarge (unit 6). Solid lines and dots are computed effects from the kinetic model given in the figure. Open dots are experimentally registered. Broken line represents computed effects omitting units 5 to 7.

3. Regional Fractional Turnover Rate of Noradrenaline and Dopamine after Morphine Administration

Many studies have suggested a possible relationship between morphine analgesia and the effect of this drug on brain monoamine metabolism (see ref. 7, for key references). However, the results are highly conflicting; some authors considering noradrenaline, dopamine or 5-HT, respectively, to be the most decisive ones.

After administration of a low analgesic dose, we investigated the fractional turnover rate of noradrenaline and dopamine in regions of the rat brain that were connected with the physiological modulation of the threshold for vocalisation and vocalisation-afterdischarge (7). The turnover rate of the two catecholamines was determined from the slope of the monoexponential decline of noradrenaline and dopamine at 2-5 hr after inhibition of tyrosine hydroxylase with α-methyl-p-tyrosine (H44/68) according to Brodie <u>et al</u>. (8). Morphine (5 mg/kg s.c.) given 135 min after H44/68 increased the turnover rate of dopamine in the telencephalic cortex by about 90% and in the diencephalon-mesencephalon-striatum portion by about 40%. The turnover rate of noradrenaline was unchanged in all regions except in the medulla oblongata-pons brain portion where a slight but significant increase was found (7).

4. Morphine Analgesia and Central Catecholaminergic Activity

To be able to obtain some evidence for a potential relationship between morphine analgesia and the described changed activity of noradrenaline and dopamine neurotransmission, we have studied the effects of morphine on the threshold for vocalisation and vocalisation-afterdischarge after different drug treatments known to interfere with the monoaminergic and cholinergic activities of central neurones (7). Parts of these studies are summarized in Table 1.

TABLE 1.

The Effects of Different Drug Treatments on the Activity of Morphine (5 mg/kg s.c.) on the Threshold for Vocalisation and Vocalisation-afterdischarge

Pretreatment (Drug, dose, time before morphine injection)	Vocalisation	Vocalisation-afterdischarge
H44/68 250 mg/kg, 3 1/4 hr	Increased	Decreased
FLA 63 10 mg/kg, 3 3/4 hr	Increased	Unchanged
Chlorpromazine 5 mg/kg, 1 hr	Increased (Prolonged)	Decreased
Pimozide 0.5 mg/kg, 2 1/2 hr	Increased	Decreased
Phenoxybenzamine 10 mg/kg, 2 1/2 hr	Increased	Increased
Yohimbine 2 mg/kg, 0 hr	Decreased	Increased
Ro 4-4602 plus l-Dopa 75 mg/kg, 1 hr	Decreased	Increased
Atropine 1 mg/kg, 1 1/2 hr	Unchanged	Unchanged

Morphine given subcutaneously in a dose of 5 mg/kg increased the threshold for vocalisation and vocalisation-afterdischarge, leaving the threshold for motor response unchanged.

Pretreatment of the animals with α-methyl-p-tyrosine (H44/68) decreased the activity on the threshold for vocalisation-afterdischarge while the dopamine β-oxidase inhibitor FLA 63 left this morphine effect unchanged. Blockade of dopamine receptors by chlorpromazine and pimozide reduced the effect of morphine on this threshold while phenoxybenzamine, yohimbine and Ro 4-4602 plus l-Dopa, respectively, all enhanced the activity. Pretreatment with atropine left the threshold unchanged (Table 1).

Taken these results into account together with the previously described studies on the turnover of brain noradrenaline and dopamine, we have suggested that the effect of morphine on the threshold for vocalisation-afterdischarge (assumed to reflect the emotional component of pain reactions) is closely related to an increased turnover of dopamine in the limbic structures of the brain. Most probably this effect is induced by an increased release of dopamine. This conclusion is further supported by our studies on theophylline (1,9). This drug has the ability to increase the pain sensitivity and thus produces a dose-dependent decrease of the threshold for vocalisation and vocalisation-afterdischarge, after both intraperitoneal and intravenous administration. Furthermore, this drug decreases the turnover rate of dopamine in the limbic structures (9). The theophylline-induced decrease of the threshold for vocalisation-afterdischarge can be reversed by pretreatment with apomorphine as well as Ro 4-4602 plus l-Dopa. Moreover, apomorphine per se dose-dependently increases the threshold for vocalisation-afterdischarge, an effect which is completely antagonized by pimozide.

The effects of morphine on the threshold for vocalisation are not as evidently explained as the effect on the threshold for vocalisation-afterdischarge. A dopaminergic influence on this threshold cannot be disregarded since decreased brain levels of this transmitter after H44/68 or blockade of dopamine receptors by pimozide or by chlorpromazine, respectively, both increase the activity of morphine on this threshold (Table 1). Furthermore, Ro 4-4602 plus l-Dopa pretreatment decreases the activity of morphine, while apomorphine per se in low doses decreases the normal threshold for the vocalisation response. Thus, a decreased activity of dopamine neurotransmission before morphine results in two opposite effects; a decreased activity on the vocalisation-afterdischarge and an increased activity on the vocalisation response.

Morphine was found to give a slight increase in the turnover of noradrenaline in the medulla oblongata-pons region. On the other hand, decreased noradrenaline levels brought about by FLA 63 and H44/68 produced a slight but significantly increased activity of morphine on the threshold for vocalisation. Furthermore, pretreatment of the animals with the noradrenaline receptor blocking agent phenoxybenzamine increased the activity on this threshold.

Clonidine, a drug considered to be a noradrenaline receptor stimulating agent, has been found to increase the threshold for vocalisation and vocalisation-afterdischarge (10). Pretreatment of the animals with phenoxybenzamine and chlorpromazine markedly increased the activity of clonidine on the threshold for vocalisation. Thus, a decreased noradrenaline neurotransmission could increase the activity of clonidine and morphine, respectively. Recently, Bolme et al. (11) have suggested that clonidine acts by stimulating adrenaline receptors, assuming an inhibitory function of adrenaline, which should result in a decreased activity of noradrenergic neurons. One attractive explanation for the effect of morphine on the threshold for vocalisation could therefore be that morphine increases the activity of adrenergic neurons or acts on a receptor which decreases the activity of ascending noradrenaline pathways. However, before any definitive conclusions can be drawn as to the effect of morphine on the threshold for vocalisation, it must be emphasized that in the present study we have investigated the importance of the neuronal activity of noradrenaline and dopamine only, but it is necessary to consider the complexity of intraneuronal relationships and that other putative transmitters such as e.g. serotonin have also been accredited a role in morphine analgesia.

The experimental model used by us for studying nociceptive responses opens the possibility of studying actions of drugs producing effects at different levels of the central nervous system. Therefore, when comparing our results with those of other authors it is important to realize that different techniques for studying antinociceptive activity can give different results, depending upon the level of central nervous system at which nociceptive responses can be modulated. The importance of this implication was evident from our studies with the catecholamine releasing drug 4,α-dimethyl-metatyramine (H77/77). This drug has been shown to be a potent displacer of dopamine and especially of noradrenaline stores in the central nervous system (12), leaving 5-HT neurons essentially unchanged. H77/77 increases both the threshold for vocalisation and vocalisation-afterdischarge, and these effects were all decreased by pretreatments decreasing the endogenous level of noradrenaline or blockade of noradrenaline receptors. Our explanation for the mechanism of action of this catecholamine releasing drug is that, possibly, it inhibits the sensory input at spinal cord level, which leads to an increased threshold for vocalisation and vocalisation-afterdischarge. Such a mechanism has also been suggested as the mechanism of action of morphine by Shiomi and Takagi (13).

To summarize parts 3 and 4: The ability of morphine to increase the threshold for vocalisation-afterdischarge (emotional component of pain reactions) was found to be closely related to an increased turnover of dopamine in regions of the brain including the limbic structures (thalamus-hypothalamus-rhinencephalon). It is suggested that this increased turnover of dopamine is related to an increased release of this transmitter. The effect of morphine on the threshold for vocalisation remains to be elucidated in greater detail, but our studies indicate that the decreased dopaminergic and noradrenergic neurotransmission in ascending neuronal pathways increases the effects of morphine on this threshold.

References

1. G. PAALZOW and L. PAALZOW, Acta Pharmacol. Toxicol. 32 22-32 (1973).
2. G. PAALZOW, L. PAALZOW and B. STALBY, Europ. J. Pharmacol. 27 78-88 (1974).
3. M.N. CARROLL and R.K.S. LIM, Arch. Int. Pharmacodyn. 125 383 (1960).
4. F. HOFFMEISTER and G. KRONEBERG, in Methods in Drug Evaluation p. 370 North Holland Publ. Co., Amsterdam (1966).
5. B. DAHLSTRÖM and L. PAALZOW, J. Pharm. Pharmacol. 27 172-176 (1975).
6. M. BERMAN, E. SHAHN and M.F. WEISS, Bioph. J. 2 275-288 (1962)
7. G. PAALZOW and L. PAALZOW, Psychopharmacologia In press (1975).
8. B.B. BRODIE, E. COSTA, A. DLABAC, N.H. NEFF and H.H. SMOOKLER, J. Pharmacol. exp. Ther. 154 493-498 (1966).
9. G. PAALZOW and L. PAALZOW, Acta Pharmacol. Toxicol. 34 157-173 (1974).
10. L. PAALZOW, J. Pharm. Pharmacol. 26 361-363 (1974).
11. P. BOLME, H. CORRODI, K. FUXE, T. HÖKFELT, P. LIDBRINK and M. GOLDSTEIN, Europ. J. Pharmacol. 28 89-94 (1974).
12. A. CARLSSON, M. LINDQVIST, J. WYSOKOWSKI, H. CORRODI and U. JUNGGREN, Acta Pharm. Suecica 7 293-302 (1970).
13. H. SHIOMI and H. TAKAGI, Brit. J. Pharmacol. 52 519-526 (1974).

RESEMBLANCE OF MORPHINE ANTINOCICEPTION TO THE CENTRAL
DEPRESSANT ACTIONS OF NOREPINEPHRINE

Eddie Wei

School of Public Health, University of California
Berkeley, California 94720

(Received in final form May 24, 1975)

Intraventricular administration of catecholamines can produce a depressed
and analgesic condition in animals which grossly resembles the acute effects
of morphine in some species (1). The relationship of norepinephrine to pain
mechanisms and morphine analgesia is poorly understood; however, most studies
indicate that manipulations which elevate brain norepinephrine produce analgesia or enhance morphine analgesia (2). In this investigation, I compared the
central pharmacological activities of norepinephrine and morphine in a antinociception test which is based on the ability of chemicals to inhibit the
shaking response of rats to a variety of noxious stimuli.

Morphine, injected intracerebrally in microgram quantities, inhibits the
shaking response of pentobarbital-anesthetized rats to ice water (3). The
periaqueductal gray and areas surrounding the fourth ventricle (PAG4) are especially sensitive to this morphine effect, the median inhibitory dose (ID50)
of morphine sulfate in the PAG4 being 0.07(0.02-0.21) µg/rat (3). 1-Norepine-
phrine hydrochloride (NE) injected into the PAG4, under the same experimental
conditions as morphine (3), will also inhibit shaking. The inhibitory effect
is dose-dependent, the ID50 for NE being 1.1(0.81-1.48) µg/rat. In additional
experiments, the following parameters of the NE effect on shaking were
characterized:

1. There are regional differences in the sensitivity of the rat brain to
the inhibitory effects of NE on the shaking response of anesthetized animals to
ice water. Norepinephrine hydrochloride (2 µg/rat) inhibited shaking when it
was injected into the lower brain stem (ventrolateral tegmentum, PAG4, locus
ceruleus) and the medial preoptic area, but not when it was injected into
anterior amygdala, substantia nigra, ventromedial hypothalamus or reticular
nucleus of the thalamus. Thus, the neuroanatomical specificity of the NE
effect resembles that of morphine (3).

2. A variety of noxious stimuli can provoke shaking in the anesthetized
rat. The inhibitory action of NE on shaking appears to be a generalized antinociceptive phenomenon because shaking provoked by ice water, xylene,
thyrotropin-releasing hormone (TRH) and naloxone-precipitated withdrawal were
all inhibited by NE (Fig. 1). Further studies showed that a) TRH-induced
shaking was blocked by subcutaneous (10 mg/kg) or intracerebral (5 µg/rat) administration of morphine sulfate and b) the i.p. ED50 for naloxone-precipitated
shaking in pentobarbital-anesthetized rats (40 mg/kg s.c.) pre-implanted with 1
morphine pellet for 3 days, was elevated from 0.36 mg/kg to 1.47 mg/kg of naloxone HCl when 5 µg/rat of NE was injected into the PAG4 10 min before
naloxone (see also 4,5).

3. A peripheral α-adrenergic blocking agent, phentolamine HCl when
administered at a dose of 20 mg/kg s.c., or 15 µg/rat in the PAG4, or 15 µg/
rat in the medial preoptic area, did not block the inhibitory effects of NE or
morphine on the shaking response to ice water. However, a higher dose of
phentolamine HCl, 40 µg/rat in the PAG4, appeared to antagonize some of the
inhibitory effects of NE. A peripheral β-adrenergic blocking agent, racemic

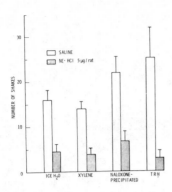

Fig. 1. <u>Inhibition of Shaking by Norepine-phrine.</u> Male rats were anesthetized with sodium pentobarbital (40 mg/kg s.c. for dependent rats and 50 mg/kg i.p. for non-dependent rats) and 30 min later, saline or 5 μg of norepinephrine was bilaterally injected at a volume of 0.5 μl/hemisphere into the PAG4. Ten minutes after NE, shaking behavior was stimulated by a) immersion in ice water b) application of .05 ml xylene on each pinna c) naloxone HCl 5 mg/kg i.p. in animals made dependent on morphine by implantation of 1 pellet for 74 hr (8) or d) 0.5 μg TRH/rat into the PAG4 (9). Shakes were counted for 5 min in (a) and (b), 10 min for (c) and 15 min in (d). N=8 for each group.

propranolol HCl, at doses up to 60 mg/kg s.c., did not prevent the inhibitory effects of NE and morphine on shaking.

4. The effects of different adrenergic agents on shaking behavior were studied (see 6). 1-Isoproterenol HCl, dopamine HCl and d-amphetamine sulfate injected intracerebrally at doses equimolar to 5 μg of NE did not inhibit the shaking response to ice water. By contrast, 1-epinephrine bitartrate and clonidine HCl completely suppressed shaking at the 0.026 μmol dose. Phenylephrine HCl was partially active.

DISCUSSION. Conceptually, morphine may exert its antinociceptive actions by mimicking or potentiating an endogenous agent with analgesic effects or by antagonizing the actions of an agent which signals the presence of noxious stimuli. The anatomical specificity and pharmacological sensitivity of the PAG4 to the inhibitory effects of NE on shaking behavior suggests that adrenergic pathways are involved in pain mechanisms and that NE actions and morphine effects in the PAG4 may be interrelated. However, it should be noted that cholinergic agents administered into the brain also have antinociceptive properties (7). Another observation made in these experiments was that TRH-induced shaking was blocked by NE and by morphine. The possibility that morphine and NE can antagonize the endogenous actions of TRH merits further investigation.

Acknowledgment- These studies were supported by USPHS Grant DA-00091.

References

1. E. MARLEY and J.D. STEPHENSON, In: <u>Catecholamines</u>, H. Blaschko and E. Muscholl, eds., pp. 463-536. Springer Verlag, Berlin (1972).
2. E.L. WAY and F.H. SHEN, In: <u>Narcotic Drugs: Biochemical Pharmacology</u>, D.H. Clouet, ed., pp. 229-253. Plenum Press, New York (1971).
3. E. WEI, S. SIGEL AND E.L. WAY, <u>J. Pharmacol. exp. Ther.</u> 193, 56-63 (1975).
4. A. HERZ, J. BLASIG and R. PAPESCHI, <u>Psychopharmacologia (Berl.)</u> 39, 121-143 (1974).
5. L.F. TSENG, H.H. LOH and E.T. WEI, <u>Europ. J. Pharmacol.</u> 30, 93-99 (1975).
6. E. MARLEY, In: <u>The Scientific Basis of Medicine, Annual Reviews</u>, pp. 359-382. Athlone Press, London (1968).
7. J. METYS, N. WAGNER, J. METYSOVA and A. HERZ, <u>Int. J. Neuropharmacol.</u> 8, 413-425 (1969).
8. E. WEI, <u>Life Sci.</u> (Part 1) 12, 385-392 (1973).
9. E. WEI, S. SIGEL, H.H. LOH and E.L. WAY, <u>Nature</u> (London) 253, 739-740 (1975).

EFFECT OF MORPHINE ON INTRACRANIAL SELF-STIMULATION BEHAVIOR FOLLOWING BRAIN AMINE DEPLETION

Agu Pert and Robert Hulsebus

Biomedical Laboratory, Edgewood Arsenal, APG, MD 21010.

(Received in final form May 24, 1975)

Morphine sulfate was found to facilitate intracranial self-stimulation 3 hrs after administration. Pretreatment with alpha-methyl-para-tyrosine reversed this facilitation whereas para-chlorophenylalanine was ineffective in modifying the actions of morphine.

Opiates have been reported to have a biphasic effect on intracranial self-stimulation (ICSS) behavior in rats. An acute administration of 10 mg/kg of morphine produces an initial depression of response rates which is followed by an increase 3-5 hrs later (1). The facilitatory effect is of special interest since several investigators have postulated that ICSS circuits may mediate rewarding and hedonistic behavior in animals and man (2). It is conceivable that activation of such circuitry may also underlie the reinforcing properties of opiates.

The purpose of this study was to examine the role of brain amines in morphine induced facilitation of ICSS. Briefly, the effects of morphine were re-assessed following depletion of brain serotonin and catecholamines with para-chlorophenylalanine (PCPA) and alpha-methyl-para-tyrosine (AMPT) respectively. Brain amines, of course, have been implicated both in the action of opiates (3) and in ICSS (4).

Methods

Fourteen rats were implanted stereotaxically with bipolar platinum self-stimulation electrodes (0.025 cm at the tip) aimed for the medial forebrain bundle at the caudal extent of the posterior hypothalamus. Following recovery, the animals were trained, in a small plexiglass chamber, to press a lever to stimulate electrically the area described above. Each lever response produced a 0.2 sec train of square wave pulses (0.2 msec in width at 100 cps). Each ICSS session lasted for 30 min.

When performance was stabilized, the animals were tested under the following drug conditions: 10 mg/kg of morphine sulfate or saline 3 hrs before testing, 50 mg/kg of AMPT 4 hrs or 5 days prior to testing followed by either saline or 10 mg/kg of morphine 3 hrs prior to testing, and PCPA 1 or 3 days prior to testing followed by either saline or morphine 3 hrs prior to testing. All animals received all drugs and drug combinations. At least two weeks were allowed to elapse between injections of the amine depleters.

Results and Discussion

The findings, in terms of mean ICSS response rates, appear in Figure 1. Briefly, it was found that pretreatment with a relatively low dose of AMPT

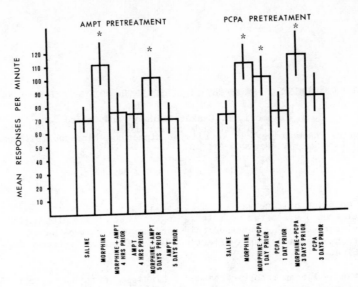

Figure 1. Effects of CA and 5-HT depletion on the facilitation of ICSS by morphine. Asterisks indicate drug effects found to be significantly different (p < .05) from the saline control with t-tests for correlated samples.

4 hrs prior to testing and 1 hr prior to morphine completely prevented the morphine induced facilitation of ICSS. Five days following the administration of AMPT, when catecholamine levels had recovered, it was no longer effective in preventing the morphine induced response increase. Depletion of brain 5-HT with PCPA, on the other hand, had no effect on the morphine response at the time point of maximal inhibition (i.e., 3 days).

The findings seem to be consonant with the notion that morphine induced facilitation of ICSS is due to an activation of CA circuits which are known to mediate such behavior (4). Such activation is consistent with the majority of biochemical findings regarding the interaction of CA with morphine (3).

It is conceivable that the activation of ICSS circuits by morphine underlies the reinforcing (drug seeking) properties of this compound. In this regard, it is interesting to note that Davis and Smith (5) have found AMPT pretreatment to block morphine self-administration in the rat.

References

1. S.A. LORENS and C.L. MITCHELL, Psychopharmacol. 32, 271-277 (1974).

2. R.G. HEATH, ed., The Role of Pleasure in Behavior, Harper and Row,NY(1964).

3. E.L. WAY and F.H. SHEN, in D.H. CLOVET, ed., Narcotic Drugs: p. 229, Plenum Press: NY (1971).

4. D.C. GERMAN and D.M. BOWDEN, Brain Res., 73, 381-419 (1974).

5. W.M. DAVIS and S.G. SMITH, Life Sci. 12, 185-191 (1973).

DIFFERENTIAL EFFECTS ON MORPHINE ANALGESIA AND NALOXONE ANTAGONISM BY BIOGENIC AMINE MODIFIERS[1]

A. E. Takemori, F. Cankat Tulunay[2] and Ichiro Yano[3]

Department of Pharmacology, University of Minnesota, Minneapolis, Minnesota 55455.

(Received in final form May 24, 1975)

Summary

The stimulation of dopaminergic receptors, inhibition of serotonin synthesis or blockade of muscurinic receptors by various modifiers led to inhibition of morphine analgesia in mice. Blockade of dopaminergic receptors or the increase in serotonergic or cholinergic activity resulted in the enhancement of morphine analgesia. Serotonergic and cholinergic systems are proposed as positive and the dopaminergic system as negative modulators of morphine analgesia. The modulation of naloxone antagonism was much more complicated than that of morphine analgesia and often the effect of biogenic amine-modifiers on antagonism differed from that on analgesia. The fact that biogenic amine-modifiers do not affect morphine analgesia and naloxone antagonism by a similar pattern suggest that interaction of narcotics and narcotic antagonists with analgesic receptors may not be exactly the same.

Numerous attempts have been made to link the pharmacologic effects of morphine with putative neurotransmitters in the central nervous system. Serotonin (5-HT), acetylcholine (Ach), dopamine (DA) and norepinephrine (NE) have been studied extensively with respect to their possible roles in the acute and chronic actions of morphine (vide rev. 1-4). However, the relationship between the putative neurotransmitters and narcotic antagonism has heretofore received very little attention. In earlier studies (5,6), we proposed that the narcotic antagonists may interact with analgesic receptors differently from the narcotic analgesics. In the present study, several neurotransmitter agonists and antagonists were employed to evaluate the roles of the central biogenic amines on morphine analgesia as well as its antagonism by naloxone.

Material and Methods

Male Swiss-Webster mice (Sasco Co.) weighing between 20 to 28 g were used in all experiments. A modification of the tail-flick assay of D'Amour and Smith (7) was employed. The animal responses were made quantal by establishing an end point at the mean peak effect which represented an increase in the reaction time of an individual animal of greater than 3 S.D. of the control mean reaction time for all animals used in the group. The usual control mean reac-

---

[1]This investigation was supported by U.S. Public Health Service Grant DA-00289.

[2]Visiting Postdoctoral Fellow from The Department of Pharmacology, University of Ankara, Faculty of Medicine, Ankara, Turkey.

[3]Visiting Research Fellow from the Department of Pharmacology, Wakayama Medical College, Wakayma, Japan.

tion time was 1.50 ± 0.03 (S.E.) seconds. At least 30 animals were used to determine each dose-response curve and ED50. The peak effect of morphine in this assay occurred 30 minutes after s.c. administration. The data were analyzed by the parallel line assay (8) with the aid of a computer program.

The ED50 of morphine after various treatments with biogenic amine-modifiers was considered significantly different from the control ED50 of morphine if the experimental ED50 lay outside the 95% confidence interval of the control ED50 and also the control ED50 lay outside the 95% confidence interval of the experimental ED50. Values significantly different from control values are designated by asterisks in the tables.

Drugs and Treatment

The various drugs and the treatments with them are listed in the individual Tables. Most of the drugs were made in saline solution such that 10 ml/kg was injected into each animal. Phenoxybenzamine was dissolved in 2 parts of acidified ethanol and diluted with 8 parts of distilled water. Haloperidol and pimozide solutions were made in 3% citric acid. 5-Hydroxytryptophan was dissolved in 1 part of 0.01 N HCl and diluted with 5 parts of distilled water. None of the latter three vehicles altered the reaction times of the mice or the response of the animals to morphine.

Naloxone hydrochloride was a gift from Endo Laboratories. It was used at a dosage of 0.16 mg/kg s.c. and administered simultaneously with various doses of morphine. The ED50 of morphine was determined in the presence of naloxone and compared with that in the absence of naloxone. The ratio of Morphine ED50 with naloxone/Morphine ED50 without naloxone and its 95% confidence interval was determined by aid of a computer program and designated as naloxone potency. Significant differences among the naloxone potencies were determined as described above for ED50 values and are indicated by asterisks in the Tables.

Determination of the concentration of morphine and naloxone in the brain.

The animals were treated with biogenic amine modifiers as indicated in Tables 1-4. Thirty min after the s.c. injection of 10 mg/kg of ^{14}C-labeled morphine (2 μCi/mouse) or 0.16 mg/kg of ^{3}H-naloxone (5.6 μCi/mouse), the animals were sacrificed and the brains rapidly removed. The brains were homogenized in 4 volumes of distilled water. One ml of the homogenate and 1 ml of 0.5M glycine buffer, pH 9.0 were mixed and this mixture was extracted three times with 10 ml portions of 10% ethanol in chloroform. The combined solvent extract was evaporated to dryness in an extraction tube. The residue was dissolved in 0.4 ml of methanol and an aliquot was mixed with 10 ml of Aquasol (New England Nuclear) to determine the radioactive content by liquid scintillation spectrometry. When the extract was submitted to thin layer chromatographic analysis, only one radioactive peak resulted which corresponded with a peak at the same R_f of either authentic morphine or naloxone. Recoveries of added morphine by this method averaged 96.2 ± 1.4% and that of naloxone was 83.5 ± 1.9%.

Results

The effect of adrenergic blockers on morphine analgesia and naloxone antagonism.

Blockade of α- or β-adrenergic receptors by phenoxybenzamine and propranolol respectively did not alter the ED50 of morphine significantly (Table 1).

We demonstrated earlier that 0.16 mg/kg of naloxone shifted the dose-response curve of morphine to the right and increased the ED50 of morphine by about 8.6 to 8.8 fold (5,6). This was confirmed in this study and taken as the control value for naloxone potency in this and all subsequent tables. While phenoxybenzamine had no effect on the naloxone potency, propranolol increased it by over two fold.

Table 1

Treatment of Mice	ED50 (95% C.L.[b]) of MS[a]	ED50(95% C.L.) of MS + Naloxone	Naloxone Potency (95% C.L.)
None	4.2(3.1-5.7)	35.8(26.0-48.3)	8.5(5.7-13.1)
Phenoxybenzamine HCl, 10 mg/kg i.p. 2 hr prior to MS[a]	4.7(3.7-5.9)	36.5(28.9-45.8)	7.8(5.6-10.8)
Propranolol, 5 mg/kg i.p. 1 hr prior to MS	3.7(2.9-4.7)	74.8(58.7-94.9)	20.0(14.3-28.4)*

[a]MS = morphine sulfate; [b]C.L. = confidence limits

The effect of stimulators and blockers of dopaminergic receptors on morphine analgesia and naloxone antagonism.

Agents which stimulate dopaminergic receptors directly or indirectly such as apomorphine and L-dopa significantly increased the ED50 of morphine by 4- and 2.5-fold, respectively (Table 2). On the other hand, dopamine receptor blocking agents, haloperidol and pimozide, significantly decreased the ED50 of morphine by about one-half.Both apormorphine and L-dopa lowered slightly the potency of naloxone. Although haloperidol failed to alter naloxone potency, pimozide increased it by nearly three-fold.

Table 2

Treatment of Mice	ED50(95% C.L.[b]) of MS[a]	ED50(95% C.L.) of MS + Naloxone	Naloxone Potency (95% C.L.)
None	4.2(3.1-5.7)	35.8(26.0-48.3)	8.5(5.7-13.1)
Apomorphine, 10 mg/kg s.c. simultaneously with MS[a]	16.7(13.1-21.0)*	84.9(67.5-107.3)	5.1(3.7-7.1)*
L-Dopa methyl ester HCl, 100 mg/kg s.c. 15 min after MS	10.6(8.1-14.0)*	59.5(44.4-78.2)	5.6(3.7-8.2)*
Haloperidol, 2.5 mg/kg i.p. 5 min prior to MS	1.9(1.5-2.3)*	17.3(14.0-21.2)	9.1(6.9-12.4)
Pimozide, 0.25 mg/kg i.p. 2 hr prior to MS	1.9(1.3-2.5)*	46.3(34.5-63.4)	24.4(16.4-39.9)*

The effect of inhibitors of serotonin synthesis and a serotonin precursor on morphine analgesia and naloxone antagonism.

Parachlorophenylalanine (pCPA) and parachloroamphetamine (pCA), more than doubled the ED50 of morphine (Table 3). In contrast the serotonin precursor, 5-hydroxytryptophan decreased the ED50 of morphine by a little less than one-half. pCPA and pCA did not alter the naloxone potency however 5-hydroxytryptophan nearly doubled the potency.

The effect of atropine and physostigmine on morphine analgesia and naloxone potency.

Atropine significantly raised the ED50 of morphine by 2.4-fold. In contrast, physostigmine significantly potentiated the morphine analgesia as seen by the decrease in the ED50 of morphine by over one-half (Table 4).
Both atropine and physostigmine decreased the potency of naloxone by over one-half.

The effect of biogenic amine modifiers on the concentration of morphine and naloxone in the brain.

Table 3

Treatment of Mice	ED50(95% C.L.[d]) of MS[b]	ED50(95% C.L.) of MS + Naloxone	Naloxone Potency (95% C.L.)
None	4.2(3.1-5.7)	35.8(26.0-48.3)	8.5(5.7-13.1)
pCPA[a] methyl ester HCl, 3 x 100 mg/kg i.p. 72 hr prior to MS[a]	9.4(8.1-10.9)*	64.2(55.1-74.2)	6.8(5.5-8.3)
pCA[c] HCl, 5 mg/kg i.p. 24 hr prior to MS	10.0(8.1-12.3)*	96.8(78.7-120.8)	9.7(7.2-13.2)
5-Hydroxytryptophan, 25 mg/kg i.p. 2.5 min after MS	2.3(1.9-2.7)*	37.5(39.7-44.3)	16.3(12.6-20.3)*

[a]pCPA = p-chlorophenylalanine; [b]MS = morphine sulfate; [c]pCA = p-chloroamphetamine; [d]C.L. = confidence limits.

Table 4

Treatment of Mice	ED50(95% C.L.[b]) of MS	ED50(95% C.L.) of MS + Naloxone	Naloxone Potency (95% C.L.)
None	4.2(3.1-5.7)	35.8(26.0-48.3)	8.5(5.7-13.1)
Atropine sulfate, 10 mg/kg s.c. simultaneously with MS[a]	10.0(7.9-12.6)*	37.7(29.8-47.4)	3.8(2.7-5.2)*
Physostigmine, 0.2 kg s.c. 10 min after MS	1.6(1.4-1.9)*	4.7(4.0-5.4)	2.9(2.3-3.5)*

[a]MS = morphine sulfate; [b]C.L. = confidence limits

None of the treatments with biogenic amine modifiers listed in Table 1-4 altered the concentrations of morphine or naloxone in the brain of mice. The average amount of free morphine and naloxone were 280 ± 27 and 6.7 ± 0.4 ng/g, respectively and 74.8 and 72.1%, respectively of the total radioactivity in the brain was determined to be the parent compounds.

Discussion

In our hands, using Swiss-Webster mice, the tail-flick assay and the treatment schedule of modifiers indicated in the Tables, stimulation of dopaminergic receptors, inhibition of serotonin synthesis or blockade of muscurinic receptors resulted in inhibition of morphine analgesia. On the other hand blockade of dopaminergic receptors or the increase in serotonergic or cholinergic activity resulted in enhanced analgesic activity of morphine. The finding that inhibition of α- and β-adrenergic systems did not modify the analgesic action of morphine is in accord with data of other investigators (9-15). There is also good agreement in the literature concerning the role of the cholinergic system in analgesia. Several authors have reported that physostigmine not only potentiates morphine analgesia but has analgesic properties itself (10, 16-21). We have also found that cholinergic blockade by atropine inhibits the analgesic action of morphine.

The roles which the dopaminergic and serotonergic systems may play in morphine analgesia are more controversial. A number of investigators have reported that L-dopa and apomorphine inhibit morphine analgesia in mice and rats (14,19,20,22-26) whereas others have shown that DL-dopa potentiates morphine analgesia (10,27). We have found that L-dopa and apomorphine inhibit morphine analgesia and in agreement with others (14), dopaminergic receptor blocking agents haloperidol and pimozide potentiate morphine analgesia. Recently we found that the stimulation of dopaminergic receptors with apomorphine or L-dopa produces hyperalgesia and this effect is blocked by dopaminergic receptor blocking agents (28). We also showed that the hyperalgesic effect of dopaminergic agonists was partially responsible for the inhibitory effect on morphine analgesia (29). Aside from this factor, there are several others such as differences in species, strain, assay methods, time of treatment with modifiers and steady-state levels of monamines which should be taken into account when one compares the data of conflicting reports. Additionally, drugs used to modify the concentration of biogenic amines may not be truly specific e.g. haloperidol and pimozide may affect the adrenergic systems as well as the dopaminergic system (vide rev. 30).

Regarding the serotonergic system, there is a vast amount of evidence which indicate that morphine analgesia is enhanced by increased serotonergic activity and reduced by decreased serotonergic activity (10,11,13,31-39). In contrast, Way's group (40,41) and Herz's laboratory (42,43) showed that decreased serotonergic tone does not inhibit morphine analgesia. In our study, the analgesic action of morphine was shown to be inhibited by the serotonin synthesis inhibitors, pCPA and pCA and potentiated by 5-hydroxytryptophan. Some of the conflicting reports in the case of the serotonergic system could be explained by differences in strain of rats (39), in serotonin turnover rate in various strains of mice (44) or in analgesic assay methods (11).

In summary with respect to the effects of biogenic amine-modifiers on analgesia, we can classify the serotonergic and cholinergic systems as positive and the dopaminergic system as negative modulators of the analgesic action of morphine. Our data together with those in the literature indicate that the reaction to a nociceptive stimulus and the modulation of analgesia is not dependent on a single monoamine.

Whereas modifiers with opposing effects on a biogenic amine system modulated morphine analgesia uniformly in an opposing manner, there is no predictable pattern of the effects of modifiers on naloxone antagonism. Neither α- nor β-adrenergic blockers altered morphine analgesia yet propranolol but not phenoxybenzamine enhanced the naloxone potency. Dopaminergic receptor stimulation inhibited both morphine analgesia and naloxone potency. However, with the use of haloperidol and pimozide, only the latter dopaminergic blocker increased naloxone potency. Inhibition of serotonin synthesis with pCPA and pCA inhibited morphine analgesia but were without effect on naloxone potency. On the other hand potentiation of morphine analgesia with 5-hydroxytryptophan also enhanced naloxone potency. Atropine and physostigmine, which had opposing effects on morphine analgesia, both lessened naloxone potency.

The changes in anticociceptive action of morphine and the antagonistic action of naloxone by the various biogenic amine modifiers could not be accounted for by an alteration of the uptake of morphine or naloxone into the brain. None of the treatments with the modifiers altered the concentration of either morphine or naloxone in the brain.

The data reveal that the modulation of naloxone antagonism is much more complicated than that of morphine analgesia and in addition to the dopaminergic, serotonergic and cholinergic systems, the β-adrenergic system may be involved in the modulation of antagonism. The findings also indicate that certain drugs which alter the analgesic effect of morphine can have similar effects, no effect or opposing effects on the antagonistic activity of naloxone. Earlier we proposed that although relatively pure antagonists such as naloxone may display an apparent competitive-type antagonism of narcotic analgesia, they may interact with analgesic receptors in a slightly different manner than the narcotic analgesics (4,6). The data in the present study support this proposal.

Acknowledgements

The capable technical assistance of Miss Joan Naeseth is gratefully acknowledged. We are also grateful to Ayerst Laboratories (propranolol), Endo Laboratories (naloxone), Janssen Pharmaceutica (pimozide), McNeil Laboratories (haloperidol) and Smith, Kline and French (phenoxybenzamine) for gifts of drugs indicated in the parentheses.

References

1. E. L. Way and F. H. Shen, in Narcotic Drugs Biochemical Pharmacology, p. 229 Plenum Press, New York (1971).
2. M. Weinstock, in Narcotic Drugs Biochemical Pharmacology p. 254 Plenum Press, New York (1971).
3. C. B. Smith, in Chemical and Biological Aspects of Drug Dependence p. 495 CRC Press, Cleveland (1972).
4. A. E. Takemori, Ann. Rev. Biochem. 43, 15 (1974).
5. F. C. Tulunay and A. E. Takemori, J. Pharmacol. Exp. Ther. 190, 395 (1974).
6. F. C. Tulunay and A. E. Takemori, J. Pharmacol. Exp. Ther. 190, 401 (1974).
7. F. E. D'Amour and D. L. Smith, J. Pharmacol. Exp. Ther. 72, 74 (1941).
8. D. J. Finney, Statistical Method in Biological Assay, 2nd ed. Hafner Publishing Co., New York (1964).
9. M. W. Nott, Eur. J. Pharmacol. 5, 93 (1968).
10. W. L. Dewey, L. S. Harris, J. F. Howes and J. A. Nuite, J. Pharmacol. Exp. Ther. 175, 435 (1970).
11. M. R. Fennesy and J. R. Lee, J. Pharm. Pharmacol. 22, 930 (1970).
12. H. N. Bhargava, S. L. Chan and E. L. Way. Proc. West. Pharmacol. Soc. 15, 4 (1972).
13. B. D. Görlitz and H. H. Frey, Eur. J. Pharmacol. 20, 171 (1972).
14. C. VanderWende and M. T. Spoerlein, Res. Commun. Chem. Path. Pharmacol. 5, 35 (1973).
15. R. E. Chipkin, W. L. Dewey and L. S. Harris, Pharmacologist 16, 204 (1974).
16. L. S. Harris, W. L. Dewey, J. F. Howes, J. S. Kennedy and H. Pars, J. Pharmacol. Exp. Ther. 169, 17 (1969).
17. J. F. Howes, L. S. Harris, W. L. Dewey and C. L. Voyda, J. Pharmacol. Exp. Ther. 169, 23 (1969).
18. J. D. Ireson, Brit. J. Pharmacol. 40, 92 (1970).
19. B. J. Pleuvry and M. A. Tobias, Brit. J. Pharmacol. 43, 706 (1971).
20. C. R. Calcutt and P. S. J. Spencer, Brit. J. Pharmacol. 41, 401P (1972).
21. H. N. Bhargava and E. L. Way, J. Pharmacol. Exp. Ther. 183, 31 (1972).
22. E. Contreras and L. Tamayo, Arch. Int. Pharmacodyn. Ther. 160, 312 (1966).
23. C. T. Major and B. J. Pleuvry, Brit. J. Pharmacol. 42, 512 (1971).
24. C. G. Sparkes and P. S. J. Spencer, Brit. J. Pharmacol. 42, 230 (1971).
25. C. VanderWende and M. T. Spoerlein, Res. Commun. Chem. Path. Pharmacol. 3, 37 (1972).
26. K. Nakamura, R. Kuntzman, A. Maggio and A. H. Conney, Neuropharmacology 12, 1153 (1973).
27. E. Contreras, L. Quijada and L. Tamayo, Psychopharmacologia 28, 319 (1973).
28. F. C. Tulunay and A. E. Takemori, Pharmacologist 16, 248 (1974).
29. F. C. Tulunay, S. B. Sparber and A. E. Takemori, Eur. J. Pharmacol. in press (1975).
30. B. K. Koe, in Industrial Pharmacology, vol. 1, Neuroleptics p. 131, Futura Publishing Co., New York (1974).
31. E. B. Sigg, G. Caprio and J. A. Schneider, Proc. Soc. Exp. Biol. Med. 97, 97 (1958).
32. F. Mercier, P. Etzensperger and J. Mercier, Anesth. Analg. 16, 70 (1959).
33. L. Tamayo and E. Contreras, Arch. Biol. Med. Exp. 2, 70 (1965).
34. S. S. Tenen, Psychopharmacologia 12, 278 (1968).
35. R. Samanin, W. Gumulka and L. Valzelli, Eur. J. Pharmacol. 10, 339 (1970).
36. T. H. Gardiner and G. Eberhart, Fed. Proc. 29, 685 (1970).

37. C. R. Calcutt, S. L. Handley, C. Q. Sparkes and P. S. J. Spencer, in Agonist and Antagonist Actions of Narcotic Analgesic Drugs p. 176 University Park Press, Baltimore (1973).
38. E. Genovese, N. Zonta and P. Mantegazza, Psychopharmacologia 32, 359 (1973).
39. H. A. Tilson and R. H. Rech, Psychopharmacologia 35, 45 (1974).
40. I. K. Ho, H. H. Loh, S. E. Lu and E. L. Way, Proc. West. Pharmacol. Soc. 15, 16 (1972).
41. I. K. Ho, S. E. Lu, S. Stolman, H. H. Loh and E. L. Way, J. Pharmacol. Exp. Ther. 182, 155 (1972).
42. J. Bläsig, K. Reinhold and A. Herz, Psychopharmacologia 31, 111 (1973).
43. K. Reinhold, J. Bläsig and A. Herz, Naunyn-Schmiedeberg's Arch. Pharmacol. 278, 69 (1973).
44. Y. Maruyama, G. Hayashi, S. E. Smits and A. E. Takemori, J. Pharmacol. Exp. Ther. 178, 20 (1971).

A COMPARISON OF NARCOTIC ANALGESICS WITH NEUROLEPTICS
ON BEHAVIORAL MEASURES OF DOPAMINERGIC ACTIVITY

Harbans Lal, Gerald Gianutsos, Surendra K. Puri

Department of Pharmacology & Toxicology, University of Rhode Island,
Kingston, R.I. 02881
(Received in final form May 24, 1975)

Because of many practical difficulties which are encountered in obtaining
direct evidence for the involvement of brain neurotransmitters in the action of
narcotic drugs, several indirect procedures are often employed. One such
method is to compare on the same measures of drug action the narcotic drugs
with a non-narcotic drug having a known mechanism of action. Haloperidol is a
prototype non-narcotic drug which blocks dopamine receptors and many of its
actions are believed to be associated with this receptor blockade. In this
paper we compare various actions of haloperidol or other neuroleptics with morphine or other narcotic analgesics using the same testing parameters. We hope
that such a comparison would evaluate the role of dopamine receptors in narcotic action and narcotic dependence. This discussion is limited only to the
behavioral measures as a comparison of neurochemical measures was recently reviewed in another paper (1).

I. ACUTE ACTIONS

A. Catalepsy: Catalepsy is a state of behavioral immobility accompanied by either muscular hypotonia as with neuroleptics, or by muscle rigidity
as with narcotics. Both, haloperidol and morphine cause catalepsy in most
animal species and in human subjects, with ED_{50} in rats, 1.5 and 20 μmol/kg
respectively. We combined a threshold dose (0.42 μmol/kg) of haloperidol with
three different doses of morphine and found that the morphine action in causing catalepsy was increased. With the ED_{50} of morphine in combination all of
the animals showed catalepsy. Also, apomorphine (8 μmol/kg) or benztropine
(6 μmol/kg) effectively counteracted catalepsy which was induced either by
haloperidol or by morphine.

B. Jumping: Dihydroxyphenylalanine (L-DOPA) injected in mice pretreated with amphetamine reliably elicits upward jumping (2,3). Haloperidol,
pimozide, chlorpromazine, thioridazine, and clozapine block the mouse jumping
(2,4) suggesting that the jumping behavior is a measure of dopaminergic stimulation. Like neuroleptics, morphine also blocks mouse jumping in a dose dependent manner. Dexitimide, a centrally acting anticholinergic drug, reversed
the pimozide induced blockade of jumping (5) without reversing the morphine-
induced blockade (Table 1), suggesting that the narcotics block dopamine receptors but through a different brain site which does not involve dopaminergic-
cholinergic interaction.

C. Stereotypy and Vomiting: Drugs which directly or indirectly stimulate dopamine receptors cause stereotypy in rats. As is seen from low ED_{50}
values (Table 2) all of the narcotics tested so far are potent antagonists of
apomorphine and amphetamine in the stereotypy test. Likewise they are also
potent antagonists of apomorphine—induced vomiting in dogs. When compared
with two prototype neuroleptics in these antidopamine tests (Table 3) morphine
shows marked activity which corresponds well with its analgesic potency.

D. Aggression: In laboratory animals, aggression can be elicited by

183

a variety of treatments. We compared haloperidol with morphine in four of the laboratory models of aggression.

(i) Apomorphine-induced aggression: Apomorphine causes aggression in a dose dependent manner and both haloperidol as well as morphine effectively blocked that aggression in the rat (Table 4).

(ii) Aggression elicited by amphetamine-DOPA: When mice are treated first with amphetamine (4 mg/kg) and then with DL-DOPA (400 mg/kg), intense aggression results upon grouping of the animals (Fig. 1). Both haloperidol and morphine effectively blocked all of the aggressive responses thus produced (Fig. 2).

Table 1. Effect of pimozide and morphine on mouse-jumping elicited by combined treatment with amphetamine and L-DOPA

Drug	mg/kg	Median Jumps/30
Saline	0	358
Pimozide	0.63	0
Morphine	20	0
Pimozide+Dexitimide	0.63+5	302
Morphine+Dexitimide	20+5	0

(iii) Shock-induced aggression: Paw shock is known to elicit aggressive responses in paired rats. We found that haloperidol blocks shock induced aggression (Fig. 3). Since haloperidol is devoid of any analgesic activity, the antiaggression action is not an artifact due to analgesia. Similarly, morphine pretreatment also blocks shock induced aggression in a dose-dependent manner (Fig. 4).

Table 2. Effectiveness of narcotic analgesics in blocking stereotypy and vomiting induced by dopaminergic stimulation (5,6,7)

	Blocking ED_{50}		
	Stereotypy (rat)		Apomorphine
	Amphetamine	Apomorphine	Vomiting (dog)
Morphine	1.7	5.9	0.55
Methadone	8.7	10.7	0.56
Demerol	20	14	15
Dextromoramide	0.5	1.	0.04
Phenoperidine	0.3	1.3	0.25

Table 3. A comparison of neuroleptics and narcotics in tests designed to measure inhibition of dopamine receptors (8)

	ED_{50} (95% fiducial limits)		
	Morphine	Chlorpromazine	Haloperidol
Apomorphine gnawing (rat)	6 (2.9-12)	6.4 (4.2-9.7)	0.17 (0.13-0.21)
Amphetamine gnawing (rat)	1.7 (.78-3.7)	1.1 (0.6-1.9)	0.03 (0.02-0.04)
Apomorphine vomiting (dog)	1	1.3	0.02

(iv) Morphine-withdrawal aggression: Animals undergoing withdrawal from narcotic drugs exhibit marked irritability and aggression (9). These signs of withdrawal are blocked by narcotics such as methadone (10). Data summarized in table 5 compare the effects of haloperidol and morphine and show that both drugs effectively blocked this aggression in relatively low doses.

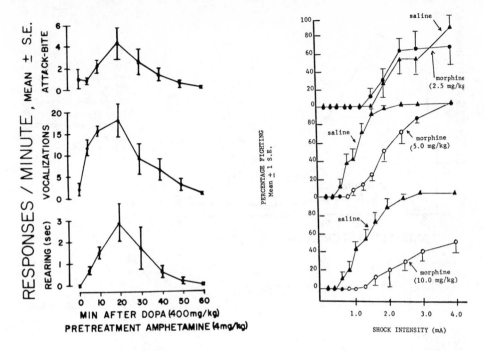

Fig. 1 (left)   Agression elicited in mice by a combined treatment with
d-amphetamine (4 mg/kg) and DL-DOPA (400 mg/kg).

Fig. 4 (right)   Reduction of shock induced aggression by morphine.

Table 4.   Effect of morphine or haloperidol on apomorphine-induced aggression.

Drug[1]	Dose	Aggressive Response/hour (mean ± S.E.)		
		Attacks	Rearing (secs)	Vocalization
Saline	– –	50 ± 9	1729 ± 246	1213 ± 152
Morphine	10	0	0	0
Haloperidol	2.5	2 ± 2	46 ± 46	33 ± 33

[1]Apomorphine (20 mg/kg) was given to 5 groups of 4 rats each for each treatment

Table 5.   Effect of haloperidol or morphine on morphine withdrawal aggression.

Drug	Dose (mg/kg)	Responses/h, Mean ± S.E.[1]		
		Attacks	Rearing	Vocalization
Saline	– –	30 ± 2	3319 ± 110	1575 ± 371
Morphine	10	0	0	0
Haloperidol	0.63	0	0	0

[1]Based upon 5 groups of rats tested for each treatment

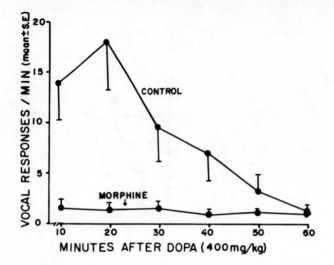

Fig. 2. Blockade by haloperidol (1 mg/kg, not shown) and morphine (20 mg/kg), of aggression elicited by amphetamine-DOPA. Attacks and rearing not shown but completely blocked.

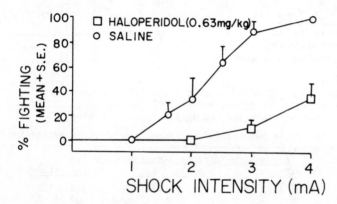

Fig. 3. Reduction of shock induced aggression by haloperidol.

II. CHRONIC ACTIONS

A. <u>Tolerance to cataleptic action</u>: Tolerance development to most of the actions of narcotic analgesics is well known. In a comparative study we treated rats with gradually increasing doses of either haloperidol or morphine (11). These rats were then maintained at the terminal doses (morphine, 400 mg/kg/day; haloperidol, 20 mg/kg/day for 4-7 days and subsequently withdrawn. Data summarized in table 6 show that, in morphine tolerant rats, there was tolerance

Table 6. Tolerance to cataleptogenic effect of morphine and haloperidol in morphine-dependent rats

		% of rats showing catalepsy	
Experimental Group	Days of Withdrawal	Morphine[1]	Haloperidol[2]
Naive	--	100	100
Morphine dependent	1	0	0
	14	80	60
Chronic haloperidol	3	100	100

[1] 40 μmol/kg injected 1 hr before test. [2] 1.3 μmol/kg injected 2 hr before test.

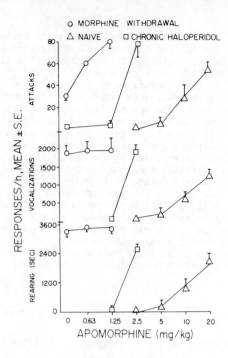

○ MORPHINE WITHDRAWAL
△ NAIVE □ CHRONIC HALOPERIDOL

RESPONSES/h, MEAN ± S.E.

APOMORPHINE (mg/kg)

Fig. 5. Aggression induced by apomorphine in rats withdrawn from chronic morphine or chronic haloperidol.

development to the catalepsy-inducing action of both morphine and haloperidol. However, in the rats chronically treated with haloperidol, there was no tolerance to either morphine or haloperidol.

B. Withdrawal signs: When an animal is treated with high doses of potent drugs for a long time, invariably, there are signs of withdrawal when the drug administration is discontinued. Withdrawal from chronic morphine produces "wet-dog"-like body-shakes, ptosis, weight loss, hyperactivity and aggression consisting of attacks, rearing and vocalization (table 7). Two of those signs were observed after haloperidol withdrawal. In both cases, there were body shakes at 24 h and increased locomotor activity at 3-7 days of withdrawal. Only with morphine-withdrawal was there loss of body weight and aggression-related behaviors. In both cases, aggression eliciting effects of apomorphine are markedly increased (Figure 5). However, whereas treatment of morphine-withdrawn rats with amphetamine elicits intense and sometimes lethal aggression (12), similar amphetamine treatment fails to elicit aggression in haloperidol withdrawn rats (table 8).

Table 7. Withdrawal signs in rats after chronic treatment with large doses of either morphine or haloperidol.

		Morphine withdrawal		Haloperidol withdrawal	
	Controls	24 hrs	72 hrs	24 hrs	168 hrs
Wet Shakes	1	7 ± 1	6 ± 1	5 ± 1	1 ± 0.7
Ptosis (seconds)	0	282 ± 38	72 ± 42	31 ± 21	0 ± 0
Weight change (g)	-	-13 ± 1.1	-36 ± 2.8	+5 ± 2.7	+21 ± 2.4
Attacks	0	-	32 ± 2	0	0
Rearing	0	-	3216 ± 118	0	0
Vocalizations	0	-	1864 ± 150	0	0
Activity (%)	100	97	125	95	175

Table 8. Failure of amphetamine but not of apomorphine in inducing aggression to haloperidol-withdrawn rats[1]

Drug	Dose (mg/kg)	Attacks	Rearing[2]	Vocalization
apomorphine	2.5	72 ± 19	3016 ± 341	1801 ± 295
d- or l-amphetamine	4,8 or 16	0	0	0

[1] 7 days after last dose of haloperidol. [2] duration in seconds

III. CONCLUSION

In the past, many behavioral tests have been developed in order to evaluate the activity of dopamine-receptor agonists and antagonists. The behavioral responses so selected are those which are increased by drugs which directly or indirectly stimulate dopamine receptors and which are depressed by the drugs which block dopamine receptors. In these tests, as is illustrated in this paper, both morphine and haloperidol resemble each other in their acute actions, suggesting that morphine also causes blockade of dopamine receptors. This conclusion is further supported by many neurochemical studies in which both haloperidol and morphine are shown to increase dopamine turnover in caudate, nucleus accumbens and olfactory tuberculum. However, many other drug-interaction studies show that haloperidol and morphine do not act at the same site. The maximum effect of morphine on striatal dopamine turnover can be further increased by haloperidol (1) and morphine induced increase in the firing rate of dopaminergic cells in the zona compacta of the substantia nigra can be further stimulated by haloperidol (13). Anticholinergic drugs reverse many of the haloperidol actions but not the morphine effects and the reverse is true of naloxone. We therefore conclude that whereas blockade of dopamine receptors by haloperidol is by direct interaction with the receptors, the blockade of the same receptors by narcotics is indirect, possibly through trans-synaptic mechanisms by which input into the dopaminergic systems is reduced.

REFERENCES

1. H. Lal, S. K. Puri, and L. Volicer, *Tissue Responses to Addiction Drugs*, Spectrum, New York, in press.

2. H. Lal, F. C. Colpaert, and P. Laudron, *Europ. J. Pharmacol.*, in press, 1975.

3. S. Fielding, M. Marky and H. Lal, *Pharmacologist* (1975), in press.

4. F. C. Colpaert, A. Wauquier, C. Niemegeers and H. Lal, *J. Pharmac. Pharmacol.* (1975) in press.

5. J. M. VanNueten, *Doctor of Science Thesis*, Paris University (1962).

6. C. J. E. Niemegeers, C. Schellekens, and P. A. J. Janssen, personal communication.

7. C. Niemegeers, *Doctor of Science Thesis*, Paris University (1960).

8. C. J. E. Niemegeers, F. J. Verbruggen, J. M. VanNueten, and P. A. J Janssen, *Int. J. Neuropharmacol.* 2, 349-354 (1964).

9. H. Lal, *Methods in Narcotic Research*, Marcel Dekker, New York (1975) in press.

10. S. K. Puri and H. Lal, *Psychopharmacologia* 32, 113-120 (1973).

11. S. K. Puri and H. Lal, *Naunyn-Schmiedeberg's Arch. Pharmacol.* 282, 155-170 (1974).

12. H. Lal, J. O'Brien and S. K. Puri, *Psychopharmacologia* 22, 217-223 (1971).

13. B. S. Bunney, personal communication.

DOPAMINE-SENSITIVE ADENYLATE CYCLASE OF THE CAUDATE NUCLEUS OF RATS TREATED WITH MORPHINE[1]

Doris H. Clouet and Katsuya Iwatsubo

New York State Drug Abuse Control Commission Testing and Research Laboratory, Brooklyn, New York 11217

(Received in final form May 24, 1975)

The addition of narcotic analgesics in vitro to nerve ending preparations from rat caudate nucleus in an assay of adenylate cyclase activity (AC) resulted in an inhibition of basal AC only at drug concentrations of 10^{-4}M or higher, and no inhibition of dopamine-stimulated (DA) AC at these drug concentrations. The acute administration of morphine at a moderately high dose (60 mg/kg) produced an increase in striatal cAMP levels, and increases in basal and DA-AC in caudate nerve-endings. In morphine-tolerant rats, striatal cAMP levels and basal AC were similar to control values, while DA-AC was elevated. These results suggest: (1) that opiates do not act directly on DA-AC, the 'dopamine receptor', and (2) that the observed behavioral DA sensitivity in tolerant animals may be produced by the DA-AC supersensitivity.

The acute or chronic administration of narcotic analgesic drugs to experimental animals produces effects on the levels of biogenic amines in brain (reviewed in 1), and on the rates of their biosynthesis (2-5). The effects of exposure to narcotics of another class of related regulator hormones, the cyclic nucleotides, have been examined indirectly for the most part. The discovery that the AC-cAMP system of brain is sensitive to norepinephrine and DA, both in vitro (6-8), and in vivo (9), suggested to us that a study of the effects of morphine and related compounds on the rates of biosynthesis and on the levels of cAMP might be rewarding.

In other reports (10, 11), we have described the effects of opiate administration on the AC-cAMP system in discrete areas of rat brain. In the present report we describe effects in one brain region: the caudate nucleus of the striatum, because the most prominent increase in neurohormone turnover after acute morphine administration was in striatal DA turnover (2, 12). One mechanism by which the turnover of DA may be increased is by a compensatory activation of DA synthesis in nerve terminals following post-synaptic DA receptor blockade. A DA-sensitive AC, found in the caudate, has been suggested as the 'dopamine receptor' (8). Since the stimulation of AC by DA can be inhibited in vitro by neuroleptic receptor blockers (which also increase DA turnover in striatum), the effects of narcotic analgesics on basal and DA-AC in striatal nerve-ending preparations in vitro have been examined in order to determine whether opiates have a direct effect on the 'dopamine receptor'. We have also examined the DA-AC from striatal nerve-endings after morphine administration to rats.

[1]K.I. is a visiting scientist from the University of Osaka, Osaka, Japan. This research was supported in part by grant DA-00087 from NIDA.

Methods

Tissue Preparation for Adenylate Cyclase Assay

Male Wistar rats (130-160 g) were killed by decapitation. Bilateral caudate nuclei were separated from the internal capsule and removed. The tissue was homogenized in 50 volumes of 0.32 M sucrose and the crude synaptsomal-mitochondrial fraction was sedimented by centrifugation at 5000 x g for 10 minutes. The sedimented particles were suspended in hypotonic 2 mM Tris-maleate buffer, pH 7.5 containing 2 mM EGTA, to give a protein concentration of 35 to 50 $\mu g/\mu l$. The protein content was measured by the Lowry method (13).

Adenylate Cyclase Assay

The formation of $cAMP^{32}$ from ATP^{32} was measured as described in our earlier papers (10, 11). Fifty μl of striatal disrupted nerve-endings were incubated for 3 minutes at $30°C$ with 200 μl of reaction mixture containing 0.5 mM ATP (about 0.2 μC of αP^{32}-ATP), 50 mM Tris-maleate buffer at pH 7.5, 2mM $MgSO_4$, 0.2 mM EGTA, 10mM theophyllin, 1 mM cAMP, 10 μg phosphatidylserine, and where indicated, 100 μM dopamine and drugs. The reaction was terminated by boiling for 2 minutes. One ml of buffer containing about 10,000 CPM of H^3-cAMP was added before centrifugation in order to calculate recovery of cAMP. cAMP was separated by alumina column chromatography (14) and barium sulfate precipitation (15) techniques, and H^3 and P^{32} radioactivities were measured in a liquid scintillation spectrometer.

cAMP Determination

At various times after drug administration rats were placed in a microwave oven while positioned in a styrofoam holder, and irradiated for 38 seconds. The whold striati were dissected out and cAMP levels were measured by the protein binding assay described by Gilman (16), except that binding protein was isolated from rabbit muscle instead of beef muscle.

Results

Effects of Analgesics Added to the Assay on Adenylate Cyclase

The effect of adding morphine or related compounds to assays for AC are shown in Table 1. At 10^{-4}M concentration, d-methadone inhibited AC. At 10^{-3}M concentration, levorphanol, l-methadone and dextrorphan inhibited basal AC. While morphine at 10^{-3}M concentration did not inhibit striatal AC, it was inhibitory at this concentration in other brain areas (10).

The addition of 100 μM DA increased AC about 50% above basal AC (Figure 1). The addition of the neuroleptic drug, haloperidol, prevented DA-stimulation at 3 μM concentration. However, morphine did not inhibit DA-AC in concentrations as high as 0.3 mM (Figure 1). Levorphanol, l-methadone and naloxone also had no effect on DA-AC (11).

Effect of Morphine Administration on cAMP Levels

The administration of 10 mg/kg morphine s.c. in rats had no effect on cAMP levels in the whole striatum (Table 2). A dose of 60 mg/kg morphine, however, increased cAMP levels thirty minutes after drug administration. In striatum from morphine-tolerant rats challenged with an 100 mg/kg dose of morphine, cAMP levels were also increased (Table 2). The administration of naloxone at a dose of 2 mg/kg s.c. showed a tendency to increase cAMP levels in naive rats, but not in tolerant rats.

TABLE 1

Effect of Narcotic Analgesic Drugs and Related Compounds on Adenylate Cyclase Activity in Striatal Nerve-endings _in vitro_

ADDED DRUGS	ADENYLATE CYCLASE ACTIVITY (pmol/min/mg protein)	
	1 mM Concentration	0.1 mM Concentration
None	430 + 50	
Morphine	390 + 35	415 + 45
Levorphanol	*210 + 55	435 + 45
Dextrorphan	*245 + 50	455 + 50
l-methadone	*290 + 30	400 + 35
d-methadone	*310 + 35	*360 + 40
Naloxone	450 + 40	470 + 35

Each value is the average of three observations + S.D.
*Different from control values at $p < 0.05$.

FIGURE 1

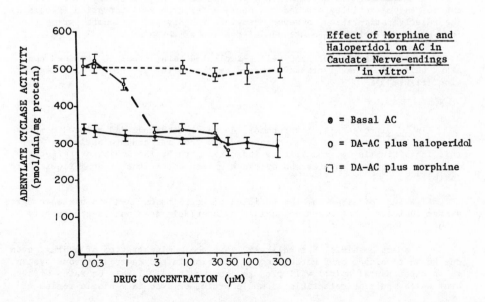

Effect of Morphine and Haloperidol on AC in Caudate Nerve-endings 'in vitro'

● = Basal AC

○ = DA-AC plus haloperidol

◨ = DA-AC plus morphine

TABLE 2

Effect of Morphine Treatment on cAMP levels in Rat Striatum

Treatment	cAMP LEVELS (pmol/mg protein)	
ACUTE MORPHINE Dose:	10 mg/kg	60 mg/kg
Zero-time control	14.6 ± 2.6	13.2 ± 1.4
30 minutes	16.2 ± 1.8	*20.2 ± 1.8
60 minutes	15.8 ± 2.6	15.4 ± 0.8
120 minutes	15.2 ± 1.0	17.0 ± 1.2
CHRONIC MORPHINE	No naloxone	Naloxone
Sham-implanted	16.2 ± 0.8	19.2 ± 2.2
Morphine pellet-implanted	*21.4 ± 0.3	14.0 ± 0.8

Morphine pellets (75 mg morphine base) were implanted s.c. on days one and five. Rats were killed on the eleventh day two hours after an 100 mg/kg morphine challenge. Naloxone was injected s.c. 0.5 hr before sacrifice at a dose of 2 mg/kg. *Different from control values at $p < 0.05$.

Effect of Morphine Treatment on Adenylate Cyclase Activity

One hour after the administration of 60 mg/kg morphine, basal AC was increased (Figure 2). A 15 mg/kg dose of levorphanol had a similar effect while the inactive isomer, dextrorphan, had no effect at the same dose (10).

DA-AC in caudate nerve-endings was increased significantly over zero-time control enzyme activity one and two hours after drug administration (Figure 2). The relative stimulation, however, remained roughly proportionate during the four hours following the acute administration of morphine.

In contrast, in morphine pellet-implanted rats, basal AC remained constant while DA-AC was increased twofold by the third day after pellet implantation (Figure 3).

Discussion

In in vitro assays, levorphanol, d- and l-methadone and related compounds inhibited AC in crude ruptured nerve-endings from rat caudate nucleus. That this inhibition is not specific is indicated both by the inhibitory effects of inactive isomers of opiates and by the high concentrations of drug required for inhibition.

The lack of effect of the addition of morphine on DA-AC in the same assay system indicates that morphine, unlike haloperidol, does not react directly with the 'dopamine receptor'.

It seems possible, but unlikely, that the administration of a drug, even one known to affect cAMP metabolism or function in the central nervous system, to an experimental animal will produce changes in cAMP levels or rates of turnover which would be detectible in whole brain, or even in a single region of

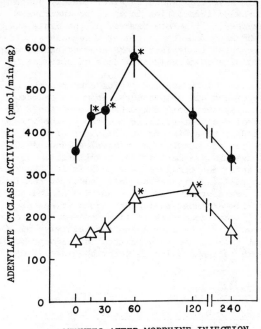

FIGURE 2

Striatal AC after acute
Morphine Treatment in Rats

The dose of morphine was 60 mg/kg
s.c. The vertical bars are S.E.
of the mean AC activities.

● = Basal AC
△ = Difference between DA-AC and
basal AC

*Significantly different from zero-
time control values at $p < 0.05$.

MINUTES AFTER MORPHINE INJECTION

FIGURE 3

Striatal AC in
Morphine-tolerant Rats

● = Basal AC

▲ = Diff. between DA-AC and
Basal AC in control rats

△ = Diff. between DA-AC and
basal AC in morphine pellet
implanted rats

*Significantly different from
control values at $p < 0.05$

DAYS OF MORPHINE PELLET IMPLANTATION

brain. Because cAMP levels in brain have been shown to alter rapidly postmortem, we sacrificed the rats by microwave irradiation in order to inactivate cAMP synthetic and degradative enzymes (17), before removal of the brain and dissection into gross areas for cAMP measurements in tissue homogenates. It was not surprising that transient changes in striatal cAMP concentrations were found only after the administration of a relatively high dose of morphine.

On the other hand, AC was measured in a smaller tissue compartment, a fraction containing ruptured synaptosomes and mitochondria from the caudate. In this preparation, which contained synaptosomal contents and membranes, including pre-synaptic and a portion of the post-synaptic membranes, specific drug-influenced AC might be expected to be an important component of total AC. Shortly after the acute administration of morphine, both basal AC and DA-AC were increased proportionately, suggesting an activation, translocation or other mobilization of both the receptor and catalytic elements in AC. However, in morphine-tolerant rats, caudate DA-AC was increased while basal AC remained constant, suggesting that only the neurohormone-sensitive portion of the AC complex was activated. An alternative explanation is that acute or chronic morphine treatment affect AC in different compartments (i.e. pre-synaptic cytoplasmic AC vs post-synaptic membrane AC). The increased DA sensitivity of AC in the caudate of morphine-tolerant rats is probably related to the supersensitivity to dopaminergic agonists such as apomorphine or methylphenidate found in behavioral experiments (18).

References

1. E.L. WAY and F.H. SHEN, in Narcotic Drugs: Biochemical Pharmacology, pp229-255, Plenum Press, New York (1971)
2. D.H. CLOUET and M. RATNER, Science 168 854-855 (1970)
3. C.B. SMITH, M.I. SHELDON, J.H. BEDNARCZYK and J.E. VILLARREAL, J. Pharmacol. Exp. Therap. 180 547-557 (1972)
4. H.A. SASAME, J. PEREZ-CRUET, G. DICHIARA, A. TAGLIAMONTE, P. TAGLIAMONTE and G.L. GESSA, J. Neurochem. 19 1953-1957 (1972)
5. C. GAUGHY, Y. AGID, J. GLOWINSKI and A. CHERAMY, Eur. J. Pharmacol. 22 311-319 (1973)
6. S. KAKIUCHI and T.W. RALL, Mol. Pharmacol. 4 379-388 (1968)
7. J.W. DALY, M. HUANG and H. SHIMAZU, in Advances in Cyclic Nucleotide Research, pp 375-387, Raven Press, New York (1972)
8. J.W. KEBABIAN, G.L. PETZOLD and P. GREENGARD, Proc. Nat. Acad. Sci. 69 2145-2149 (1973)
9. W.P. BURKARD, J. Neurochem. 19 2615-2619 (1972)
10. K. IWATSUBO and D.H. CLOUET, Fed. Proc. 32 536 (1973)
11. K. IWATSUBO and D.H. CLOUET, Biochem. Pharmacol. (In Press) (1975)
12. J.C. JOHNSON, M. RATNER, G.L. GOLD and D.H. CLOUET, Res. Comm. Chem. Path. Pharmacol. 9 41-53 (1974)
13. O.H. LOWRY, N.J. ROSEBROUGH, A.L. FARR and R.J. RANDALL, J. Biol. Chem. 193 265-275 (1951)
14. A.A. WHITE and T.V. ZENSER, Anal. Biochem. 41 372-396 (1971)
15. G. KRISHNA, B. WEISS and B.B. BRODIE, J. Pharmacol. Exp. Therap. 163 379-386 (1968)
16. A.G. GILMAN, Proc. Nat. Acad. Sci. 67 305-312 (1970)
17. M.J. SCHMIDT, J.T. HOPKINS, D.E. SCHMIDT and G.A. ROBINSON, Brain Res. 42 465-477 (1972)
18. G. GIANUTSOS, M.D. HYNES, S.K. PURI, R.B. DRAWBAUGH and H. LAL, Psychopharmacol. 34 37-44 (1974)

DOPAMINERGIC MECHANISMS IN WITHDRAWAL HYPOTHERMIA IN MORPHINE DEPENDENT RATS

Barry Cox[1], Marylouise Ary[2] and Peter Lomax

Department of Pharmacology, School of Medicine and the Brain Research Institute, University of California, Los Angeles, California 90024.

(Received in final form May 24, 1975)

The role of several putative neurotransmitters in the development of tolerance and dependence to the narcotic analgesics has been the subject of a recent review (1), which demonstrated the lack of a consensus on the precise role of the catecholamines in this syndrome. A definitive role for brain dopamine in withdrawal aggression and withdrawal hypothermia has been suggested (2,3,4), although in the case of the hypothermia few details are available. We therefore decided to assess the importance of dopamine in withdrawal using apomorphine and pimozide, drugs claimed to be specific for dopamine receptors.

Methods

Male Sprague Dawley rats weighing 210-230 g were rendered dependent by subcutaneous implantation of a 75 mg morphine pellet. Withdrawal was induced by injection of naloxone (1 mg/kg i.p.) 72 hr later. Hypothermia was measured in rats placed in restraining cages at an ambient temperature of 18°C using rectal thermistor probes inserted to a depth of 6 cm. Some rats had been implanted with stainless steel cannula guides into the preoptic/anterior hypothalamic (PO/AH) nuclei 7 days before receiving the morphine pellet. Withdrawal hypothermia was measured in rats receiving either pimozide (0.5 mg/kg i.p.), apomorphine (1.25 mg/kg i.p.) or vehicle (1 ml/kg i.p.), the systemic group; and rats receiving either morphine (25 µg) pimozide (0.5 µg) or vehicle (1 µl) intracerebrally, the central group. Withdrawal behavior was assessed for 1 hr before and 1 hr after naloxone. For chewing, licking, teeth chatter, facial tremor, grooming, sneezing and writhing each 1 hr observation period was divided into 20 3 min sessions and the number of sessions in which each sign occurred were counted. The proportion of rats in the group with diarrhea was calculated and head shakes and wet dog shakes were counted individually. The withdrawal score was corrected by subtracting the pre-naloxone score for apomorphine, pimozide or vehicle pretreated groups.

Results

Fig. 1 illustrates the temperature changes. Naloxone caused a 1.37°C fall in morphine dependent rats which was similar in magnitude to that seen after apomorphine. Pimozide produced only a small, non-significant, fall in morphine dependent rats. When apomorphine and naloxone were injected together a fall in rectal temperature occurred which was not significantly different from the effect when either was injected alone. Pimozide pretreatment caused a significant (p < 0.05) antagonism of the withdrawal hypothermia. Injection of morphine (25 µg) or pimozide (0.5 µg) into the PO/AH nuclei immediately before systemic naloxone caused a significant antagonism of the hypothermia. Apomorphine (1.25 mg/kg) significantly reduced wet dog shakes, teeth chatter and

[1]Supported by USPHS Fellowship 1, F05, TWO 2130-01
[2]Supported by USPHS MH-6415

FIG. 1

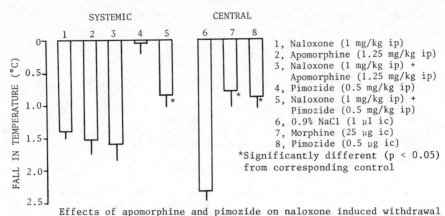

1, Naloxone (1 mg/kg ip)
2, Apomorphine (1.25 mg/kg ip)
3, Naloxone (1 mg/kg ip) +
   Apomorphine (1.25 mg/kg ip)
4, Pimozide (0.5 mg/kg ip)
5, Naloxone (1 mg/kg ip) +
   Pimozide (0.5 mg/kg ip)
6, 0.9% NaCl (1 μl ic)
7, Morphine (25 μg ic)
8, Pimozide (0.5 μg ic)
*Significantly different (p < 0.05)
from corresponding control

Effects of apomorphine and pimozide on naloxone induced withdrawal

writhing and gave an almost significant reduction in chewing. Pimozide (0.5 mg/kg) significantly increased chewing, headshakes and writhing. Diarrhea, facial tremor, grooming, licking and sneezing were unaffected by either pimozide or apomorphine.

Discussion

By using rats which had developed a medium degree of dependence it was possible to demonstrate dopaminergic involvement in naloxone precipitated withdrawal in both directions. Thus, whilst the hypothermia appeared to be dopamine mediated (blocked by pimozide), other signs - chewing, head shakes and writhing - appeared to be under a dopaminergic inhibitory influence (potentiated by pimozide). Apomorphine significantly antagonized the writhing, and reduced the chewing, providing further evidence for a dopamine inhibitory mechanism. Although wet dog shakes and teeth chatter were not affected by pimozide, they were markedly reduced by apomorphine suggesting that stimulation of dopamine receptors can also reduce these signs.

The fact that central injection of morphine antagonized naloxone precipitated withdrawal hypothermia indicated that not only was this a centrally mediated response but probably that it occurred in the PO/AH region. Pimozide was also an effective antagonist at this central site confirming the peripheral studies and implicating a dopaminergic mechanism in the PO/AH area. For a number of the signs there was no evidence of any dopaminergic involvement.

These results emphasize the need to be specific about the particular sign under study when discussing the mechanisms of withdrawal. They further demonstrate that not only may different neurotransmitters be involved but that the same neurotransmitter can exert either a facilitatory or inhibitory influence depending on the sign measured.

References

1. A. E. TAKEMORI, Ann. Rev. Biochem. 43: 15-33 (1974).
2. H. LAL, S. K. PURI, and Y. KARKALAS, Pharmacologist 13: 263 (1971).
3. S. K. PURI and H. LAL, Psychopharmacologia 32: 113-120 (1973).
4. G. GUINUTSOS, M. D. HYNES, S. K. PURI, R. B. DRAWBAUGH and H. LAL, Psychopharmacologia 34: 37-44 (1974).

DOPAMINE RECEPTOR SENSITIVITY AFTER REPEATED MORPHINE ADMINISTRATIONS TO RATS

Klaus Kuschinsky

Dept. of Biochemical Pharmacology, Max-Planck-Institute for Experimental Medicine, D-34 Göttingen, Hermann-Rein-Str. 3, F.R. Germany

(Received in final form May 24, 1975)

It was studied in rats, if chronic morphine treatment induces a supersensitivity of dopamine receptors in brain. The rats were treated twice daily for 8-11 days with single doses of morphine, increasing from 10 to 20 mg/kg i.p. The experiments were carried out 16-20 hours after the last injection of morphine. After chronic morphine treatment, the potency of apomorphine in lowering the striatal dopamine turnover was increased. On the other hand, apomorphine was not more potent in inducing stereotypies (sniffing, licking, gnawing) after chronic morphine administration than in saline controls. Finally, dopamine activated the adenylate cyclase in striatal homogenates of rats after chronic morphine treatment to a similar extent as in homogenates of control rats. The results suggest that a supersensitivity of dopamine receptors in brain is not necessarily involved in symptoms of an increased dopaminergic activity after chronic morphine application.

Obviously, narcotic analgesics have various, more or less independent sites of action in the central nervous system. One of these sites is the nigro-striatal dopaminergic system. In vivo, morphine and other narcotics induce symptoms of a decreased dopaminergic neurotransmission, e.g. catalepsy and muscular rigidity, in rats. These symptoms are accompanied by an increase of striatal dopamine turnover (1,2,3,4). Furthermore, in vitro studies showed that morphine slowed the K^+-induced release of labeled dopamine from striatal slices (5). All these effects can be inhibited by narcotic antagonists. The in vitro observations strongly suggest that narcotics decrease the central dopaminergic neurotransmission mainly at a presynaptic site in nigro-striatal dopaminergic neurons.

After repeated morphine administrations, the cataleptic effects decrease, while symptoms of locomotor stimulation and of stereotypies, particularly of gnawing activity, become predominant (6). This suggests that now the dopaminergic neurotransmission in brain is enhanced. Similarly, in narcotic withdrawal, symptoms of a dopaminergic hyperactivity seem to predominate, as shown by Puri and Lal (7). These authors postulated that chronic morphine treatment induces a supersensitivity of postsynaptic dopamine receptors, as a consequence of the chronically decreased dopaminergic neurotransmission. In a more general theory, Collier (8) had postulated that a supersensitivity against the effects of neurotransmitters might be an important feature of the development of tolerance to and physical dependence on drugs. It was, therefore, our aim to test this hypothesis in the nigro-striatal dopaminergic system. Three criteria were used to assess the sensitivity of the dopamine receptors in controls and rats after repeated morphine administrations: 1) the potency of apomorphine to induce stereotyped behavior, 2) the potency of apomorphine to decrease the dopamine turnover in vivo, and 3) the potency of dopamine to activate an adenylate cyclase (EC 4.6.1.1.) in striatal tissue in vitro.

Pretreatment of animals

Male albino Wistar rats (F. Winkelmann, D-4791 Borchen) of 120-160 g were used. Chronic morphine treatment was as follows: day 1 and 2: two injections of 10 mg/kg each, day 3 and 4: 15 mg/kg each, then two injections of 20 mg/kg each were given for further 4-7 days. All morphine injections were given i.p., the morphine doses were calculated as the free base. The applied schedule of chronic morphine treatment induced hyperkinesia and gnawing movements after each injection. Furthermore, naloxone (2-4 mg/kg i.p.) after this treatment induced symptoms of morphine withdrawal (e.g. teeth-chattering, salivation, wet dog shaking, grubbing up the ground like a pig etc.). The rats were compared with control animals, treated chronically with saline during the same time period. In all experiments, the sensitivity of the dopamine receptors was tested 16-20 hours after the last injection of morphine or saline, respectively, i.e. in the early withdrawal state.

Stereotypies after apomorphine

The stereotypies after apomorphine were assessed as described by McKenzie (9) in a slightly modified form for 40 min (cf. 10). Apomorphine directly stimulates dopamine receptors (11,12) and, therefore, seems to be a good indicator of the sensitivity of these receptors. In the case of a supersensitivity of dopamine receptors, apomorphine should have an increased potency in inducing stereotypies (13).

Chronic morphine treatment did not increase the apomorphine-induced stereotypies, but it seemed to slightly decrease them (FIG. 1). This result, therefore, does not suggest a postsynaptic supersensitivity of dopamine receptors in the rat striatum.

Decrease of dopamine turnover after apomorphine

The effect of apomorphine on dopamine turnover was studied by measuring the striatal homovanillic acid (HVA) concentration after pretreatment with probenecid (FIG. 2). Chronic morphine treatment did not affect the dopamine turnover, and 0.5 mg/kg apomorphine were ineffective in morphine - as well as control groups. 1.0 mg/kg apomorphine i.p., however, significantly ($P < 0.025$, Student's t-test) reduced the dopamine turnover in the rats, treated chronically with morphine but not in the

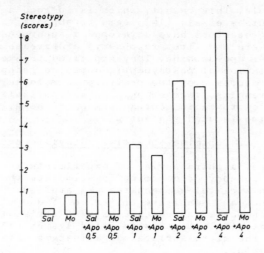

FIG. 1

Effects of chronic morphine treatment on stereotypies, induced
by various doses of apomorphine. The rats were observed for 40
40 min after apomorphine or saline application. The test was performed 16-20 hours after the last morphine injection. The sum of
the scores during the whole observation time (sniffing, licking,
gnawing) is given (mean of 8 animals). Mo = chronic morphine
treatment, Sal = chronic saline treatment, Apo = apomorphine
treatment.

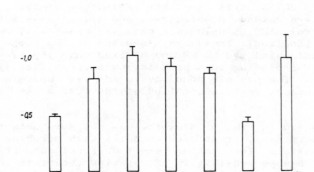

FIG. 2

Effects of apomorphine on homovanillic acid (HVA) concentrations
in striata of rats, treated either chronically with morphine or
with saline. The last of these injections was given 16-20 hours,
probenecid (200 mg/kg) 90 min and apomorphine 60 min before
sacrifice. HVA [μg/g wet weight ± S.E.] , N = 3-6

saline controls. This result, which is in good agreement with
that of Gianutsos et al. (14) seems to support the idea that
the dopamine receptors have developed a supersensitivity: Andén
et al. (11) were the first to observe a decrease of dopamine
turnover after apomorphine. They explained this effect by a
direct stimulation of postsynaptic dopamine receptors and a
compensatory decrease of the presynaptic release and utiliza-
tion. These results, suggesting a supersensitivity of dopamine
receptors, seem to be in contradiction to those, obtained with
the apomorphine-induced stereotypies.

Dopamine-sensitive adenylate cyclase

Therefore, a third series of experiments were performed,
in which the potency of dopamine to stimulate the synthesis of
cyclic AMP in striatal homogenates was studied. This seems to be
the most direct and sensitive criterion of dopamine receptor
sensitivity, since a supersensitivity of striatal dopamine receptors is detectable in this in vitro system (15) after destruction of the nigro-striatal dopaminergic pathways with
6-hydroxydopamine.

The rats were decapitated and the striata were quickly
prepared, homogenized in 50 volumes (weight to volume) of 2 mM
tris-(hydroxymethyl)aminomethane maleate buffer (pH = 7.4) +
2 mM EGTA, as described by Clement-Cormier et al. (16) (slightly modified). 50 µl of this homogenate were pipetted into
400 µl of a medium (end concentrations = mM): tris(hydroxymethyl)aminomethane maleate, 80.2; $MgSO_4$, 6.0; theophylline, 10;
EGTA, 0.6, dopamine in various concentrations. 40 sec. after
shaking and incubating the samples at 37° C, 50 µl of ATP were
added (final concentration: 1.5 mM), and the samples were incubated for further 2.5 min. The reaction was terminated by putt-
ing the samples into boiling water for 2 min. Then they were
stored at -20° C until used. For estimation of cycl. AMP, the
samples were thawed, homogenized, and aliquots were taken to
measure cycl. AMP by using a cyclic AMP assay kit, purchased at
Amersham (England). This assay is based on the competition
between unlabeled cycl. AMP and a fixed quantity of ^{3}H-labeled
compound for binding to a protein, which specifically binds
cycl. AMP. The protein bound cycl. AMP was separated from the
unbound nucleotide by adsorption of the free nucleotide to
charcoal.

As shown in FIG. 3, dopamine was not more potent in striatal tissue of rats, treated chronically with morphine than in
saline controls. This latter result does not support the assump-
tion that a supersensitivity of dopamine receptors in brain is
necessarily involved in symptoms of an increased dopaminergic
activity after chronic morphine application. However, the
results do not exclude the possibility that in other brain
regions, the development of a supersensitivity to neurotransmitters, different from dopamine, might be of importance for
the occurrence of some symptoms of tolerance and physical
dependence.

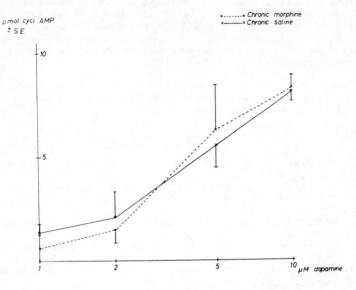

FIG. 3

Stimulation by dopamine of the synthesis of cyclic AMP in homogenates of rat striata. Tissues of rats, treated chronically with morphine (16-20 hours after the last injection) were compared with tissues of the corresponding saline controls. Abscissa: dopamine concentration [µM], ordinate: p mol cycl. AMP per 0.1 mg tissue ± S.E. N = 5.

Discussion

It is not yet clear, why apomorphine was more potent in rats, treated chronically with morphine than in control rats in lowering the striatal dopamine turnover. This decrease of dopamine turnover might, at least under some conditions, not be due to a stimulation of postsynaptic dopamine receptors, but to some other, unknown effects, occurring presynaptically. In any case, it does not seem to be a very reliable criterion of the dopamine receptor sensitivity, at least under some conditions.

The shift from a decreased dopaminergic activity in rats after a single dose of morphine to an increase of dopaminergic neurotransmission after chronic morphine treatment cannot be explained as yet. One possibility is that by some, still unknown mechanism, the concentration of dopamine at its receptors is increased after chronic morphine treatment. In this context, it seems to be interesting that Iwamoto et al. (17) observed a sudden elevation of brain dopamine in morphine-dependent rats, after being treated with naloxone. Another possibility might be that a mechanism, counteracting dopaminergic actions (e.g. a cholinergic or serotoninergic one), decreases during chronic morphine treatment. As a consequence, the antagonistic balance between dopaminergic on the one hand and cholinergic and/or serotoninergic mechanisms on the other hand (18) should be shifted in favor of the dopaminergic ones. The - relative or absolute - activation of dopaminergic mechanisms after chronic morphine treatment, in any case, seems to be an important factor in inducing symptoms of psychological and/or physical dependence on narcotics, since haloperidol, which predominantly blocks dopamine receptors, suppresses the craving for the narcotic drug in heroin-dependent patients (19).

Acknowledgements: I am indebted to Mrs. H. Kügler for her skilful technical assistance. Probenecid was kindly donated by Sharp & Dohme GmbH, München.

References

1. L.M. GUNNE, J. JONSSON, and K. FUXE, Europ. J. Pharmacol. 5, 338-342 (1969).
2. H. A. SASAME, J. PEREZ-CRUET, G. DI CHIARA, A. TAGLIAMONTE, P. TAGLIAMONTE, and G.L. GESSA, J. Neurochem. 19, 1953-1957 (1972).
3. K. KUSCHINSKY and O. HORNYKIEWICZ, Europ. J. Pharmacol. 19, 119-122 (1972).
4. L. AHTEE and I. KÄÄRIÄINEN, Europ. J. Pharmacol. 22, 206-208 (1973).
5. B. CELSEN and K. KUSCHINSKY, Naunyn-Schmiedeberg's Arch. Pharmacol. 284, 159-165 (1974).
6. E. JOEL and A. ETTINGER, Naunyn-Schmiedeberg's Arch. exp. Path. Pharmakol. 115, 334-350 (1926).
7. S. K. PURI and H. LAL, Psychopharmacologia 32, 113-120 (1973).
8. H.O.J COLLIER, Nature 220, 228-231 (1968).
9. G.M. MC.KENZIE, Psychopharmacologia 23, 212-219 (1972).
10. K. KUSCHINSKY, Psychopharmacologia, in the press.
11. N.-E. ANDÉN, A. RUBENSSON, K. FUXE, and T. HÖKFELT, J. Pharm. Pharmacol. 19, 627-629 (1967).
12. A.M. ERNST, Psychopharmacologia 10, 316-323 (1967).
13. D. TARSY and R.J. BALDESSARINI, Neuropharmacol. 13, 927-940 (1974).
14. G. GIANUTSOS, M.D. HYNES, S.K. PURI, R.B. DRAWBAUGH, and H. LAL, Psychopharmacologia 34, 37-44 (1974).
15. R.K. MISHRA, E.L. GARDNER, R. KATZMAN, and M.H. MAKMAN, Proceed. Nat. Acad. Sci. USA 71, 3883-3887 (1974).
16. Y.C. CLEMENT- CORMIER, J.W. KEBABIAN, G.L. PETZOLD, and P. GREENGARD, Proceed. Nat. Acad. Sci. USA 71, 1113-1117 (1974).
17. E.T. IWAMOTO, I.K. HO, and E.L. WAY, J. Pharmacol. Exp. Ther. 187, 558-567 (1973).
18. R. HASSLER, Parkinson's Disease - Rigidity, Akinesia, Behavior. J. Siegfried (ed.), Vol. 1, p. 333, Hans Huber Publishers, Bern, Stuttgart, Wien (1972).
19. J. KARKALAS and H. LAL, Internat. Pharmacopsychiat. 8, 248-251 (1973).

MECHANISM OF DEVELOPMENT OF TOLERANCE TO INJECTED MORPHINE
BY GUINEA PIG ILEUM[1,2]

Seymour Ehrenpreis, Joel Greenberg and Joseph E. Comaty

New York State Research Institute for Neurochemistry and Drug Addiction
Ward's Island, New York, New York 10035

(Received in final form May 24, 1975)

Injection of a large dose of morphine into a guinea pig
results in a block of electrically-induced contractions of the
ileum in vitro. A similar dose is almost ineffective in guinea
pigs given morphine chronically. The time course for development of this tolerance has been determined in guinea pigs
injected twice daily with morphine 100 mg/kg and challenged on
various days with 750 mg/kg of the drug. Animals similarly
injected but not challenged served as controls. The inhibitory
effect of the challenging dose on electrical stimulation of
longitudinal muscle decreased with successive days of morphine
administration; by the 10th day there was almost complete
tolerance to the challenging dose. Sensitivity of the tissues
of chronically morphinized unchallenged controls towards
acetylcholine, serotonin, histamine and norepinephrine was
essentially the same as that of naive animals. The potency of
morphine in vitro in blocking electrical stimulation was also
unchanged by chronic morphine administration in the above
manner. Thus tolerance to injected morphine cannot be explained
by reduced affinity of the drug for the opiate receptor.
Tissues of chronically morphinized animals gave a contracture
with naloxone, the extent of the contracture increasing with
time of drug administration. This naloxone effect is attributed
to displacement of morphine from a new opiate receptor site
induced during morphine administration. It is suggested that
this new receptor is involved in tolerance to injected morphine
as well as some aspects of the withdrawal syndrome.

Beginning with the pioneering studies of Paton on electrically stimulated
guinea pig ileum (1), it has been recognized that this tissue is uniquely
favorable for studying many aspects of the actions of opiates. Among the
properties of the tissue which have a direct bearing on this field the following may be cited: 1. An almost perfect correlation between potency of a
large series of opiates in blocking cholinergic transmission and effectiveness
as analgesics in man and other species (2,3,4). 2. Ability of known
antagonists to act in a similar way on the ileum. This includes both pure
and mixed type antagonists (5,6). 3. Demonstration that the tissue can show

---

[1]Experimental studies in this laboratory were supported by USPHS grants
DA 00496 and NS 03226.
[2]A preliminary report of these results was presented at the FASEB meeting,
Atlantic City, April, 1975.

tolerance to the effects of morphine on transmission (1,6,7,8). To this list of similarities between ileum and CNS actions of opiates we have added two others: 1. Development by the ileum of tolerance to injected morphine by guinea pigs administered morphine chronically and 2. in vitro demonstration of a type of withdrawal from morphine which can be precipitated by exposing ilea of tolerant animals to naloxone in vitro. Preliminary evidence along these two lines has been presented (9,10); the present paper explores the underlying mechanism of these phenomena.

The paradigm for studying tolerance and withdrawal has been provided by our previous studies (9,10): If a naive guinea pig is administered a very large dose of morphine, 500-750 mg/kg, and the ileum removed 2 hours later, electrical stimulation fails to cause a contraction even if the tissue is washed for many hours. The injected drug evidently causes a change in the tissue which is essentially irreversible. On the other hand, this same dose administered to guinea pigs maintained for 1-2 weeks on morphine (200 mg/kg/day) is almost ineffectual in causing blockade of the response. Thus chronic administration of morphine can produce a change in the tissue which is clearly a manifestation of tolerance. In this paper we explore the conditions for this type of tolerance as well as the properties of ilea removed from animals administered morphine chronically, including sensitivity to acetylcholine (ACh), serotonin (5-HT), histamine, norepinephrine (NE) and morphine in vitro. In this way we could test the concept developed by Collier (11) that supersensitivity to one or more neurotransmitters is involved in tolerance development.

In addition, the relationship was determined between duration of administration of morphine and naloxone-induced contracture (9). It had previously been suggested (9) that this effect of naloxone, observed only in ilea exposed to morphine in vivo or in vitro can provide insight into the mechanism of tolerance and withdrawal.

Materials and Methods

The longitudinal muscles of naive and chronically morphinized guinea pigs were set up in the manner described by Rang (12) using the apparatus devised in this laboratory (9,13,14) for electrical stimulation. Tyrode's solution gassed with 95% O_2 and 5% CO_2 was used; bath temperature was 37C. For studying morphine and (NE), the tissue was stimulated at a current duration of 0.4 msec., 0.1 Hz, 60 volts. This gives about 80% of the maximum contraction height. To determine maximum contraction, current duration was increased to 2-4 msec.

Both morphine and NE block contractions. ED_{50} to both drugs was determined by the cumulative method as previously described (9,13,14). A small volume of the drug was added at a concentration which produced a measurable block of contractions; when this leveled off, additional drug was added to give a final concentration 2-3 times that of the initial. The procedure is repeated until height of contraction was less than 50% of the control (pre-drug) value. The tissue was washed several times for at least 30 minutes before being used for subsequent testing.

Cumulative dose-response curves to ACh and 5-HT were determined in the manner described by Ariens et al (15). Contraction was considered to be maximum when two successive concentrations of the drug produced essentially the same contraction height. The tissue was washed for at least 30 minutes before being used again.

Injection schedule: For chronic administration of morphine the following procedure was used: On day 1 the animals were injected i.p. twice with 30mg/kg on day 2 with 60 mg/kg, and thereafter with 100 mg/kg twice daily. Food and water was given ad lib. Animals were weighed each day and were found to lose significant weight with time of morphine administration. Two animals given morphine for 3, 7 and 10 days were sacrificed. One of the two was injected with 750 mg/kg morphine i.p., sacrificed 1 1/2 hours later and ileum removed; this was the challenged animal. The other animal was killed at the same time but given no additional drug; this served as the unchallenged control. In some experiments an unchallenged control and a naive animal were sacrificed at the same time for direct comparison of properties.

Naloxone-induced contracture: Pieces of whole ilea were used for this determination since the results with longitudinal muscle varied greatly. 4-5 cm of ileum from naive and chronically morphinized animals were set up for measuring contractions. After equilibration for 1 hour, 40 ng/ml naloxone was added. Contracture, when it occurred, was allowed to proceed to completion, i.e., until the tension returned to base line. The outline of the tracing was traced on weighing paper, cut out and weighed.

Cross tolerance to methadone: It was determined that methadone, 100 mg/kg, given to a naive guinea pig produced almost complete block of electrically-induced contractions. This same dose was injected into guinea pigs injected for 10 days with morphine as described above.

RESULTS

Effect of the challenging dose of morphine: Fig. 1 shows the effect of injecting 750 mg/kg of morphine into a naive guinea pig and into one which had been injected with morphine for 10 days. It is apparent that the injected drug caused a complete block of electrically-induced contractions of the ileum of the naive animal whereas large contractions could be elicited from the ileum of the chronically morphinized guinea pig. These responses could be elicited despite the fact that this was a lethal dose. This is therefore a clear indication that tolerance had developed to injected morphine as a result of the chronic administration of the drug. The figure also shows that naloxone, 40 ng/ml causes a very different response in both tissues: a marked contracture of the ileum from the tolerant animal but only a reversal of block of contractions in the naive animal. Naloxone contractures could also be elicited from ilea removed from unchallenged animals (see below).

The only major effect on the naive ileum of the challenging dose is inhibition of electrically-induced contractions. Response to ACh was unaffected. Thus the site of action of the drug is neuronal and those changes which occur during tolerance arise within the nerve and not within the muscle.

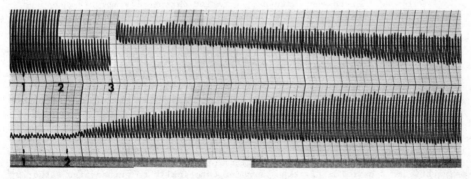

Fig. 1

Effect of challenging dose of morphine (750 mg/kg) on responses of longitudinal muscle of naive (lower panel) and 10 day chronically morphinized guinea pig (lower panel). Lower panel: 1. stimulator on; 2. naloxone, 40 ng/ml added to bath. Upper panel: 1. stimulator on; 2. sensitivity reduced; 3. naloxone added to bath.

<u>Time-course for development of tolerance</u>: Maximum contraction elicited by electrical stimulation in ilea of unchallenged and challenged animals are shown in Table 1. By day 10 the challenging dose is essentially ineffectual in causing an effect on transmission, i.e., contraction height in challenged and unchallenged ilea are almost the same. It may be noted that contraction height of the unchallenged tissue reaches a maximum on day 3 and then reverts back almost to normal (day zero) by day 10.

TABLE 1

Properties of Ilea from Chronically Morphinized Guinea Pigs*

Day	Max. Cont. mm		ED_{50} Morph. ng/ml		ED_{50} ACh ng/ml		ED_{50} 5HT ng/ml		ED_{50} NE μg/ml		Naloxone Contraction ‡
	Unch.	Chal.	Unch.	Chal.	Unch.	Chal.	Unch.	Chal.	Unch.	Chal.	
0	29	5	9	--	7	7	36	92	.3	--	0
3	45	20	11	72	6	12	34	33	1.1	0.8	22.2
7	41	16	14	132	5	6	19	46	.5	1.0	36.8
10	40	30	17	400	6	8	22	79	.9	2.0	68.2

* Average of 6-10 longitudinal muscles for unchallenged, 2-6 for challenged.
‡ Determined by weighing tracing of complete contraction. Average of 8-10 pieces of whole ileum.

<u>In vitro morphine responses</u>: Unchallenged ilea show essentially no change in sensitivity to morphine given <u>in vitro</u> over the entire time period of chronic administrations of the drug (Table 1). However, the challenging dose of morphine does cause a marked decrease in morphine effectiveness; by day 10 an ED_{50} could not be determined and thus all the data in Table 1 are plotted as ED_{30}.

<u>Acetylcholine responses</u>: ED_{50} data for ACh, shown in Table 1, reveal that chronic morphine treatment causes very little if any change. Some desensitization to ACh by the challenging dose is apparent but only with the day 3 ileum.

<u>Serotonin responses</u>: Once again, little if any change in responsiveness of the tissue of chronically morphinized, unchallenged guinea pigs was discerned (Table 1). Some changes were noted in the challenged tissues, primarily a diminished response in the naive, challenged.

<u>Responses to norepinephrine</u>: Chronic morphinization caused fairly minimal changes in potency of NE in blocking electrically-induced contractions (Table 1, NE, unchal.). Although the ED_{50} did increase perhaps 3-fold on day 3, sensitivity returned essentially to normal by day 10. On the other hand, the challenged tissue showed a progressively increasing resistance to NE.

<u>Naloxone-induced contractures</u>: Data for chronically morphinized, unchallenged tissues exposed to naloxone (40 ng/ml) <u>in vitro</u> are compiled in Table 1. It is evident that the extent of contracture closely parallels the development of tolerance. Naloxone does not cause any overt effect on ileum of naive guinea pig.

<u>Cross tolerance with methadone</u>: Methadone, 100 mg/kg, injected into guinea pigs maintained for 10 days on morphine, caused little effect on transmission of the ileum <u>in vitro</u>. This same dose completely blocked transmission when administered to a naive guinea pig.

Discussion

The present results show that it is possible to demonstrate development of tolerance and cross-tolerance to the depressant effect of injected opiates on cholinergic transmission in the ileum of the guinea pig. Several other investigators have administered morphine chronically to guinea pigs either by pellet implantation (16) or chornic injection (3,17) and have examined the properties of ilea <u>in vitro</u>. In some instances it has been shown that this treatment results in a decreased sensitivity to morphine. However, an <u>in</u>

vitro effect does not necessarily shed light on the mechanism of tolerance when the drug is administered to the animal. The implication of decreased sensitivity to morphine _in vitro_ is that tolerance results from a reduced affinity of the opiate for the receptor and thus larger and large doses are required to produce the initial effect. Our results, in agreement with those of Fennessy et al (3), reveal that this most likely is not the case since chronic administration of morphine does not in itself produce a change in the opiate receptor. Direct determination of affinity of opiates to receptors, using stereospecific binding, has shown that such binding increases with little if any change in affinity (18).

Our results provide a possible explanation for the lack of agreement of the effect of chronic morphine administration on the affinity of the drug for its ileal receptors _in vitro_. The potency of morphine _in vitro_ apparently depends greatly on the level of morphine administered to the animal. Our unchallenged controls are comparable to those of Fennessy et al (3), i.e., we both gave 200 mg/kg/day. Such ilea, which are tolerant to the challenging dose, have receptors which show their normal affinity for morphine. On the other hand, Schulz et al (16) and Haycock and Rees (17) actually gave massive doses of morphine to their animals, the former by means of pellets (4-75 mg pellets/animal) the latter by injection of up to 1 gm/kg/day. Such doses correspond to those of our challenging dose which, as noted in Fig. 3, results in an ileum that is indeed highly resistant to morphine _in vitro_. Our results in effect show that it is unnecessary to resort to such massive amounts of the drug in order to achieve total tolerance to the blocking action of morphine on cholinergic transmission and that tolerance to injected morphine is not necessarily associated with an altered affinity of the drug for its receptors.

The finding that the challenged ileum _in vitro_ is resistant to morphine would not explain tolerance to the injected drug. Tolerance must be related to changes occurring under the influence of chronic exposure to morphine, and this must be related to the properties of the unchallenged morphinized ilea. This increased resistance may reflect an exaggeration of the acute tolerance or tachyphylaxis shown by a naive ileum exposed to morphine (1,6,7,8). Such an effect most likely is not related to tolerance development _in vivo_ since _in vitro_ tolerance develops rapidly and is readily reversible. It is doubtful that the _in vitro_ exposure imparts any kind of permanant change in properties of the ileum as is the case of chronic morphinization.

At one time or another, the following transmitters, putative transmitters or modulators have been implicated in development of tolerance to opiates: ACh (7,11), NE (19), 5-HT (16,20), dopamine (21), and cyclic AMP (22). With our demonstration that tolerance to injected morphine could be shown in an _in vitro_ system, it became relatively straightforward to test at least some of these proposals. It is evident from the data presented on the time-course for development of tolerance that ACh, NE and 5-HT are not involved since, although some changes in affinity of these for their receptors were noted, in general these were minor and showed no correlation with tolerance development. At the present time we have not tested dopamine's possible involvement since this compound has relatively unimpressive effects on transmission in the ileum. With regard to cyclic AMP, we have obtained evidence that the adenylate cyclase system plays little if any role in effects of opiates on transmission in the ileum.

The excitatory action of naloxone on ilea of chronically morphinized guinea pigs, manifested as a contracture, increases progressively with time on morphine. This phenomenon, not observed with normal ileum, was first described by Ehrenpreis and coworkers (9); evidence was presented that this effect is due to liberation of ACh from the tissue. It has been proposed (9) that this type of release of ACh in the CNS and periphery could give rise to opiate withdrawal symptoms, many of which are cholinergic in nature. However, there are conflicting reports concerning the effect of cholinergic blocking agents in altering symptoms of withdrawal. Crossland (23), Brase et al (24), Jhamandas and coworkers (25,26) reported that atropine attenuates several such symptoms, whereas Collier et al (27) contend that atropine both depressed and enhanced some of the signs of withdrawal.

One possible explanation for tolerance is provided by the effect of naloxone. It has been suggested (9) that the contracture which this antagonist causes in ilea of animals injected with morphine is due to displacement of morphine from a secondary receptor site with concomitant release of ACh. It is possible that this receptor, which may be present on synaptic vesicles, is induced during the course of chronic morphine administration. As a result, the drug which enters the nerve terminals is strongly bound to this secondary receptor thereby being prevented from combining with the primary morphine receptor which is involved in the coupling between electrically-induced excitation and ACh release. Hence transmission may be normal, as in the ileum from guinea pigs injected for 10 days with morphine, despite the presence of very large amounts of drug in the tissue.

References

1. D.M. PATON, Brit. J. Pharmac. 11 119-127 (1957.
2. B.M. COX and M. WEINSTOCK, Brit. J. Pharmacol. 27 81-92 (1966).
3. M.R. FENNESSY, R.L.H. HEIMANS and M.J. RAND, Brit. J. Pharmacol. 37 436-449 (1969).
4. L.S. HARRIS and W.L. DEWEY, Agonist and Antagonist Actions of Narcotic Analgesic Drugs, pp. 198-206 University Park Press, Baltimore (1973).
5. H.W. KOSTERLITZ and A.J. WATT, Brit. J. Pharmacol. 33 266-276 (1968).
6. E.A. GYANG and H.W. KOSTERLITZ, Brit. J. Pharmacol. 27 514-521 (1966).
7. S. SHOHAN and M. WEINSTOCK, Brit. J. Pharmacol. 52 597-603 (1974).
8. H.W. KOSTERLITZ and A.A. WATERFIELD, Brit. J. Pharmacol. 53 131-138 (1975).
9. S. EHRENPREIS, I. LIGHT and G.H. SCHONBUCH, Drug Addiction: Experimental Pharmacology, pp. 319-342 Futura Pub. Co., Mt. Kisco, N.Y. (1972).
10. S. EHRENPRETS, J. GREENBERG and J. COMATY, Fed. Proc. 34 736 (1975).
11. H.O.J. COLLIER, Nature 220 228-231 (1968).
12. H.P. RANG, Brit. J. Pharmacol. 22 356-365 (1964).
13. S. EHRENPREIS, Methods in Narcotics Research, M. Dekker, New York (1975) (in press).
14. S. EHRENPREIS, Advances in General and Cellular Pharmacology, Plenum Pub. Co., New York (1975) (in press).
15. E.J. ARIENS, A.M. SIMONIS and J.M. VAN ROSSUM, Molecular Pharmacology, p. 119 Academic Press, New York (1964).
16. R. SCHULZ, C. CARTWRIGHT, and A. GOLDSTEIN, Nature 251 329-331 (1974).
17. V.K. MAYCOCK and J.M.H. REES, J. Pharm. Pharmacol. 24 47-52 (1972).
18. R.J. HITZEMANN, B.A. HITZEMANN and H.H. LOH, Life Sci. 14 2393-2402 (1974).
19. M. WEINSTOCK, Brit. J. Pharmacol. 17 433-442 (1961).
20. A. GOLDSTEIN and R. SCHULZ, Brit. J. Pharmacol. 48 655-666 (1973).
21. K. FUKUI and H. TAKAGI, Brit. J. Pharmacol. 44 45-51 (1972).
22. I.K. HO, H.H. LOH, E.L. WAY, J. Pharmacol. Exp. Ther. 185 347-357 (1973).
23. J. CROSSLAND, Agonist and Antagonist Actions of Narcotic Analgesic Drugs, pp. 235-239 University Park Press, Baltimore (1973).
24. D.A. BRASE, L. TRENG, H.H. LOH and E.L. WAY, Eur. J. Pharmacol. 26 1-8 (1974).
25. K. JHAMANDAS and G. DICKINSON, Nature New Biol. 245 219-221 (1973).
26. K. JHAMANDAS, M. SUTAK and S. BELL, Eur. J. Pharmacol. 24 296-305 (1973).
27. H.O.J. COLLIER, D.L. FRANCIS and C. SCHNEIDER, Nature 237 220-223 (1972).

POSSIBLE ROLE OF BRAIN HISTAMINE IN MORPHINE ADDICTION
(Received in final form May 24, 1975)

R. W. Henwood[1] and I. M. Mazurkiewicz-Kwilecki[2,3]
Department of Pharmacology, Faculty of Medicine, Ottawa University
275 Nicholas Street, Ottawa, Ontario, Canada.

Several biogenic amines have been suggested to play a possible role in opiate addiction. While some reports indicated changes in brain norepine-phrine and dopamine concentrations and/or synthesis (1,2,3), others have demonstrated the involvement of serotonin or acetylcholine (4,5,6,7). In view of recent reports suggesting a possible role for histamine in brain function as another putative neurotransmitter (8), we have investigated whether this bio-genic amine might also participate in morphine addiction and withdrawal.

Materials and Methods

In acute experiments, male Sprague Dawley rats (200-225 g) were injected intraperitoneally (i.p.) with morphine, methadone, or naloxone and sacrificed one hour after the morphine or methadone and 20 minutes following naloxone injection. In chronic studies the rats (starting weights 150-160 g) were treated i.p. with increasing doses of morphine according to the method of Takemori (9) and killed 18 hours after their last injection.

Histamine was determined by the double isotope technique of Taylor and Snyder (10) using ^{14}C-S-adenosylmethionine as the methyl donor and adding tracer quantities of ^{3}H-histamine to correct for the varying degree of hista-mine methylation in different samples. ^{14}C-^{3}H-methylhistamine and ^{14}C-methyl-histamine were separated from ^{3}H-histamine and ^{14}C-S-adenosylmethionine by extracting into chloroform from a salt-saturated alkaline solution.

Results and Discussion

Endogenous histamine concentrations of the hypothalamus, brain stem, or cortex were not significantly changed after acute treatments with morphine (30mg/kg), methadone (5mg/kg), or with naloxone (0.4mg/kg), however chronic treatment with increasing doses of morphine for 21 days resulted in a signifi-cant decrease in the endogenous brain histamine concentration in the hypo-thalamus (71.5±4.6% of control). Decreases in the brain stem (92.3±8.3% of control) and cortex (77.6±16.7% of control) were also noted although they were not statistically significant.

The naloxone-induced withdrawal syndrome in rats treated with morphine for 21 days as judged by wet dog shakes, teeth chattering, weight loss, and temperature decline, resulted in a further decrease in the endogenous histamine concentrations in the hypothalamus (64.0±5.5% of control), brain stem (84.6±10.3% of control) and cortex (66.7±5.1% of control), which were, however, not significantly greater than the decrease seen in the morphine-treated rats.

Abrupt withdrawal of morphine after 21 days of chronic morphine treatment and replacement with saline injections for an additional 2 days, induced a further significant decrease in the histamine concentrations in the hypo-thalamus (53.5±2.9% of control), brain stem (67.7±9.7% of control), and cortex (50.0±4.5% of control).

[1] Ontario Mental Health Foundation Research Student.
[2] This project was supported by OMHF grant # 379-71 D.
[3] Requests for reprints to be addressed to I.M. Mazurkiewicz-Kwilecki.

These changes were statistically significant not only when compared with control rats treated with saline for an identical period of time but also with rats chronically treated with morphine for 21 or 23 days.

Replacement of morphine, after 21 days of chronic treatment, with methadone (15mg/kg), for an additional 2 days, resulted in histamine values not different from those seen in the hypothalamus, brain stem, or cortex of rats chronically treated with morphine alone for 21 or 23 days. The morphine-methadone treated rats however, had significantly higher histamine concentrations in the three brain regions studied, than those seen in animals abruptly withdrawn from morphine.

The presently observed decrease in histamine concentration induced by chronic morphine administration was most intense in the hypothalamus. This coincides with the highest concentration and a very rapid turnover of histamine in this brain region (11). The decrease in histamine concentration occurred only after chronic treatment which could indicate a slowly developing process which might have been due to an induced imbalance between the rate of synthesis and metabolism or release of this biogenic amine. Morphine is known to release histamine from the rat peripheral tissues (12) and chronic histamine administration influences catecholamine concentrations in the brain and peripheral tissues of rat (13). The already reported changes in the concentration or synthesis of other biogenic amines after morphine administration could have been triggered by, associated with, or secondary to, a decrease of brain histamine.

It seems now acceptable that not one biogenic amine but the interaction between several of them may play an important role in the complicated processes linked with tolerance development and addiction. Our present data indicates that in addition to other biogenic amines, histamine may be involved in the mechanism of morphine addiction.

References

1. Narcotic Drugs, Biochemical Pharmacology, Ed. D.H. Clouet, Plenum Press New York (1971).

2. K. KUSCHINSKY, Experientia, 29, 1365-1366, (1973).

3. J.C. JOHNSON, M. RATNER, G.T. GOLD, D.H. CLOUET, Res. Comm. in Chem. Path. and Pharm., 9, 41-53, (1974).

4. A. HERZ, J. BLASIG, R. PAPESCHI, Psychopharm. (Berl), 39, 121-143 (1974).

5. S. KNAPP, A.J. MANDELL, Science, 177, 1209-1211, (1972).

6. F.H. SHEN, H.H. LOH, E.L. WAY, J. Pharm. Expt. Ther., 175, 427-434, (1970).

7. E.F. DOMINO, A. WILSON, J. Pharm. Expt. Ther., 184, 18032, (1973).

8. S.H. SNYDER, K.M. TAYLOR, p. 43-73 in Perspectives in Neuropharmacology Ed. S.H. Snyder, Oxford University Press, Toronto (1972).

9. A.E. TAKEMORI, J. Pharm. Expt. Ther., 130, 370-374, (1960).

10. K.M. TAYLOR, S.H. SNYDER, J. Neurochem., 19, 1343-1358, (1972).

11. K. DISMUKES, S.H. SNYDER, Brain Res., 78, 101-109, (1974).

12. A.M. ROTHSCHILD, P. 386-430 in Handbook of Experimental Pharmacology Ed. O. Eichler and A. Farah, Springer-Verlag, New York (1966).

13. I.M. MAZURKIEWICZ-KWILECKI and D.A.V. PETERS, Biochem. Pharm., 22, 3225-3235, (1973).

SINGLE NEURON STUDIES OF OPIATE ACTION IN THE GUINEA PIG MYENTERIC PLEXUS

Raymond Dingledine and Avram Goldstein

Department of Pharmacology, Stanford University, and Addiction Research Foundation, Palo Alto, California 94304.[1]

(Received in final form May 24, 1975)

Summary

The action of narcotics and other drugs on electrical activity of neurons in the guinea pig myenteric plexus was examined by extracellular recording with a suction electrode. Morphine, in a stereospecific and naloxone-sensitive action, inhibits spontaneous electrical activity of many neurons, and antagonizes an increased firing rate caused by serotonin or nicotine. The inhibition by morphine of spontaneous electrical activity occurs under conditions of synaptic transmission blockade, which renders unlikely several possible synaptic mechanisms in the primary effect of opiates. Morphine was found not to alter conduction velocity of myenteric neurons. It is concluded that morphine probably acts to reduce the excitability of a class of myenteric plexus neurons, perhaps by hyperpolarizing or stabilizing the membrane potential.

The myenteric plexus of the guinea pig ileum is a network of nonmyelinated nerve fibers with ganglia (containing cell bodies) at intersections of the net, and is situated between the circular and longitudinal muscle layers of the gut. This tissue was developed, initially by Paton and Kosterlitz, as a peripheral system to study the effects of narcotic opiates. The relevancy of this tissue to the central actions of opiates has been reviewed by Ehrenpreis et al. (1).

Over the last decade the neuronal organization of this tissue has been extensively studied. It has become clear that the myenteric plexus is not merely a parasympathetic "relay station" in the classic sense, but rather presents a fairly complex synaptic organization. In addition to the well-recognized parasympathetic pathway, there is now solid histochemical evidence for a dense network of adrenergic and serotoninergic fibers that seem to terminate on or near myenteric ganglion cells (2-6). Catecholamine-containing nerve cell bodies are absent in the myenteric plexus of the guinea pig ileum (2-4,6), but scattered groups of serotonin-containing cell bodies have recently been reported (7). There is also evidence for non-adrenergic inhibitory intrinsic neurons that innervate the longitudinal muscle layer (8).

The longitudinal muscle with adherent myenteric plexus can be stripped from the ileum, mounted in an organ bath and driven by electrical field stimulation to contract. The electrically-induced contraction is inhibited by morphine (9-11) and by catecholamines via an α-adrenergic receptor (12,13). In both cases this inhibition is a result of interference with acetylcholine

---

[1] Experimental studies in this laboratory were supported by National Institute on Drug Abuse grants DA-972 and DA-249. R.D. is a National Science Foundation Pre-doctoral Fellow.

release from myenteric neurons, but the primary site and nature of the morphine effect are unknown. Exogenous serotonin and nicotine cause a contraction of the longitudinal muscle that is blocked by atropine or scopolamine
(14,15), and is therefore probably due to excitation of cholinergic motor
neurons in the plexus. Morphine also antagonizes contraction induced by serotonin (14,16) or nicotine (17,18). The above evidence has led to the model
of synaptic organization of the myenteric plexus shown in Figure 1 (19,20).
This model postulates that cholinergic, serotoninergic and adrenergic neuronal
pathways all converge on the cholinergic motor neuron. Pre-synaptic inhibition by presumed adrenergic neurons has recently been postulated (21). The
complex neural circuitry proposed for the myenteric plexus, and the several
actions of morphine on this tissue, provide many possibilities for the primary
site of narcotic action. Morphine might act directly on cholinergic nerve
terminals to exert "pre-synaptic" inhibition of acetylcholine release (1).
Alternatively, opiates may oppose excitatory transmission at serotoninergic
synapses, as suggested by Schulz and Cartwright (19). Although Kosterlitz
and Wallis have shown that morphine does not disrupt axonal conduction in
fibers of the rabbit vagus or cat saphenous and hypogastric nerves (22), it is
possible that opiates exert a local anesthetic effect on the very fine unmye-
linated nerve fibers of the myenteric plexus. It is unlikely that opiates act
to block nicotinic receptors, or to stimulate release of norepinephrine, since
morphine is still active in the guinea pig ileum in the presence of hexamethonium, phenoxybenzamine and propranolol (23).

We have investigated various electrophysiologic aspects of opiate action
in the myenteric plexus, with the aim of describing at the neuronal level the
nature and primary site of narcotic action.

Methods

Male guinea pigs, 300-500 g., were decapitated, the ileum was removed,
and the longitudinal muscle with attached myenteric plexus was stripped off
and mounted in a 1 ml organ bath set up for extracellular recording with a

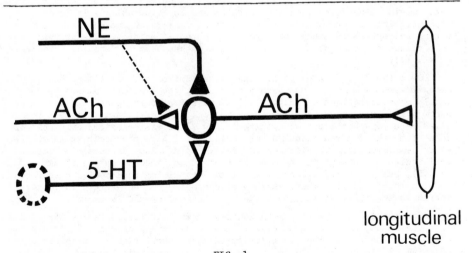

FIG. 1
Possible synaptic organization of the myenteric plexus. Excitatory synapses
(open) made by cholinergic (ACh) and serotoninergic (5HT) neurons, and inhibitory synapses (solid) made by adrenergic neurons (NE) are shown. The non-
adrenergic inhibitory system, although recognized, is not shown in this figure.

suction electrode, as described previously (20). To minimize spontaneous muscle movement an area of approximately 1 mm^2 was cut out and pinned to a thin layer of silicone rubber (Sylgard #184) at the base of the organ bath. When required a second suction electrode used for point stimulation was positioned near the recording electrode, on the same or on an adjacent ganglion. Following single stimuli, both directly driven ("antidromic") and synaptically driven spikes were observed. During point stimulation atropine (10^{-7}M) was present to reduce local muscle twitches.

A Krebs-bicarbonate buffer (20) was continuously perfused over the preparation at 36-37°C. and removed by continuous aspiration. Drug solutions were prepared in separate reservoirs of buffer and washed into the bath through a three-way valve. Electrical signals were amplified and displayed as described previously (20). Action potentials were separated from background noise by a voltage gating circuit and converted to pulses of constant size. They were then integrated over 5-sec intervals and the neuron firing rate displayed on a polygraph. Drug effects were measured as a change in unit firing rate.

Results

Effect of drugs on spontaneous electrical activity

Most units fired irregularly at rates of 1-10/sec, although occasionally a "burst-type" unit (24) was seen (but not studied further). The firing rate of a majority of units tested was decreased by norepinephrine and increased by serotonin and nicotine (Table 1). Most cells were inhibited by morphine (Table 1), although two neuronal populations could be distinguised, based on relative sensitivity to morphine. The observation that hexamethonium was without effect on firing rate (Table 1) indicates that the electrical activity

TABLE 1

Drug Effects on Spontaneous Firing of Myenteric Neurons

Drug	Concentration (µM)	Units responding with [1]			Firing rate in presence of drug [2]	Number of units tested
		+	–	0		
Serotonin	1.0	69%	8%	23%	410% ± 25%	119
Nicotine	6.0	96	0	4	330 ± 28	23
morphine	0.1	0	50	50	18.5 ± 4.2	32
morphine	0.3	0	73	27	15.2 ± 2.3	33
morphine	0.6	0	100	0	30.3 ± 10.7	8
levorphanol	0.3	5	80	15	9.7 ± 3.2	20
dextrorphan	0.3	4	0	96	––	22
norepinephrine	3.0	0	71	29	30.0 ± 8.9	14
naloxone	0.3 - 1.0	0	5	95	––	19
hexamethonium	10-30	0	10	90	81	10

1. "+" defined as an increased firing rate (>115% of control), "–" as a decreased firing rate (< 85% of control) and "0" as no effect (85-115% of control.

2. Drug-induced firing rate, as per cent of spontaneous firing rate preceding drug addition. Data refer only to units stimulated by serotonin or nicotine, or inhibited by morphine, levorphanol, norepinephrine, or hexamethonium. Data are mean ± SEM.

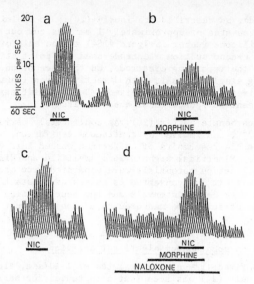

FIG. 2.
Effects of nicotine and morphine on the firing rate of a myenteric neuron.
Drugs were added to the tissue chamber in the order shown by a–d, 10–30 min
being allowed between each test. Nicotine excited this unit (a,c), and morphine, although having little effect of its own, partially antagonized this
nicotine effect (b). Naloxone antagonized the ability of morphine to reduce
nicotine-induced excitation (d). Drugs are $6 \cdot 10^{-6}$M nicotine (NIC), 10^{-6}M
morphine and 10^{-6}M naloxone.

observed was not a result of tonic excitation by cholinergic inputs to cells
under study. The inhibition by morphine of spontaneous activity is stereospecific (Table 1) and blocked by naloxone (20), and is therefore considered
a "typical opiate effect". We have previously reported that morphine, in a
stereospecific and naloxone sensitive action, antagonizes the increase in firing rate induced by serotonin (20). Morphine also antagonized a nicotine-
induced elevation in firing rate in seven of eight cells tested. Pre-exposure
of units to $6-10 \cdot 10^{-7}$M morphine for 60 sec reduced nicotine-induced firing to
$47.4\% \pm 8.4\%$ (mean $\pm$ SEM; n=7) of the rate in the presence of nicotine alone.
An example is shown in Figure 2. This effect of morphine was antagonized by
10^{-6}M naloxone in both cases tested (e.g., Figure 2), and was stereospecific.
That is, nicotine-induced elevation in unit firing rate was reduced to 6.7%
$\pm 5.0\%$ (n=6) of control rate in the presence of $6 \cdot 10^{-7}$M levorphanol, but in the
same cells was $95\% \pm 3.5\%$ of control rate in the presence of $6 \cdot 10^{-7}$M dextrorphan. The nicotine-induced excitation was also blocked by $1-3 \cdot 10^{-5}$M hexamethonium in seven of eight units tested.

These data provide no evidence for a unique relation between morphine and
serotoninergic synapses in the myenteric plexus, as suggested earlier (19,20).

Effect of morphine under synaptic transmission blockade

Evidence is presented elsewhere (25) that in the presence of Ca-free
Ringer containing 4.8 mM Mg and 2.4 mM EGTA, synaptic transmission in the myenteric plexus is eliminated or greatly reduced. The ability of morphine to
inhibit spontaneous activity was determined on the same neuron in normal Ringer and in Ca-free, high-Mg Ringer. The data, shown in Table 2, indicate that
the ability of morphine to inhibit spontaneous activity is only slightly reduced under conditions of synaptic transmission blockade.

Effect of morphine on axonal conduction

Single pulses applied by point stimulation elicited compound action potentials with constant latency in the range 0.5-6 msec. These spikes could follow stimuli at frequencies up to 30 Hz, and are considered to be the result of antidromic invasion of myenteric neurons. Conduction velocity of these fibers was very low, in the range 0.07-0.5 m/sec, in agreement with the findings of Nishi and North (26). Morphine, in a concentration which markedly inhibits spontaneous activity ($3 \cdot 10^{-7}$M), had no effect on conduction velocity or antidromic spike size, while lidocaine (10^{-3}M) decreased conduction velocity and spike amplitude of the same cells. These findings confirm extensive observations made by Kosterlitz and Wallis (22) that morphine has no local anesthetic properties at normal pharmacologic concentrations.

Discussion

Morphine, which inhibits release of acetylcholine from myenteric neurons, inhibits the spontaneous electrical activity of many neurons in the plexus. Furthermore, morphine is able to inhibit spontaneous activity of myenteric neurons that are receiving no synaptic input. Assuming a single site of morphine action in the myenteric plexus, this finding makes it unlikely that the primary effect of opiates is to stimulate release of an inhibitory transmitter, to prevent release of an excitatory transmitter, or to block the post-synaptic receptor for an excitatory transmitter. The antagonism by opiates of the increase in firing rate caused by serotonin or nicotine is therefore probably post-synaptic, although not due to receptor blockade. We found no evidence that morphine disrupts axonal conduction of myenteric neurons. Morphine

TABLE 2

Morphine Effect in Normal Ringer and in Ca-free Ringer[1]

morphine	% inhibition [2]		ratio
	normal Ringer	Ca-free Ringer	Ca-free / normal
$1 \cdot 10^{-8}$M	7%	7%	1.00
$4 \cdot 10^{-8}$M	76	70	0.92
	97	88	0.91
	100	88	0.88
$9 \cdot 10^{-8}$M	85	85	1.00
	95	88	0.93
	48	33	0.69
	68	31	0.46
	92	92	1.00
$3 \cdot 10^{-7}$M	91	100	1.10
	82	56	0.68
	100	100	1.00
		mean ±	0.88 ±
		SEM	0.05

1. "Ca-free Ringer" also contains four times the normal Mg concentration and 2.4 mM EGTA.

2. Inhibition of spontaneous electrical activity, as per cent of pre-drug firing rate. Each line gives data from one unit. Each value is the average of 1-3 determinations.

probably decreases the excitability of a class of myenteric neurons, perhaps by hyperpolarizing or stabilizing the membrane potential. This hypothesis can best be tested by intracellular recording. It is not clear whether this hypothesis is sufficient to account for all opiate actions in the myenteric plexus. In several cells (e.g., Figure 2) morphine antagonized excitatory effects of serotonin or nicotine while having little or no effect on spontaneous firing rate.

References

1. S. Enrenpreis, I. Light and G. H. Schonbuch, in Drug Addiction, Experimental Pharmacology. J. H. Singh, L. H. Millerand and H. Lal (eds). Futura Pub. Co., Mount Kisco, N.Y. (1972).

2. K.A. Norberg, Int. J. Neuropharmacol., 3, 379–382 (1964).

3. J.B. Read and G. Burnstock, Histochemie, 17, 263–272 (1969).

4. R.G. Robinson and M.D. Gershon, J. Pharmacol. Exp. Ther., 178, 311–324 (1971).

5. L.L. Ross and M.D. Gershon, J. Cell Biol., 55, 220a (1972).

6. M. Costa and J.B. Furness, Histochem. J., 5, 343–349 (1973).

7. M.D. Gershon and C.F. Dreyfus, Fed. Proc., 34, 810 (1975).

8. G. Burnstock, Pharmacol. Rev., 24, 509–581 (1972).

9. W. Schaumann, Brit. J. Pharmacol., 12, 115–118 (1957).

10. W.D.M. Paton, Brit. J. Pharmacol., 12, 119–127 (1957).

11. W.D.M. Paton and A. Zar, J. Physiol. (London), 194, 13–33 (1968).

12. W.D.M. Paton and E.S. Visi, Brit. J. Pharmacol., 35, 10–28 (1969).

13. H.W. Kosterlitz, R.J. Lydon and A.J. Watt, Brit. J. Pharmacol., 39, 398–413 (1970).

14. G.H. Gaddum and Z.P. Picarrelli, Brit. J. Pharmacol., 12, 323–328 (1957).

15. G. Brownlee and E.S. Johnson, Brit. J. Pharmacol., 21, 306–322 (1963).

16. R. Schulz and C. Cartwright, J. Pharmacol. Exp. Ther., 190, 420–430 (1974).

17. H.W. Kosterlitz and J.A. Robinson, Brit. J. Pharmacol., 13, 296–303 (1958).

18. G.P. Lewis, Brit. J. Pharmacol., 15, 425–431 (1960).

19. R. Schulz and A. Goldstein, Nature, 244, 168–170 (1973).

20. R. Dingledine, A. Goldstein and J. Kendig, Life Sci., 14, 2209–2309 (1974).

21. G.D.S. Hirst and H.C. McKirdy, Nature, 250, 430–431 (1974).

22. H.W. Kosterlitz and D.I. Wallis, Brit. J. Pharmacol., 22, 499–510 (1964).

23. E.A. Gyang and H.W. Kosterlitz, Brit. J. Pharmacol., 27, 514–527 (1966).

24. J.D. Wood, Am. J. Physiol., 225, 1107–1113 (1973).

25. R. Dingledine and A. Goldstein, J. Pharmacol. Exp. Ther., submitted for publication (1975).

26. S. Nishi and R.A. North, J. Physiol. (London), 231, 471–491 (1973).

ACTION OF MORPHINE ON GUINEA-PIG MYENTERIC PLEXUS AND
MOUSE VAS DEFERENS STUDIED BY INTRACELLULAR RECORDING

R. Alan North[1] and Graeme Henderson

Unit for Research on Addictive Drugs, University of Aberdeen,
Aberdeen, Scotland.

(Received in final form May 24, 1975)

Morphine reduces the output of transmitter from the myenteric
plexus-longitudinal muscle preparation of the guinea-pig ileum and
from the mouse vas deferens.   Intracellular recordings were made
from ganglion cells of the myenteric plexus and smooth muscle cells
of the vas deferens.   Synaptic transmission within the myenteric
plexus was blocked by hexamethonium.   Morphine did not change the
properties of the ganglion cells, nor did it affect synaptic
potentials.   5-Hydroxytryptamine inhibited acetylcholine release
at intraganglionic synapses by an action which was unaffected by
morphine.   In the vas deferens, excitatory junction potentials
were elicited by stimulation of postganglionic adrenergic nerve
fibres.   The junction potentials were depressed by morphine and
levorphanol but not by dextrorphan.   This depression was reversed
by naloxone.   The results indicate that morphine acts directly to
reduce transmitter release at the neuro-effector junctions in the
myenteric plexus-longitudinal muscle preparation and in the vas
deferens in these species.

Narcotic analgesics have been shown to affect transmission at several
autonomic neuro-effector junctions (1).   Some of the effector organs are
difficult to isolate from ganglionic elements and it has been proposed that the
primary action of narcotics is on transmission within intramural ganglia (2)
rather than at the neuro-effector junction proper.   Morphine inhibits the
contraction of the longitudinal muscle of the guinea-pig ileum by depressing
the release of acetylcholine from the myenteric plexus (3).   The contractile
response of the mouse vas deferens and the output of noradrenaline from this
preparation have also been shown to be sensitive to narcotics (4).   The
receptors involved in these actions appear to be identical with those which
mediate analgesia in man (5).   The aim of the present experiments was to
elucidate the site and nature of these actions of morphine by intracellular
recording techniques.

Myenteric plexus ganglion cells

Intracellular recordings were made from ganglion cells by the method
previously described (6).   Individual ganglion cells were impaled under direct
vision and stable recordings were obtained for periods of up to 7 hours.
Neuronal elements were stimulated by means of a focal micro-electrode, the tip
of which was placed on the surface of the ganglion within 100 μm of the impaled
cell.   Two types of neuron are found in the myenteric plexus (6,7).   Type 1

[1]Present address: Department of Pharmacology, Loyola University Medical
Center, Maywood, Illinois 60153.

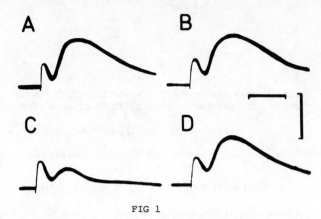

FIG 1

Absence of effect of morphine on a nicotinic e.p.s.p. in
a single myenteric plexus neuron.   A single focal stimulus
was applied to the surface of the ganglion at a distance of
40 μm from the impaled neuron.   This excited neuronal
elements which synapsed on the soma of the impaled ganglion
cell.   In this experiment, one of the processes of the
ganglion cell was also excited by the stimulus; this conducted to the soma and was recorded as an all-or-nothing
response of rapid time course (for further explanation, see
ref. 6).   A, Control.   B, after 10 min morphine (1 μM).
The e.p.s.p. is unaffected.   C, after 3 min hexamethonium
(100 μM).   The e.p.s.p. is depressed.   D, after 8 min
wash-out.   Calibrations: horizontal 20 ms, vertical 20 mV.

cells have properties similar to other autonomic ganglion cells and can be
excited synaptically.   Type 2 cells receive no synaptic input, are character-
ised by a slow after-hyperpolarisation following a single action potential and
are probably afferent (6-9).

　　Type 1 cells.   The excitatory postsynaptic potentials (e.p.s.p.) were
blocked by hexamethonium (10 - 400 μM), greatly prolonged by physostigmine (9)
and could be mimicked by iontophoretic application of acetylcholine to the cell
soma.   Morphine (1 - 10 μM) did not affect the e.p.s.p., nor did it alter
neuronal membrane potential or input resistance.   In several cells it was
possible to show that morphine had no action on a synaptic potential that could
be reversibly abolished by hexamethonium (Fig. 1) and by noradrenaline.   The
action of noradrenaline has been shown to be presynaptic (10).   Naloxone
(100 nM)did not change the amplitude of the e.p.s.p.

　　In most cells, 5-hydroxytryptamine (5-HT) (25 nM - 1 μM) reversibly depressed the e.p.s.p. without changing membrane potential or input resistance.
A depolarisation of time course similar to the e.p.s.p. produced by iontophoretic application of acetylcholine was not depressed by 5-HT; therefore this
action of 5-HT is presynaptic.   The action of 5-HT was not affected by
morphine (Fig. 2) but was antagonised by cyproheptadine, methysergide and
lysergic acid diethylamide.   In a few experiments, 5-HT produced an irreversible depolarisation and an increase or decrease in input resistance; these
findings were usually associated with, and probably caused by, an increase in
movement of the underlying muscle fibres which often accompanied the addition
of 5-HT.

Type 2 cells.   Morphine (1 - 10 μM) did not change the resting potential, action potential, input resistance or slow after-hyperpolarisation of Type 2 cells.   5-HT often caused a depolarisation associated with muscle movement. In preparations which did not move, 5-HT (1 μM) produced a hyperpolarisation and concomitant fall in input resistance.   This action of 5-HT reversed on washing and was not affected by morphine.   Noradrenaline (1 μM) had a similar action.

These experiments on myenteric neurons provide no evidence for non-cholinergic transmission within the plexus.   Morphine does not affect acetylcholine release at intraganglionic synapses, although release is depressed by 5-HT and by noradrenaline.   The absence of any effect of morphine on transmission

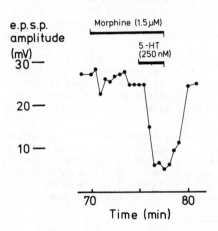

FIG 2

Effects of morphine and 5-HT on the amplitude of the e.p.s.p. in a single myenteric neuron.   The e.p.s.p. was elicited at 30 s intervals.   The e.p.s.p. in this cell was also reversibly abolished by 5-HT alone and by hexamethonium.

between neurons suggests that its action must be at the neuro-effector junction. This conclusion accords with the observation that morphine depresses the contractile response of the longitudinal muscle to field stimulation even in the presence of hexamethonium (11).

Extracellular recording has shown that 5-HT increases the firing rate of a proportion of neurons within the myenteric plexus, and that this effect is prevented by morphine (2,12).   But intracellular recording reveals no excitatory effects of 5-HT upon ganglion cell somata or upon intraganglionic synaptic transmission.   This disparity might be resolved by postulating that the excitatory effects of 5-HT and the inhibitory effect of morphine occur only at the varicose cell processes from which acetylcholine is released towards the muscle.   Spike activity in such processes would be recorded by extracellular but not necessarily by intracellular techniques.   This action of 5-HT could be mediated by Gaddum's M-receptors (13).

Mouse vas deferens

Intracellular recordings were made from single smooth muscle cells of the mouse vas deferens for periods of up to 4 hours.   The intramural nerves were stimulated with platinum ring electrodes at a distance of about 5 mm from the point of recording.   Each stimulus (0.033 Hz) was followed by an excitatory junction potential (e.j.p.).   The short latency of the e.j.p. (less than 10 ms) indicated direct stimulation of postganglionic neurons.

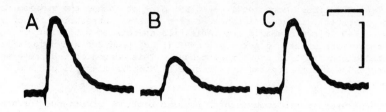

FIG 3

E.j.p.s in a single muscle cell of the mouse vas deferens.
A, control.   B, after 8 min exposure to morphine (1 μM).
The e.j.p. was depressed.   C, after 5 min exposure to
morphine (1 μM) and naloxone (100 nM).   The depression was
reversed.   Calibrations: horizontal 100 ms, vertical 20 mV.

Normorphine and morphine (50 nM - 5 μM) depressed the amplitude of the
e.j.p. in a dose-dependent manner.   Their action was antagonised by naloxone
(Fig. 3) and reproduced by levorphanol though not be a ten-fold higher concentration of dextrorphan.   Normorphine did not affect the resting membrane
potential of the smooth muscle cells, nor did it alter their sensitivity to
exogenous noradrenaline.

The mouse vas deferens receives an intimate innervation (14), the varicose
adrenergic fibres making close contacts with individual muscle cells.   Intracellular recording of e.j.p.s offers a sensitive method of studying factors
which affect transmitter release in this preparation.   Our findings strongly
support the conclusion (4) that morphine acts in the mouse vas deferens by
directly depressing the release of noradrenaline at the neuro-effector junction.

Acknowledgements

Supported by a grant to Dr. H. W. Kosterlitz from the U.S. National
Institute on Drug Abuse (DA 00662).   G.H. is an I.C.I. Research Fellow.

References

1. G.M. LEES, H.W. KOSTERLITZ and A.A. WATERFIELD, in Agonist and Antagonist
    Actions of Narcotic Analgesic Drugs, eds. H.W. Kosterlitz, H.O.J. Collier
    and J.E. Villarreal.   pp. 142-152.   Macmillan, London (1972).
2. R. DINGLEDINE, A. GOLDSTEIN and J. KENDIG, Life Sciences 14, 2299-2309
    (1974).
3. W.D.M. PATON, Brit. J. Pharmacol. 12, 119-127 (1957).
4. G. HENDERSON, J. HUGHES and H.W. KOSTERLITZ, Brit. J. Pharmacol. 46,
    764-766 (1972).
5. H.W. KOSTERLITZ and A.A. WATERFIELD, Ann. Rev. Pharmacol. 15, 29-47 (1975).
6. S. NISHI and R.A. NORTH, J. Physiol.,Lond. 231, 471-491 (1973).
7. G.D.S. HIRST, M.E. HOLMAN and I. SPENCE, J. Physiol.,Lond. 236, 303-326
    (1974).
8. R.A. NORTH, Brit. J. Pharmacol. 49, 709-711 (1973).
9. R.A. NORTH and S. NISHI, in Proc. IV Intern. Symp. Gastro-intestinal
    Motility, pp. 667-676.   Mitchell Press, Vancouver (1974).
10. S. NISHI and R.A. NORTH, J. Physiol.,Lond. 231, 29-30P (1973).
11. H.W. KOSTERLITZ and A.A. WATERFIELD, Brit. J. Pharmacol. 46, 569-570P
    (1972).
12. T. SATO, I. TAKAYANAGI and K. TAKAGI, Japan. J. Pharmacol. 23, 665-667
    (1973).
13. J.H. GADDUM and Z.P. PICARELLI, Brit. J. Pharmacol. 12, 323-328 (1957).
14. A. YAMEUCHI and G. BURNSTOCK, J. Anat. 104, 17-32 (1969).

EFFECTS OF MORPHINE, L-DOPA AND TETRABENAZINE ON THE
LAMINA V CELLS OF SPINAL DORSAL HORN

Hiroshi Takagi, Takayuki Doi and Kazuo Kawasaki

Department of Pharmacology, Faculty of Pharmaceutical Sciences
Kyoto University, Kyoto 606, Japan

(Received in final form May 24, 1975)

Summary

Experiments were performed to clarify the adrenergic
mechanism of morphine action in the spinal cord. Unit
activity of lamina V cell of spinal dorsal horn (L_6-L_7) of
the rabbit was recorded using microelectrode. An administration of bradykinin into the femoral artery markedly
increased in frequency of the unit activity. Morphine or
L-DOPA inhibited the bradykinin-induced response of lamina
V cell. In contrast, tetrabenazine facilitated the bradykinin-induced response. Electrical stimuli of the bulbar
reticular formation, particulary the nucleus reticularis
gigantocellularis markedly inhibited the dorsal horn response
induced by bradykinin injection. Effect of stimulation of
the bulbar reticular formation was blocked by tetrabenazine
and reversed by L-DOPA. These results support the hypothesis
that the bulbospinal catecholaminergic neuron inhibits the
pain transmission at the dorsal horn of the spinal cord and
analgesic action of morphine is mainly mediated by activation
of this neuron.

Recent microphysiological studies have shown that the lamina V cells in
the spinal dorsal horn play an important role in the integration and transmission of pain messages to brain, since they respond in a graded manner to
progressively more intense stimuli, including those at nociceptive levels
(1, 2, 3), receive visceral afferents (4, 5, 6), are activated by intra-
arterial injections of bradykinin (7, 8) and suppressed by analgesic doses
of morphine (7, 9). Moreover, we have shown that morphine depresses sensory
transmission through the spinal cord by strengthening activity of the
descending inhibitory system, particularly the noradrenergic system of brain
stem origin (7, 10, 11).
The present experiments were undertaken in order to obtain further
information on the relationship between analgesic action of morphine and
catecholaminergic neurons of the spinal cord.

Methods

This study was carried out on rabbits weighing 2 to 3 kg. The animals
were prepared under ether anesthesia, immobilized with gallamine triethiodide
(Flaxedil), artificially ventilated and placed a stereotaxic apparatus. The
vertebral column was immobilized with metal clamps. Laminectomy was carried
out, the dura mater opened and the cord exposed from L_5 to S_1, and covered
with warm paraffin oil (37-38°C). In some experiments the spinal cord

section was performed at L_2 level. Recordings were begun three hours after terminating ether anesthesia. Lidocaine was repeatedly applied to wound edges throughout the entire experiments. Extracellular unit activity was recorded from the left lamina V cells of L_6-L_7 segments using a tungsten microelectrode the tip of which was about 1 μ in diameter and the resistance of which remained between 1 and 3 megohms. The cells were selected according to the electrophysiological properties described by Wall (1) and Kitahata et al. (12). The potentials were amplified, displayed on an oscilloscope and photographed.

A polyethylene cannula of 0.9 mm diameter was introduced in a retrograding manner into the left deep femoral artery and tied into place in such a way that the tip was just distal to the bifurcation. Bradykinin (2 μg in 0.1 ml saline) was rapidly (1 sec or less) injected into the femoral artery through the cannula at intervals of 10 min. The cannula was flushed with saline (0.1-0.2 ml) 1-2 min after each bradykinin injection.

We recorded the spontaneous activity and the response to arterial bradykinin injection. In these cases we used a small computer (Nihon Koden ATAC 501-10S) to measure the number of unit activities occurring during second periods. The number of unit discharge of each neuron was counted for 60 sec before and after each bradykinin injection. To examine the effects of drugs, only those neurons in which unitary activity increased following bradykinin injection were used. The number of unit discharges after bradykinin minus the number before bradykinin is considered as bradykinin-induced. The 95% confidence limits were calculated from five values of the bradykinin-induced discharges before administration of the drug. If the values following two successive bradykinin injections after drug administration were either below or above the calculated 95% confidence limits, the effect of the drug was regarded as being inhibitory or facilitatory, respectively, and expressed as a percent change from control.

In some experiments, effects of electrical stimulation of the brain stem, particulary the nucleus reticularis gigantocellularis, on the bradykinin-induced response of lamina V cells were tested and effects of tetrabenazine and L-DOPA thereon were investigated.

After termination of experiments in which a typical response to bradykinin injection was observed, the location of the recording electrode in the spinal cord was histologically confirmed. Tips of the electrodes were located in cells which corresponded to the lamina V of cat's dorsal horn (14).

Morphine hydrochloride and L-DOPA were injected intravenously and tetrabenazine was given subcutaneously. Drug doses are given in terms of the salt.

Results

1. Morphine

Intravenous administration of morphine (0.3-2.0 mg/kg) to intact rabbits decreased the number of spontaneous activity as well as bradykinin-induced activity. Representative effects of 0.3 mg/kg and 2.0 mg/kg of morphine on the bradykinin-induced response are shown in FIG.1. When 2 mg/kg of morphine was injected, the inhibitory effects were observed in 6 out of 10 rabbits, facilitatory effect in 1 out of 10 and no change in 3 out of 10 rabbits. Their maximum inhibitory effects were obtained in 20-30 min after injections and lasted for 40-50 min. The inhibitory effects of morphine were antagonized by nalorphine (0.2 mg/kg) injected after 20-30 min. In spinal rabbits, morphine, at a dose of 2 mg/kg, did not inhibit the number of bradykinin-induced unit discharges, but at a dose of 5 mg/kg the response was inhibited. This inhibition was antagonized by nalorphine (0.5 mg/kg).

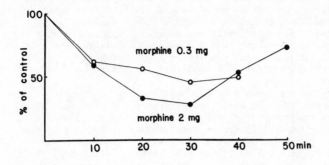

FIG. 1

Inhibitory effects of morphine on the bradykinin-
induced response of lamina V cell of the spinal
dorsal horn. Abscissa indicates time(min) after
morphine injection.

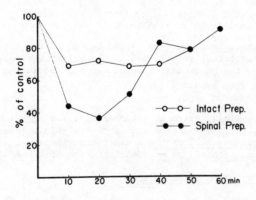

FIG. 2

Inhibitory effects of L-DOPA on the bradykinin-
induced response of lamina V cells of the spinal
dorsal horn in intact and spinal rabbits. Abscissa
indicates time (min) after L-DOPA injection.

2. L-DOPA

    Intravenous administration of L-DOPA (20 mg/kg) to intact rabbits
decreased the number of spontaneous activity as well as bradykinin-induced
activity. Typical effects of L-DOPA in intact and spinal rabbits are shown
in FIG. 2. Inhibitory effects of L-DOPA in spinal rabbits were more marked
than those in intact rabbits. Pure inhibitory effects of L-DOPA in spinal

rabbits were observed in 4 out of 8 rabbits, inhibitory effect with initial facilitation in 3 out of 8 and no change in 1 out of 8 rabbits.

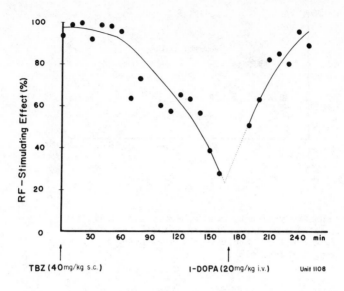

FIG. 3

Effects of tetrabenazine (TBZ) and L-DOPA on the inhibitory
effect of electrical stimulation of the bulbar reticular
formation on the bradykinin-induced response of lamina V cell.

3. Tetrabenazine

Subcutaneous administration of tetrabenazine (40 mg/kg) to intact
rabbits significantly increased the number of bradykinin-induced discharges
of the lamina V cells to 207% of the pretetrabenazine level. This effect of
tetrabenazine was antagonized by an administration of L-DOPA (20 mg/kg).

4. Electrical stimulation of brain stem

Electrical stimuli of the reticular formation of the midbrain and the
medulla oblongata inhibited bradykinin-induced reaction of lamina V cells.
The most effective area to electrical stimulation was the bulbar reticular
formation including the nucleus reticularis gigantocellularis. Tetrabenazine (40 mg/kg s.c.) blocked the inhibitory effect of bulbar reticular
formation and this effect was reversed by a subsequent administration of
20 mg/kg of L-DOPA (FIG. 3). However, the blocking effect of tetrabenazine
was not reversed by an administration of L-5-hydroxytryptophan (20 mg/kg).

Discussion

The possibilities that the descending inhibitory system from the bulbar
reticular formation to the lamina V cells of spinal dorsal horn consists of
noradrenergic neurons and that noradrenaline released from the descending
noradrenergic neuron inhibits pain transmission at the spinal level are
suggested from the present findings: 1) tetrabenazine, a monoamine depletor,

increased the number of bradykinin-induced discharge; 2) electrical stimulation of the bulbar reticular formation inhibited the bradykinin-induced response and this effect was blocked by tetrabenazine and reversed by L-DOPA, but not by L-5-hydroxytryptophan; 3) L-DOPA itself showed an inhibitory effect on the lamina V cells. Moreover, there is a definite evidence (15) that noradrenaline administered micro-electrophoretically to feline lumbar cord inhibits the activities of the dorsal horn neurons.

Previously we reported that the analgesic action of morphine was depressed by tetrabenazine pretreatment (14), that analgesic doses of morphine produced the increase in normetanephrine contents in the dorsal half of the spinal cord, without affecting its contents in the ventral half (11), and that morphine inhibited the transmission of pain at the spinal cord, through its facilitatory action on the descending inhibitory system of brain-stem origin (16).

These results support our hypothesis (11) that analgesic action of morphine is mainly mediated by activation of descending inhibitory noradrenergic neuron. However, the possibility that dopamine formed from L-DOPA in the spinal cord acts as an inhibitory transmitter at the dorsal horn cannot be ruled out. Moreover, it is interesting to note that a possible analgesic action of L-DOPA was suggested from the present results which this drug inhibited the activities of lamina V cells of the dorsal horn.

Acknowledgement

This work was supported in part by a grant from the Ministry of Education of Japan.

References

1. P.D. WALL, J. Physiol. 188, 403-423 (1967).
2. P. HILLMAN and P.D. WALL, Exp. Brain Res. 9, 284-306 (1969).
3. I.H. WAGMAN and D.D. PRICE, J. Neurophysiol. 32, 803-817 (1969).
4. B. POMERANZ, P.D. WALL and W.V. WEBER, J. Physiol. 199, 511-532 (1968).
5. M. SELZER and W.A. SPENCER, Brain Res. 14, 331-348 (1969).
6. M. SELZER and W.A. SPENCER, Brain Res. 14, 349-366 (1969).
7. M. SATOH, N. NAKAMURA and H. TAKAGI, Eur. J. Pharmacol. 16, 245-247 (1971).
8. J.M. BESSON, C. CONSEILLER, K.F. HAMANN and M.C. MAILLARD, J. Physiol. 221, 189-205 (1972).
9. L.M. KITAHATA, Y. KOSAKA, A. TAUB, K. BONIKOS and M. HOFFERT, Anesthesiol. 41, 39-48 (1974).
10. H. TAKAGI, M. MATSUMURA, A. YANAI and K. OGIU, Japan J. Pharmacol. 4, 176-187 (1955).
11. H. SHIOMI and H. TAKAGI, Brit. J. Pharmacol. 52, 519-526 (1974).
12. L.M. KITAHATA, A. TAUB and I. SATO, J. Pharmacol. Exp. Ther. 176, 101-108 (1971).
13. B. REXED, J. Comp. Neurol. 96, 415-495 (1952).
14. H. TAKAGI, T. TAKASHIMA and K. KIMURA, Arch. int. Pharmacodyn. 149, 484-492 (1964).
15. I. ENGBERG and R.W. RYALL, J. Physiol. 185, 298-322 (1966).
16. M. SATOH and H. TAKAGI, Eur. J. Pharmacol. 14, 60-65 (1970).

VIMINOL STEREOISOMERS AND LAMINA V INTERNEURONS ACTIVITY: PRELIMINARY RESULTS

Davide Della Bella* - Giancarlo Benelli* - Jean-Marie Besson**

* Zambon S.p.A. Research Laboratories, Bresso-Milan, Italy
** Laboratory of Physiology of Nervous Centers, University of Paris, Paris, France

(Received in final form May 24, 1975)

The pharmacological profile of Viminol, a pyrrylethanolamine synthetic derivative provided with central analgesic properties, and of its stereoisomers have been extensively described (1). Referring to the absolute configuration of the two sec.butyl radicals of the aminic group the biological properties of the Viminol stereoisomers can be summarized as follows: 1) the R,R configuration exhibits agonistic effects both on single and repeated administration; 2) the S,S configuration produces effects antagonistic to those of the R,R stereoisomers be they acute (analgesia) or chronic (physical dependence); 3) the R,S(S,R) or Meso configuration, on the contrary, do not modify the analgesic effects, but only oppose the R,R stereoisomers physical dependence producing capacity in rodents (2). Using the single dose suppression test in morphinized monkeys, however, the Viminol R,R stereoisomers do not appear to substitute for morphine. In the same experimental conditions the S,S stereoisomers, possessing antagonistic properties, and the Meso stereoisomers make the withdrawal signs more severe but do not precipitate directly a withdrawal syndrome in morphinized monkeys (3). To further illustrate the complex inter-relationship existing between the differently configurated Viminol stereoisomers and clarify their contribution to the resultant pharmacological profile of Viminol racemate whose analgesic activity has been assayed and proved in man by several Authors (4,5,6), some experiments were undertaken, in spinalized cats in which the lamina V interneurons activity was registered. The depressant influence of narcotic analgesics on the interneurons firing evoked by peripheral nociceptive stimulation has been widely described and its correlation with central analgesia has been proved (7,8,9). Our experiments were performed in 39 spinalized cats of both sexes, weighing 2 to 3 kg. 3 M KCl microelectrodes were used for search of extracellular characteristic lamina V interneurons activity at L 6th level and electrophoretic injection of pontamine blue was performed to determine the microelectrode tip position. The results obtained are the following: the Viminol R,R active enantiomer (R_2) intravenously administered at doses of 0.5 to 1 mg/kg reduces or abolishes the responses to nociceptive peripheral stimulation: in comparison with morphine Viminol R_2 appears 2-4 times more active, the R_1 enantiomer being on the contrary 20-40 times less active. A similar activity ratio has also been found in analgesic tests in vivo (2). In a few observations, the development of acute tolerance to the effects of R_2 second administration

FIG. 1

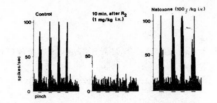

was found; a similar observation has been done also with morphine (8). As it appears from Fig. 1 intravenous naloxone, 0.1 mg/kg, completely abolishes R_2 effects. Viminol S,S configurated stereoisomer (active enantiomer S_2) shows (3 mg/kg i.v.) a full antagonism to R_2 effects. Even at higher dose (4 mg/kg) S_2 does not modify the morphine activity (1 mg/kg). Intravenous administration of Meso stereoisomers (0.5 to 4 mg/kg) neither influences the interneurons firing, nor the inhibitory effects produced by R_2 or morphine.

Conclusive remarks

The assignment of agonistic properties to the Viminol R,R configurated stereoisomers and of antagonistic activity to the S,S configurated ones appears confirmed. The correlation between the analgesic activity and the depression of the lamina V interneurons firing by nociceptive stimulation is strongly supported by the different degree of activity exhibited by Viminol R_1 and R_2 enantiomers. It is worthwhile mentioning that in contrast to the confirmed difference in the intrinsic activity of R_1 and R_2 the affinity of these two compounds for the synaptosomal binding sites has been shown to be practically of the same order of magnitude (D. Della Bella and A. Sassi, unpublished data).

References

1. D. DELLA BELLA, Boll. Chim. Farm. 111 5-19 (1972).
2. D. DELLA BELLA, V. FERRARI, V. FRIGENI, and P. LUALDI, Nature New Biology 241 282-284 (1973).
3. H.H. SWAIN, and M.H. SEEVERS, Proc. "Committee on Problems of Drug Dependence", 36th Annual Meeting, Mexico City, 10-14 March 1974, pp. 1168-1195.
4. G. BUZZELLI, M. GRAZZINI, and V. MONAFO, Curr. Therap. Res. 12 561-569 (1970).
5. L. MARTINETTI, E. LODOLA, V. MONAFO, and V. FERRARI, J. Clin. Pharmacol. 10 390-399 (1970).
6. F. NOBILI, and G.C. BERNARDI, Europ. J. Clin. Pharmacol. 3 119-122 (1971).
7. J.M. BESSON, M.C. WYON-MAILLARD, J.M. BENOIST, C. CONSEILLER, and K.F. HAMMAN, J. Pharmacol. Exp. Ther. 187 239-245 (1973).
8. C. CONSEILLER, D. MENETRY, D. LE BARS, and J.M. BESSON, J. Physiol. (Paris) 65, suppl., 220-221 A (1972).
9. L.M. KITAHATA, Y. KOSAKA, A. TAUB, K. BONIKOS, and M. HOFFERT, Anesthesiology 41, 39-48 (1974).

INTERACTION BETWEEN MORPHINE AND PUTATIVE EXCITATORY
NEUROTRANSMITTERS IN CORTICAL NEURONES IN NAIVE AND
TOLERANT RATS.

M. Satoh[+], W. Zieglgänsberger and A. Herz
Department of Neuropharmacology, Max-Planck-Institut
für Psychiatrie, Munich, Germany.

(Received in final form May 24, 1975)

Summary

Microelectrophoretically applied morphine depressed spontaneously discharging cortical neurones of rats and blocked excitation
induced by electrophoretic administrations of either acetylcholine
or l-glutamate. This depressant effect and both the anti-acetyl-
choline and the anti-glutamate effect were naloxone antagonizable
and therefore regarded as specific morphine actions. The excitatory effects of morphine were not affected by naloxone application and were classified as non-specific.

In chronically morphinized rats the depressant effect of morphine on spontaneous discharge activity and also its blocking action upon acetylcholine and l-glutamate-induced excitation were almost completely abolished. The predominant response in such pretreated animals was non-specific excitation. Acetylcholine and
l-glutamate were found to be more effective in tolerant rats
(supersensitivity).

Much data points to an involvement of putative neurotransmitters in acute and chronic opiate actions. Little is known, however, in which way opiates interfere with neurotransmitters, e.g.
whether pre- or postsynaptic mechanisms are affected. The micro-
electrophoretic method offers the possibility of studying opiate
effects at the single neurone level. A series of studies demonstrated effects of opiates and interactions with neurotransmitters in various structures of the central nervous system (1-13).
The interpretation of some of the results is hampered by the fact
that few studies have clearly separated non-specific effects from
those mediated via specific opiate receptors.

Recent electrophoretic studies on cortical neurones in rats
(11) revealed two types of opiate action: a) Inhibition of spontaneous discharge activity following applications of low doses
of morphine, and b) excitation which especially became manifest
during repeated applications or at higher dose-levels and made
the cells discharge, frequently in a burst-like manner. Only the
depressant effect, which could be antagonized by the specific
morphine antagonist naloxone, may be regarded as a specific opiate
action, while the excitatory effect which is not blocked by naloxone, was attributed to non-specific membrane effects. In morphine-

---

[+]Fellow of the Humboldt-Stiftung

tolerant rats the inhibitory action was found to be nearly abolished - and excitation became the prevailing response. The present study deals with the interaction of morphine with acetylcholine and l-glutamic acid, both of which can be considered as playing a role as transmitter in cortical neurones (14). Results obtained in naive rats were compared to those in tolerant animals.

Methods

Male Sprague Dawley rats were anesthetized with chloralose/urethane (90 mg/kg, 300 mg/kg respectively, i.p.), immobilized with gallamine and artificially respirated. The skull overlying the sensorimotor cortex was removed, the dura dissected and covered with warm paraffin. Twin electrode assemblies, consisting of a tungsten electrode and a conventional three- or four-barrelled multipipette, glued side to side, were used for recording and electrophoretic drug application respectively. The tungsten electrode protuded beyond the multipipette by 20-30 µm. Action potentials were recorded using conventional technique and were continuously monitored on an oscilloscope. Pulse gated action potentials were fed into a rate meter. Substances used for electrophoresis: morphine-HCl (50 mM, pH 5.0), naloxone-HCl (50 mM in 100 mM NaCl-solution, pH 5.0), l-mono-sodium glutamate (3 M, pH 8.0) and acetylcholine chloride (1 M, pH 5.0). Sodium chloride (3 M, pH 5.0) was used as the neutral barrel for current control.

In one set of experiments, chronically morphinized rats were used. Morphine pellets, containing 75 mg morphine base were implanted subcutaneously. Implantation schedule: 1 pellet on the 1st day, 2 pellets on the 4th day and 3 pellets on the 7th day. The experiments were performed on the 10th-12th day. By this implantation schedule a rather high degree of tolerance and dependence is induced (15). Hereafter these animals will be referred to as tolerant.

Results

The interaction between morphine and l-glutamate or acetylcholine (Ach) respectively, was studied in spontaneously discharging cortical neurones. L-glutamate or Ach was applied repeatedly for 20 sec at intervals of 1.0-1.5 min at doses which induced about a 3-fold increase in firing rate. Repeated administration of the same doses led to almost constant excitatory responses. After morphine (50 nA) was applied for 2 min the excitatory effect of the putative transmitters was again tested.

Effects of Glutamic Acid

In practically all neurones recorded glutamic acid induced a steep increase in firing rate, an effect which vanished rapidly after termination of drug application. Following electrophoretic morphine administration this excitatory effect of l-glutamate was found to be greatly reduced. In the experiment presented in Fig.1 morphine (50 nA, 2 min) causes an almost complete block of spontaneous discharge activity within 20 sec. This inhibitory effect dwindles slightly in spite of ongoing drug application. After termination of morphine application l-glutamate-induced excitation is considerably smaller than before. This blocking effect is fully reversible within about 2 min. Application of naloxone (20 nA, 4 min) prior to morphine not only abolishes morphine's inhibitory effect on spontaneous activity, but also its antagonistic effect on l-glutamate-induced excitation. The antagonistic effect of morphine on l-glutamate-induced excitation does not result from an

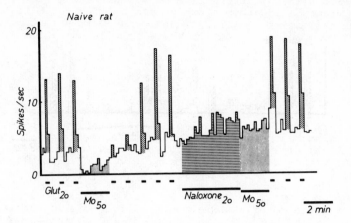

Fig.1 Effect of morphine on l-glutamate-induced excitation
on a cortical neurone and block of this morphine effect
by naloxone. The numbers indexed give the current applied
in nA.

inactivation of spikes. The anti-glutamate effect was obvious at
morphine doses which hardly affected the shape and duration of
spikes. Signs of a procaine-like effect of morphine became obvious
only at higher dosages.

A blocking of l-glutamate-induced excitation by morphine, as
shown in Fig.1, was observed in 32 out of 38 cortical neurones tested. In 6 out of 8 cells the blocking could be clearly antagonized by prior naloxone applications.

Effects of Acetylcholine

Spontaneously discharging neurones which could be activated by
Ach application were found, in contrast to glutamic acid, almost
exclusively in deeper layers of the cortex ($>$ 500 μm). At this
depth about 90 % of the neurones were excited by Ach and in most
of them an excitatory response with a short time course similar to
the response to glutamate was evoked (Fig.2). Also, the Ach-induced excitation could be blocked by morphine. In the experiment illustrated in Fig.2 this anti-Ach effect is present but no influence
upon spontaneous discharge activity is observed. Naloxone, applied
prior to morphine, antagonized in 6 out of 7 neurones this anti-
Ach effect which was observed in 31 out of 45 neurones tested.

Effects in Tolerant Rats

Experiments similar to those done in naive rats were performed
in chronically morphinized animals which had reached a rather high
degree of tolerance (see Methods). In these tolerant rats no gross
changes in the number of spontaneously discharging neurones or in
their discharge rates in comparison to naive rats were observed.
The inhibitory effect of morphine upon spontaneous firing rates
was abolished and morphine excited most cells. Furthermore, morphine no longer blocked l-glutamate- or Ach-induced excitation(Tab.1)

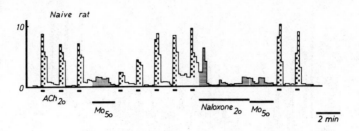

Fig.2 Effect of morphine on Ach-induced excitation in a
cortical neurone and block of this effect by naloxone.
The numbers indexed give the current applied in nA.

Table

| ANIMALS | GLUTAMATE | | ACETYLCHOLINE | |
| | BLOCK BY MORPHINE | NO BLOCK | BLOCK BY MORPHINE | NO BLOCK |
	(number of neurones)		(number of neurones)	
naive (n = 24)	32	6	31	14
tolerant (n = 10)	0	26	1	23

Table 1 Effect of morphine (50 nA) applied for 2 min on
1-glutamate- andAch-induced excitation of cortical
neurones in naive and tolerant rats.

In the course of the present study, it became obvious that in
tolerant rats the same excitatory effect of 1-glutamate and Ach
could be obtained at lower dose-levels than in naive rats. Tandem
experiments were performed in order to quantitatively compare results obtained with different micropipettes. A naive and a tolerant rat were prepared, and the response of cortical cells to
1-glutamate and Ach were tested with the same micropipette. These
experiments showed that in tolerant rats both putative transmitters induced excitations at lower dosages than in naive rats, indicating the development of supersensitivity to both transmitters.

Discussion

The present data on the interaction between morphine and putative excitatory transmitters is part of a more extensive study on
the actions of narcotic analgesics in cortical and spinal neurones (11,12,13). Both, the depressant effect of morphine upon spontaneous discharge activity and Ach- or 1-glutamate-induced excita-

232

tion was found to be antagonized by naloxone. This antagonism indicates that we are dealing with effects mediated via specific opiate receptors. It became evident from a synopsis of the most recent data reported that, depending on the structure, morphine produced either a specific inhibitory or a specific excitatory action (6,8,11).

Interactions of morphine with putative transmitters have been studied in a variety of central neurones (1,2,5,6,7,9,10), but some of these results are somewhat conflicting because they are lacking proof that they are mediated by specific opiate receptors. In brain stem neurones, where, in a way obviously similar to cortical neurones, inhibition of neuronal activity proved to be a specific opiate effect (8), Ach-induced excitation was found to be blocked in a number of neurones (5), but it is not yet known, whether or not this inhibition would be reversed by morphine antagonists. In spinal Renshaw cells, which receive cholinergic nerve endings, electrophoretic morphine application induced complex effects: an increase in latency of discharges after electric stimulation of the ventral roots is interpreted as resulting from inhibition of release of Ach from the nerve endings (2). On the other hand a direct excitation of the Renshaw cells and potentiation of Ach-induced excitation is reported (10). Interestingly, not only was the morphine effect found to be blocked by naloxone, but also Ach-induced excitation (6).

Most difficulties in interpreting the data obtained, result from the local anesthetic properties of morphine when applied to excitable membranes. Although several of the reported findings are obviously not attributable to such a procaine-like depressant effect upon the spike-generating mechanism (7), intracellular recordings are necessary to provide credence to the belief that morphine applied at low dose-levels interacts with ionic channels different from the voltage-dependent Na^+-channel.

For technical reasons we performed our intracellular recordings in cat spinal neurones, which are supposed to receive glutaminergic and cholinergic terminals (14). From these studies we learned that electrophoretically applied morphine alters neither the membrane potential nor the resistance of the postsynaptic membrane. Morphine clearly reduced the amplitude of differently evoked EPSPs and prevented depolarizations by l-glutamate by means of a blockade of the associated Na^+-influx. Naloxone antagonized the depression of the EPSP amplitude and the blockade of the Na^+-influx (19). A three- to four-fold dosage increase also blocked spike initiation which is resistant to naloxone administration (13). These results are of particular interest in view of previous data reported which was generally interpreted in terms of an impairment of transmitter release from presynaptic terminals (16,17,18). It may be deduced from the interaction between morphine and Ach or l-glutamate on cortical neurones observed in the present study that these effects are also mediated via postsynaptically located receptors.

A surprisingly fast onset and termination of the depolarizing action of Ach was obtained in almost all cortical cells studied. These actions are obviously not of such a pure muscarinic type of action as described to be the prevailing cholinergic response in cortical neurones of cat (14). The characteristics resemble more the actions of l-glutamate and may be mediated predominantly by nicotinic receptors.

233

A close coincidence between the antagonistic action of morphine on spontaneous discharge activity and electrophoretically induced excitation is also evident in tolerant animals. In these animals both, the depressant effect of morphine on spontaneously discharging neurones and its anti-Ach and anti-glutamate effect are abolished. These results provide some evidence that postsynaptic sites are involved in the development of tolerance.

In our tandem-studies using the same electrode in tolerant and naive animals we observed that in tolerant rats comparable doses of Ach and l-glutamate induce much stronger effects than in naive. Whether this development of supersensitivity to excitatory transmitters is the basic mechanism underlying the development of tolerance and closely correlated to the effects of morphine abstinence is still an open question.

References

1) CURTIS, D. R. and A. W. DUGGAN, Agents and Actions 1, 14-19 (1969).
2) DUGGAN, A. W. and D. R. CURTIS, Neuropharmacology 11, 189-196 (1972).
3) BISCOE, T. J., A. W. DUGGAN and D. LODGE, Brit. J. Pharmacol. 46, 201-212 (1972).
4) BRADLEY, P. B. and G. J. BRAMWELL, Brit. J. Pharmacol. 51, 51-52 (1975).
5) BRADLEY, P. B. and A. DRAY, Brit. J. Pharmacol. 50, 47-55 (1974).
6) DAVIES, J. and A. W. DUGGAN, Nature 250, 70-71 (1974).
7) DOSTROVSKY, J. and B. POMERANZ, Nature New Biology 246, 222-224 (1973).
8) BRAMWELL, G. J. and P. B. BRADLEY, Brain Res. 73, 167-170 (1974).
9) HENRY, J. L., Fed. Proc. 34, 3045 (1975).
10) LODGE, D., P. M. HEADLEY, A. W. DUGGAN and T. BISCOE, Europ. J. Pharmacol. 26, 277-284 (1974).
11) SATOH, M., W. ZIEGLGÄNSBERGER, W. FRIES and A. HERZ, Brain Res. 82, 378-382 (1974).
12) ZIEGLGÄNSBERGER, W. and J. BAYERL, 24th Intern. Congr. of Physiol. Sci., Satellite Symposium, Lucknow (1974) in press.
13) ZIEGLGÄNSBERGER, W. and J. BAYERL, Pflügers Arch. Suppl. to Vol. 355, R 85 (1975).
14) KRNJEVIC, K., Physiol. Rev. 54, 418-540 (1974).
15) BLÄSIG, J., A. HERZ, K. REINHOLD and S. ZIEGLGÄNSBERGER, Psychopharmacologia 32, 19-38 (1973).
16) JHAMANDAS, K., C. PINSKY and J. W. PHILLIS, Brit. J. Pharmacol. 43, 53-66 (1971).
17) MATTHEWS, J. D., G. LABRECQUE and E. F. DOMINO, Psychopharmacologia 29, 113-120 (1973).
18) MONTEL, H., H. D. TAUBE and K. STARKE, Naunyn-Schmiedeberg's Arch. Pharmacol. 283, 357 (1974).

EFFECTS OF NALOXONE AND ACETYLCHOLINE ON MEDIAL THALAMIC AND CORTICAL UNITS IN NAIVE AND MORPHINE DEPENDENT RATS

Robert C. A. Frederickson, Franklin H. Norris and Christina R. Hewes

Lilly Research Laboratories, Eli Lilly and Co., Indianapolis, Ind. 46206

(Received in final form May 24, 1975)

An important role has been suggested for acetylcholine (ACh) in both the development and the expression of dependence upon morphine (1). However, the specific nature of this role has not been established. Much recent evidence implicates the medial thalamic (m. thalamic) region in the genesis of these phenomena. In particular, Wei et al. (2) report this area to be one of the most effective brain regions for the precipitation of withdrawal (WD) in opiate dependent rats by the direct implantation of naloxone. Furthermore, electrical stimulation of the m. thalamic region of naive rats can produce a series of responses reminiscent of the morphine WD syndrome (unpublished observations). Thus naloxone may precipitate WD in opiate dependent animals by exciting neurons in the m. thalamic region which are not similarly excited in naive animals. It might do this by releasing increased stores of ACh onto receptors made supersensitive secondary to inhibition of ACh release by morphine (2,3,4). However, recent work suggests that such a simplistic mechanism is probably inadequate to explain opiate WD (1). The present experiments were performed to test this theory more directly using the technique of microiontophoresis. The results indicate that the number of neurons excited by naloxone is increased in m. thalamus, but not cerebral cortex, of dependent animals. However, this cannot be attributed simply to a release of ACh by naloxone and receptors appear subsensitive rather than supersensitive to ACh in dependent animals.

Methods

Male Sprague-Dawley rats (230-260g) were tested 48 hr after treatment with either a slow release suspension of morphine at 300 mg/kg (5) or the suspension vehicle only. The rats were anesthetized with urethane (1.4-1.7 g/kg, i.p.) and multi-barrel microelectrodes were placed into the region of the m. thalamus (tmm, tml) stereotactically according to the atlas of Konig and Klippel (6). Neurons were also studied in the cerebral cortex over the m. thalamus in order to control for regional specificity of any responses observed since Wei et al. (2) reported no WD response to implantation of naloxone in this region. Immediately before use the drug barrels were filled by pressure with the following solutions: monosodium-l-glutamate (0.2M, pH 8.5), NaCl (2M), naloxone HCl (0.2M, pH 4.0), ACh Cl (0.2M, pH 4.3), atropine SO_4 (0.15M, pH 4.5) and morphine SO_4 (0.05M, pH 4.0). The unit recording and microiontophoretic techniques have been described previously (7).

Results and Discussion

Spontaneously-firing neurons (143 in total) were examined in the m. thalamus and cerebral cortex of 9 naive and 8 morphine dependent rats. The results are summarized in Table 1.

The firing rate of m. thalamic neurons was increased by naloxone in a significantly greater proportion ($p < 0.05$, chi-squared test) in dependent rats than in naive rats. This did not occur in the cerebral cortex. The difference was not as dramatic as we had expected. At the end of iontophoretic experiments the effect of systemic naloxone was observed on the activity of m. thalamic neurons in 5 dependent rats and 3 naive rats. All 5 neurons in dependent rats

Table 1. Effects of Naloxone and ACh on Medial Thalamic Unit Activity
in Naive (n=9) and Dependent (n=9) Rats.

	A. Naloxone			B. ACh		
	Excit.	Depress.	Nil	Excit.	Depress.	Nil
Naive (39)[1]	13%(5)	23%(9)	64%(25)	54%(21)	23%(9)	23%(9)
Depend. (50)	34%(17)	28%(14)	38%(19)	38%(19)	22%(11)	40%(20)

increased their firing rate within 2-5 min following the injection of naloxone
at 1 mg/kg s.c. Similar responses were not seen with the 3 neurons in naive
rats. Two of the 5 neurons in dependent rats were also excited by naloxone
applied by iontophoresis but 2 were not. One was not tested. Thus another
site in the brain may be initiating some responses to naloxone. We studied the
anterior boundary of the region reported to be highly responsive to implanted
naloxone (2) and we may find more responsive neurons further caudal in this
m. thalamic region.

The results do not support the proposal that the responses to naloxone are
directly mediated by ACh. Only 12 of the 50 neurons tested in dependent rats
were excited by both naloxone and ACh. 30% of the neurons excited by naloxone
were not also excited by ACh. The excitations by naloxone were not sufficiently reproducible to permit an examination with anticholinergic drugs. The results with iontophoretic ACh raise serious doubts for the "cholinergic excess"
theory of WD. We found no evidence of a supersensitivity to ACh but in fact
the receptors mediating cholinergic excitation appeared subsensitive in both
medial thalamus (Table 1) and cerebral cortex, although this was not quite significant at the 0.05 level. It might be argued that the exposure to morphine
in these experiments was not of sufficient duration to allow development of
supersensitivity. However Yarbrough (8) also found no evidence for a supersensitivity to ACh in rat cortex after treatment with morphine for up to 29 days.
Labreque and Domino (9) recently reported a reduced release of ACh from cortex
of dependent cats 15 min after naloxone. Thus the early phase of WD probably
corresponds to a period of reduced rather than increased cholinergic activity
in the brain. This gains support from our recent findings that pharmacologi-
cally-induced increases in central muscarinic activity reduce rather than increase WD severity (unpublished observations).

Acknowledgements

The authors are grateful to Vigo Burgis and Carolyn E. Harrell for their
assistance in this work.

References

1. R. C. A. FREDERICKSON and C. PINSKY, J. Pharmacol. Exp. Ther. 193 44-55
    (1975).
2. E. WEI, H. H. LOH and E. L. WAY, J. Pharmacol. Exp. Ther. 185 108-115 (1973)
3. W. D. M. PATON, Can. J. Biochem. Physiol. 41 2637-2653 (1963).
4. H. O. J. COLLIER, Nature 220 228-231 (1968).
5. R. C. A. FREDERICKSON and S. E. SMITS, Res. Comm. Chem. Path. Pharmacol.
    5 867-870 (1973).
6. J. F. R. KONIG and R. A. KLIPPEL, The Rat Brain. A stereotaxis atlas of
    the forebrain and lower parts of the brain stem, The Williams and Wilkins
    Co., Baltimore (1963).
7. R. C. A. FREDERICKSON, L. M. JORDAN and J. W. PHILLIS, Comp. Gen. Pharmacol.
    3 443-456 (1972).
8. G. G. YARBROUGH, Life Sciences 15 1523-1529 (1975).
9. G. LABRECQUE and E. F. DOMINO, J. Pharmacol. Exp. Ther. 191 189-200 (1974).

[1]Numbers in brackets refer to numbers of neurons.

A SYSTEMS AND CONTROL THEORY APPROACH TO DYNAMIC NEUROTRANSMITTER BALANCE IN NARCOTIC ADDICTION AND NARCOTIC ANTAGONISM

Joyce J. Kaufman, Walter S. Koski, and David Peat[#]
(Received in final form May 24, 1975)
Department of Anesthesiology, The Johns Hopkins University School of Medicine, Baltimore, Maryland 21205 and Department of Chemistry, The Johns Hopkins University, Baltimore, Maryland 21218. #Visiting Scientist, National Research Council of Canada, Ottawa, Canada

We have formulated a pharmacological-physiological systems analysis and control theory based on interactive neuronal feedback loops (the effects of endogenous neurochemical diseases and exogenous CNS drugs on neurotransmitter synthesis and release, reuptake and metabolism) for normal, abnormal and catastrophic situations.

We set up the systems diagrams for neurotransmitter systems and in that single framework were able to describe endogenous neurochemical disorders, the effect that their drug treatment modalities had on the dynamic neurochemical balance and the effect other CNS drugs such as narcotics and narcotic antagonists had on neurochemical balance. This led to a hypothesis that narcotic addiction is caused by negative feedback induced increase in synthesis and release of certain neurotransmitters, tolerance arises in a related manner, narcotic withdrawal symptoms are caused by out-of-phase feedback and a major mechanism of antagonist action of narcotic antagonists is not merely competitive displacement of a narcotic from its "receptor site" but rather is due to an increase in the concentration of catecholamines in the synaptic cleft.

Biological Systems

A consistent picture emerges. Compounds which block postsynaptic receptor sites (or which in other ways decrease the amount of normal neurotransmitters available to the postsynaptic receptor site) apparently increase by a negative feedback process the synthesis and release of the biogenic amines whose receptor sites are blocked. Compounds which act as agonists at postsynaptic receptors cut down on the synthesis and release of these neurotransmitters whose receptor sites are being stimulated. Compounds which block the reuptake of biogenic amines reduce the turnover of biogenic amines and compounds which deplete brain biogenic amines stimulate the synthesis of these amines. Direct pharmacological stimulation of a receptor appears to decrease the neuronal firing rate as does the presence of an excess of the neurotransmitter in the synapse. Blockade of a receptor leads to an increase in neuronal firing.

Effects of Narcotics and Narcotic Antagonists

Several investigators have reported that morphine increases the incorporation of ^{14}C-tyrosine (T) (or ^{3}H-tyrosine) into ^{14}C-labelled (or ^{3}H-labelled) catecholamines (CA) in the brains of mice. The effect on 5-HT is not yet resolved; both an increased rate of synthesis and no effect have been reported. (1) Narcotics inhibit the release of acetylcholine from the presynapse.

The ^{14}C turnover data indicates that under the influence of morphine there is an increase in the synthesis and turnover of ^{14}C-DA, ^{14}C-NE and ^{14}C-5-HT indicating that not enough of these normal neurotransmitters were available at their postsynaptic receptor sites. This could arise in several ways: either that postsynaptic receptor sites were being blocked (or, as some recent evidence indicates, that at least one of the neurotransmitters, DA, was being metabolized before being released from the presynapse). This led us to postulate (1) that the addictive properties of narcotics were related to this increase in synthesis and turnover of at least some if not all of the above three of these normal neurotransmitters. Conversely, because of a linked dopaminergic-cholinergic system, while the subject is under the influence of a narcotic little or no acetylcholine is released. As long as the subject is under the influence of the narcotic, the narcotic negates the effect of the increased synthesis and release of the neurotransmitters, DA, NE and 5-HT. Withdrawing the narcotic must be a classic case of an out-of-phase positive feedback output. The feedback signal cannot turn off the synthesis and release of the neurotransmitters quickly enough to prevent a flood of at least some of the normal neurotransmitters, which cause the "withdrawal symptoms". Taking more narcotic immediately would again negate the effect of what must be increased synthesis and turnover of the above three neurotransmitters and would act to quell the withdrawal symptoms.

In our framework, the development of tolerance also becomes more clear. The longer the postsynapse is deprived of neurotransmitter, the more the presynapse will try to overcome this deficiency by synthesizing (and releasing) still more of the neurotransmitter whose postsynaptic receptor is deficient. Thus, more of the drug, D, will be necessary to retain the same concentration of D·R complex. The major mode of antagonist action of a narcotic antagonist is very unlikely to be merely competitive replacement of the narcotic at a receptor site. The antagonist effect of a narcotic antagonist is much too rapid for it to occur by immediate reversal of the feedback loop(s) that is (are) being influenced by the narcotic. We had earlier suggested (1) that narcotic antagonists do not work merely by competitive antagonism but perhaps their major mode of action was to increase the concentration of catecholamines in the synaptic cleft. In particular, we had postulated based on ^{14}C turnover studies indicating increased synthesis of DA, NE and 5-HT that a narcotic causes a decrease in availability of these several neurotransmitters at their postsynaptic receptors (which could be due either to postsynaptic receptor blockade or recent evidence points also to a possible presynaptic metabolism at least of DA prior to release), that a narcotic antagonist exerted its antagonist action by increasing the concentration of catecholamines (DA and NE) in the synaptic cleft, either by prevention of reuptake or inducing release or both.(1) Kopin, in 1972, said if our hypothesis were true then amphetamine or cocaine should mimic these effects and intensify withdrawal symptoms. Our hypothesis has recently been confirmed vividly by two different independent observations. At the Drug Dependence Meeting, March 1974, a narcotic abuse clinic, that was using ex-multiple drug abusers, now drug free, as counselors, gave them blocking doses of naloxone and asked them to describe the effects. All of the subjects said the effects resembled amphetamine or cocaine. At the opiate receptor meeting, spring 1974, Herz reported that amphetamine, cocaine and 1-dopa given to narcotic addicted animals all increase the severity of narcotic withdrawal symptoms caused by naloxone. Supported in part by NIDA Grant No. DA00539.

1. For detailed references see J. J. KAUFMAN and W. S. KOSKI. In DRUG DESIGN, pp. 251-340, Academic Press (1975), Vol. V.

PROSTAGLANDINS, CYCLIC AMP AND THE MECHANISM OF OPIATE DEPENDENCE

Harry O.J. Collier, David L. Francis, Wendy J. McDonald-Gibson
Ashim C. Roy and Sheikh A. Saeed

Research Department, Miles Laboratories Limited,
Stoke Poges, Slough, SL2 4LY, England

(Received in final form May 24, 1975)

SUMMARY

Further evidence is given that dependence arises from the agonist action of opiates. From this and our previous propositions assigning a fundamental role to neuronal cyclic AMP in (i) the agonist action of opiates and (ii) the expression of the abstinence syndrome, it follows that opiate dependence is a state of heightened potential activity of a neuronal cyclic AMP mechanism, initiated and maintained by the blockade of an adenylate cyclase. Various possible mechanisms are discussed by which this potential is heightened. New evidence is given that morphine and naloxone stimulate prostaglandin biosynthesis without mutual antagonism. Preliminary evidence also is given that (i) the formation of cyclic AMP is enhanced in brain homogenates from heroin-dependent rats, and (ii) an acidified ethylacetate extract of brains of morphine-dependent rats induces quasi-abstinence effects when injected into a lateral cerebral ventricle of naive rats.

Many of us may have asked ourselves: what is the biochemical action of morphine that leads to dependence? This generates a second question: is it the agonist action of morphine that induces dependence? If the answer is affirmative, a third question arises: what is the biochemical action of morphine that leads to its agonist effects? From this the question arises: how does this biochemical action induce dependence? To limit the answers to the last question, let us begin with the mechanism of the abstinence syndrome.

PRIMARY PROCESS OF THE ABSTINENCE SYNDROME

Do all the signs of abstinence arise from activation of a single, primary biochemical process? If this question is studied with drugs, such as atropine and hemicholinium, that interfere with a single neurohumoral transmitter, in this case acetylcholine, the answer emerges that the drug lessens some abstinence signs, but not others, or even increases others (1,2). Hence, there might be no primary process, or, if there were, it would not directly concern the neurohumoral transmitter studied. That phosphodiesterase inhibitors not only intensify most of the signs of precipitated abstinence in true morphine dependence, but also, given to naive rats shortly before naloxone, produce an almost perfect replica of the abstinence syndrome (4,5,6), argues that there is one primary biochemical process of abstinence. These observations, coupled with the finding that cyclic AMP, but not cyclic GMP, intensifies the abstinence syndrome (3), indicate that this primary process is the activation of a cyclic AMP mechanism. This is supported by the observation that the intensity of the precipitated abstinence syndrome is directly related to the level of cyclic AMP in the brain (7).

As Claude Bernard observed, the pharmacological effects of morphine are a mixture or a succession of the depressant and the stimulant. Only some of these are the drug's agonist effects, which are those readily antagonized by naloxone. Naloxone antagonizes analgesia, euphoria, respiratory depression and the inhibition by opiates of evoked responses of isolated guinea pig ileum (8) and mouse vas deferens (9). Naloxone does not antagonize the emetic effect of injecting morphine into a cerebral ventricle of the cat, although it does antagonize the more persistent anti-emetic effect of morphine (10). We have found that naloxone, likewise, does not antagonize the ability of morphine to stimulate prostaglandin biosynthesis by bull seminal vesicle homogenate.

We know that naloxone precipitates the abstinence syndrome in dependent animals; but does it antagonize the induction of opiate dependence? Martin (11), reviewing earlier work with partial antagonists, such as nalorphine and levallorphan, concluded that they do inhibit the induction of dependence; but lately there have been dissentient voices (12). It is reassuring, therefore, that Frederickson et al (13), using sustained-release naloxone, have shown that it inhibits the induction of dependence by sustained-release morphine. In our laboratory, this was shown in another way, by giving four 20mg/kg subcutaneous doses of naloxone in saline, at 2h intervals, starting 1h before the injection of 150mg/kg morphine in a sustained-release preparation to induce dependence. When abstinence was precipitated 24h later with a much smaller dose of naloxone (0.25mg/kg), the incidence of diarrhoea (P=0.012), squeak on handling (P <0.005) and the abstinence syndrome as a whole (P=0.012) were all lowered (G. Henderson and C. Schneider, unpublished).

If the agonist action of opiates produces dependence, and if opiates exert that action by inhibiting an adenylate cyclase of morphine-sensitive neurones, as we have argued (14), it follows that dependence arises in response to the inhibition of this adenylate cyclase. If our other argument also holds, that opiate withdrawal effects express increased activity of a neuronal cyclic AMP mechanism (3,4), it follows that the induction of dependence and the manifestation of abstinence express movements in opposite directions of neuronal cyclic AMP mechanisms. This conclusion accords with the hypothesis of Himmelsbach (15), that dependence arises from a homeostatic increase in excitation in brain centres to compensate for the acute depressant effects of opiates. In biochemical terms, we conceive the state evisaged by Himmelsbach as one of potential activity of a central cyclic AMP mechanism, initiated and maintained by the blockade of an adenylate cyclase of morphine-sensitive neurones.

This concept envisages the mechanism of dependence as a biochemical change to restore homeostasis after inhibition of a neuronal cyclic AMP function. There are many ways, within the framework of known biochemical processes, whereby such a compensating biochemical hypertrophy might develop. For example, there could be changes in an adenylate cyclase mechanism. The amount of this enzyme or its activity could increase, as Sharma et al (16) have suggested. Again, the amount or activity of an endogenous stimulant of adenylate cyclase, such as E prostaglandin, could increase. Yet again, the enzyme could become more responsive to the stimulant. An alternative group of processes would be a decrease in the amount, activity or sensitivity of a phosphodiesterase, or an increase in an endogenous inhibitor of this enzyme. Yet again, protein kinase activity could increase, as Clark et al (17) observed some years ago in rat brain during morphine withdrawal. This list does not exhaust all possibilities and more than one mechanism affecting cyclic AMP may operate.

Investigators agree that at least part of the adenylate cyclase inhibited by morphine responds to stimulation by E prostaglandin (14). We have therefore studied the interaction with prostaglandin synthetase of apomorphine, morphine (18, 19), codeine and naloxone. Three of these drugs stimulate prostaglandin biosynthesis in homogenate of bull seminal vesicles, with added arachidonic acid, and without added co-factors; but codeine inhibits prostaglandin synthetase more effectively in our hands than does aspirin, the IC 50 values being: codeine, 61μg/ml; aspirin, 108μg/ml (Fig.1).

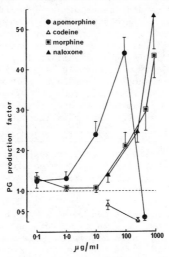

Fig. 1.

Effect of apomorphine, codeine, morphine and naloxone on prostaglandin production by bull seminal vesicle homogenate. The PG production factor is the ratio of total PG-like activity in test incubate to that in reference incubate (basal), assayed on rat stomach strip. The incubates contained added substrate (61μM arachidonic acid), but no added co-factors (19). The concentrations in μg/ml that increased PG production by 50% (SC 50) are: apomorphine, 1.7; morphine, 38; naloxone, 44. The concentration of codeine that halves PG production is 61μg/ml.

That codeine more potently than aspirin inhibits prostaglandin biosynthesis suggests that it may partly act as an analgesic by inhibiting prostaglandin synthetase. Many properties of codeine, however, indicate that it is a narcotic, and hence that its analgesic action partly arises from the same mechanism as that of morphine. Compared to morphine, codeine has about 1/2 to 1/7 the antinociceptive potency in mice (20), but about 1/100 to 1/150 the potency on isolated mouse vas deferens (9) or guinea-pig ileum (8), and only about 1/3000 the affinity for the opiate receptor (21). The possible dual analgesic action of codeine may help to explain its quite different potency in different tests, as yet attributed to its metabolic conversion to morphine.

It seems possible, even likely, that some of the stimulant effects of apomorphine and morphine may be due to their ability to increase prostaglandin production. If this ability of morphine does not induce tolerance, it might also participate in some phenomena of abstinence. We have not, however, yet succeeded in demonstrating an increased content of E or F prostaglandins in rat brain during dependence or precipitated abstinence, although measurable quantities of both prostaglandins are present.

The stimulation of prostaglandin production by naloxone, which is evident at about 10^{-4}M, finds an echo in the stimulation of PGE_1-activated cyclic AMP formation in cultured neuroblastoma cells that Traber et al (22) observed at concentrations of 3×10^{-4}M naloxone and upwards. We have seen a comparable effect in rat brain homogenate, where, in the presence of IBMX (5×10^{-4}M), naloxone at 10^{-3}M, but not at 10^{-5}M, stimulated cyclic AMP formation.

Such concentrations of naloxone far exceed those likely to occur in the brain with doses that precipitate abstinence or quasi-abstinence _in vivo_. Although $<10^{-5}$M naloxone would not be likely to stimulate adenylate cyclase or PG synthetase, it would be enough to antagonize endogenous enkephaline, if the effective concentration of naloxone _in vivo_ corresponded with that observed by John Hughes _in vitro_ (23). If enkephaline acted by inhibiting an adenylate cyclase of morphine-sensitive neurones (14), these findings suggest that, in the normal rat, there is a spontaneous tendency for cyclic AMP formation to occur in these neurones, and that this tendency is controlled by the activities of enkephaline and phosphodiesterase. When both controls are removed, spontaneous behaviour, of a type seen in abstinence, is expressed.

ENZYMES AFFECTING CYCLIC AMP

We have tried a number of times to detect changes in phosphodiesterase or adenylate cyclase activity in brain homogenates from heroin-dependent rats. Rats were given frequent, regular, automated intravenous infusions of heroin during several days, while control animals received saline instead of heroin. The rats were withdrawn from treatment and, 0 to 5.5h afterwards, they were decapitated and brain homogenates made. We found no difference in brain cyclic AMP phosphodiesterase between the heroin and saline groups, as others have reported for morphine. With adenylate cyclase, results were inconsistent and usually PGE_1 failed to increase activity. In one experiment, however, PGE_1 stimulated cyclic AMP formation to a much greater extent in the heroin than in the saline-treated homogenate. In this experiment, the factor by which cyclic AMP formation was increased by the prostaglandin (3.8 fold) exceeded that in any experiment with normal rat brain. In two other experiments, basal cyclic AMP formation was considerably greater in the heroin-treated than the saline-treated brains. These experiments therefore suggest that adenylate cyclase activity is enhanced in opiate dependence and that there may develop a supersensitivity to E prostaglandin.

EXTRACTS OF DEPENDENT BRAINS

We have also tested whether an extract, prepared by methods of prostaglandin extraction, of brain homogenate from morphine-dependent rats would produce a quasi-abstinence syndrome after intracerebroventricular injection into naive rats. To produce the extracts for test, rats received 150mg/kg of morphine subcutaneously in a sustained-release preparation. Controls received either the sustained-release vehicle or no treatment. After 24 h treatment, the rats were decapitated and the brain immediately removed, frozen and stored at -20°C. For extraction, the brains were homogenized for 30 sec at high speed in a small volume of 0.2M citric acid. The acidified homogenate was then extracted twice with ethylacetate and the solvent layer washed free of acid. After the ethylacetate had been removed _in vacuo_, the residue was redissolved in ethanol and diluted in Krebs' solution for test to a final concentration of 3% ethanol. This was tested by injection in a 25 or 30µl volume through an indwelling cannula into a lateral cerebral ventricle of naive rats. The behaviour of treated rats was then recorded, during 15 min after injection, by observers who did not know which treatment each animal had received.

In three series of observations, a total of 35 naive rats received ethyla-cetate extracts of morphine-dependent brain and 25 rats received control brain extracts. The pooled results indicated the presence of a quasi-abstinence syndrome in animals receiving the brain extract from the morphine-treated rats, but not in those receiving control extract (P <0.0002). In one of these tests, the active extract elicited jumping.

TABLE 1

Production of quasi-morphine abstinence syndrome in naive rats by intra-cerebroventricular injection of brain extract from morphine-dependent rats.

Sign	Incidence of sign after injection of brain extract		
	Morphine-treated	Vehicle-treated	P value
Jumping	0	0	-
Chattering	7	1	<0.02
Squeak on touch	1	0	-
Squeak on handling	6	0	<0.01
Diarrhoea	1	0	-
Chewing	5	0	<0.02
Ptosis	0	0	-
Body shakes	0	1	-
Head shakes	0	0	-
Paw tremor	1	0	-
Rearing	12	6	<0.01
Restlessness	10	2	<0.01
Salivation	0	0	-
Median total score	3.0	1.0	<0.0001
Interquartile range	2-5	0-1	
Number of rats	12	12	-

Three rats received 150mg/kg morphine subcutaneously in a sustained-release vehicle, and three, vehicle alone. After 24h, all were decapitated and the brains of each group pooled, quickly frozen and later homogenised in citric acid. The homogenate was extracted with ethylacetate and the extract evaporated to dryness in vacuo. The residue was taken up in ethanol and diluted 28 fold in Krebs' solution. A 30μl volume was injected through an indwelling cannula into a lateral cerebral ventricle, and behaviour was recorded for 15 min afterwards by observers who did not know which treat-ment each animal had received.

Table 1 illustrates an experiment with acidified ethylacetate extract of the pooled brains of three rats that had received morphine and of three that had received vehicle. After intracerebroventricular injection, the naive rats receiving extract from morphine-dependent brains had a significantly higher incidence of five behavioural signs and a higher total quasi-abstinence score (P <0.0001).

DISCUSSION AND CONCLUSIONS

The foregoing analysis argues, on the one hand, that opiate dependence arises as a compensation for the inhibition by opiate of adenylate cyclase in mor-phine-sensitive neurones and that abstinence effects express increased ac-tivity of a neuronal adenylate cyclase. It argues, on the other hand, that a substance is produced in the brain in morphine dependence that may mediate withdrawal effects in dependent animals. We do not know whether the active substance interacts with a neuronal cyclic AMP mechanism.

243

The role of cyclic AMP in dependence is unlike that of opiates or antagonists. Thus, heroin increases the induction of dependence and lessens the expression of abstinence (1), whereas naloxone has the opposite effect. Cyclic AMP, both enhances induction, at least in the mouse (24), and intensifies abstinence.

The question remains: whatever has happened to all the humoral neurotransmitters that have been implicated in dependence? The short answer is that involvement of cyclic AMP does not exclude the participation of neurotransmitters in dependence mechanisms, but our observations suggest that cyclic AMP has the primary role.

We thank Mr. M.A. Collins, Mr. N.J. Cuthbert and Miss. J.F. de C. Sutherland for help in observing animals; Miss J. Bennett, Mr. N.M. Butt and Mr. C. Shah for technical assistance; Mr. L.C. Dinneen for statistical advice; and Sankyo Limited for naloxone.

REFERENCES

1. H.O.J. COLLIER, D.L. FRANCIS, C. SCHNEIDER, Nature, Lond. 237, 220-223 (1972).
2. H.N. BHARGAVA, S.L. CHAN, E. LEONG WAY, Europ.J.Pharmacol. 29, 253-261 (1974).
3. H.O.J. COLLIER, D.L. FRANCIS, Nature, Lond. 255, 159-162, (1975).
4. D.L. FRANCIS, A.C. ROY, H.O.J. COLLIER. This symposium.
5. H.O.J. COLLIER, Pharmacology, 11, 58-61 (1974).
6. H.O.J. COLLIER, D.L. FRANCIS, G. HENDERSON, C. SCHNEIDER, Nature, Lond., 249, 471-473 (1974).
7. C.S. MEHTA, W. JOHNSON, Fedn.Proc., 33, 493 (1974).
8. H.W. KOSTERLITZ, A.J. WATT, Br.J.Pharmac., 33, 266-276 (1968).
9. J. HUGHES, H.W. KOSTERLITZ, F.M. LESLIE, Br.J.Pharmac., 53, 371-381 (1975).
10. D.J. COSTELLO, L.E. McCARTHY, S.J. GIDDINGS, H.L. BORISON, Pharmacologist, 16, 206 (1974).
11. W.R. MARTIN, Pharmac.Rev., 19, 463-521 (1967).
12. E. EIDELBERG, R. ERSPAMER, Arch.int.Pharmacodyn, 211, 58-63.
13. R.C.A. FREDERICKSON, J.S. HORNG, V. BURGIS, D.T. WONG, Report of Committee on Problems of Drug Dependence, 1974. pp. 411-434, Nat.Acad.Sci.
14. A.C. ROY, H.O.J. COLLIER. This symposium.
15. C.K. HIMMELSBACH, Fedn.Proc., 2, 201-203 (1943).
16. S.K. SHARMA, M. NIRENBERG, W.A. KLEE, Proc.Nat.Acad.Sci. U.S.A. 72, 590-594 (1975).
17. A.G. CLARK, R. JOVIC, M.R. ORNELLAS, M. WELLER, Biochem.Pharmac. 21, 1989-1990 (1972).
18. H.O.J. COLLIER, W.J. McDONALD-GIBSON, S.A. SAEED, Br.J.Pharmac., 52, 116P (1974).
19. H.O.J. COLLIER, W.J. McDONALD-GIBSON, S.A. SAEED, Nature, Lond., 252, 56-58 (1974).
20. H.O.J. COLLIER, L.C. DINNEEN, C.A. JOHNSON, C. SCHNEIDER, Br.J.Pharmac., 32, 295-310 (1968).
21. C.B. PERT, S.H. SNYDER, Science, 179, 1011-1014 (1973).
22. J. TRABER, K. FISCHER, S. LATZIN, B. HAMPRECHT, Nature, Lond., 253, 120-122 (1975).
23. J. HUGHES, Brain Research, 88, 295-308 (1975).
24. I.K. HOH, H.H. LOH, E. L. WAY, J.Pharmac.exp.Ther., 185, 347-357 (1973).

SOME THOUGHTS ON THE SIGNIFICANCE OF
ENKEPHALIN, THE ENDOGENOUS LIGAND

Hans W. Kosterlitz and John Hughes

Unit for Research on Addictive Drugs,
University of Aberdeen, Aberdeen, Scotland.

(Received in final form May 24, 1975)

Enkephalin is compared to morphine and its congeners with
particular regard to physico-chemical properties, biological
stability and sensitivity to narcotic antagonists.   Possible
sites of action are considered.   Interactions between endogenous
enkephalin and exogenous opiate at the opiate receptor are
discussed as a possible basis of tolerance and dependence caused
by chronic administration of opiates.

The evidence for the presence of an endogenous ligand of the opiate
receptors is now so convincing (see other papers in this volume) that it will
fulfil a useful purpose to compare known properties of this ligand to those of
the naturally occurring narcotic analgesics and their semisynthetic and synthetic surrogates.   We have proposed to give the name of enkephalin to the
natural compound, stressing its origin without presuming its structure or
physiological functions.

General Considerations

Although it is not certain whether there are natural ligands other than
enkephalin, it would appear from the data presented by several speakers
(Hughes, Terenius, Pasternak) that we are dealing with one or more closely
related small peptides which are readily destroyed by enzymatic action of
tissue extracts.   It is of interest to point out that, in contrast to
enkephalin, the plant alkaloids morphine and, to a lesser extent, codeine show
a considerable resistance to enzymatic degradation.   This different behaviour
of compounds derived from the animal and plant kingdoms is reminiscent of a
similar relationship between the muscarinic agents, acetylcholine and
muscarine.   Here, as with the narcotic analgesics, the plant alkaloids are
much more toxic than the compounds occurring naturally in animals.

The information that is available with regard to the action of narcotic
analgesics at the cellular level, indicates that transmitter release is
depressed at selective morphine-sensitive neurones (1-4).   It is essential
for the action of a neurotransmitter or neuromodulator that its onset and
offset of action be rapid.   In this connection the observation (5) is
important that in isolated preparations, namely the myenteric plexus-longitudinal muscle of the guinea-pig ileum and the vas deferens of the mouse,
the rates of onset and offset of action of narcotic analgesics are inversely
related to lipid solubility.   In contrast, in the whole animal, the rates
of onset and of recovery are directly related to lipid solubility which
facilitates drug movement to and from the brain (6).   The relationships
between lipid solubility and rates of onset and offset are shown in Table 1.

TABLE 1

Relationships of Rates of Onset and Offset of Action
to Lipid Solubility in the Guinea-Pig Ileum

Drug	Rank Order of Lipid Solubility[1]	Half-times[2] (sec) of Onset	Offset
Normorphine	1	11	22
Dihydromorphine	2	18	23
Morphine	3	23	32
Ketobemidone	4	45	109
Levorphanol	5	75	268
Etorphine	6	74	211
Methadone	7	91	619
Buprenorphine	8	623	very long

[1]From Ref. (6), except buprenorphine (P. H. McNally, personal communication).   [2]From Ref. (5).

The results obtained on the mouse vas deferens were similar to those shown in Table 1.   The rate of onset of the action of enkephalin is at least as fast as that of the most rapidly acting narcotic analgesic, normorphine. The rate of recovery from the action of enkephalin is considerably faster than that of normorphine (7), probably due to its rapid enzymatic degradation (Fig. 1).

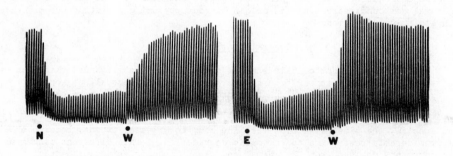

FIG. 1

Rates of onset and offset of action of normorphine (N)
and enkephalin (E) in the mouse vas deferens.
Frequency of stimulation: 0.4 Hz (F. M. Leslie).

There is no evidence of tachyphylaxis to repeated applications of enkephalin.   Thus, the kinetics of enkephalin action are consistent with its role as a putative neurotransmitter or neuromodulator.   It should be pointed out, however, that so far the only evidence for such a role is the specific pharmacological interaction with the opiate receptors of the mouse vas deferens (7) and the specific binding of factors from purified brain extracts to the opiate receptors in the brain (8,9).   Recently, it has been shown that pure enkephalin binds stereospecifically with the opiate receptors of guinea-pig brain

(Hughes, Kosterlitz and Smokcum, unpublished observations). No correlation between pharmacological action and receptor binding can be made at present, in view of the rapid enzymatic degradation in the brain homogenate.

Tests for antinociceptive and other typical effects of morphine-like drugs will have to await the synthesis of enkephalin.

It would be of great importance to be able to decide whether or not repeated administration of enkephalin would lead to tolerance and physical dependence. At present this problem cannot be investigated directly. Its rapid rates of onset and offset of action would appear to suggest that tolerance and dependence might not arise. An interesting observation is the fact that in order to antagonise a given agonist effect of enkephalin about 4 times more naloxone is required than for the agonist effect of normorphine or morphine. This is similar to the behaviour of some benzomorphans which are very potent <u>pure</u> agonists without physical dependence capacity in the morphine-dependent monkey (Table 2). In this context, it is of interest to note that enkephalin is so far the only peptide which is known to be antagonized by compounds other than peptide analogues.

TABLE 2

Dissociation Constants of Naloxone Measured against Agonists without or with Physical Dependence Capacity (PDC) in the Dependent Monkey.[1]

Agonist	Physical Dependence Capacity	Dissociation Constant of Naloxone (K_e; nM)	
		Guinea-Pig Ileum	Mouse Vas Deferens
Normorphine	high	1.89 ± 0.15 (12)	3.10 ± 0.25 (6)
Phenazocine	high	2.08 ± 0.39 (5)	4.05 ± 0.19 (3)
Ketocyclazocine	none	15.2 ± 3.1 (3)	–
Ethylketocyclazocine	none	14.9 ± 0.9 (4)	11.0 ± 0.6 (3)
Mr 1353	none	11.7 ± 1.0 (4)	–
Mr 2034	probably none	10.4 ± 1.8 (7)	9.1 ± 0.7 (3)
Enkephalin	?	–	13.4 ± 1.9 (5)

Ketocyclazocine is α-5,9-dimethyl-8-oxo-2-cyclopropylmethyl-2'-hydroxy-6,7-benzomorphan; in ethylketocyclazocine C_5 has an ethyl group (Sterling-Winthrop; Dr. S. Archer). Mr 1353 is α-5,9-dimethyl-2-(3-methylfurfuryl)-2'-hydroxy-6,7-benzomorphan and Mr 2034 is (-)-α-5,9-dimethyl-2-(L-tetrahydrofurfuryl)-2'-hydroxy-6,7-benzomorphan (C. H. Boehringer Sohn, Ingelheim; Dr. H. Merz). [1]The physical dependence data were obtained from Refs. 10-12; the other data are unpublished observations (J. Hughes, H. W. Kosterlitz, F. M. Leslie and A. A. Waterfield).

On present evidence, it is difficult to offer an interpretation for the observations shown in Table 2. It is known that all narcotic agonists with high physical dependence capacity so far investigated require lower concentrations of naloxone for antagonism than compounds with dual agonist and antagonist action and low physical dependence capacity (13). As far as interaction with the opiate receptor is concerned, the <u>pure</u> agonists shown in Table 2, namely the benzomorphans without physical dependence capacity and enkephalin, may have to be classified with the compounds of dual agonist and antagonist actions. The possibility of the existence of more than one type of opiate receptor will have to be considered.

Possible Mechanism of Tolerance and Dependence

The **presence** of a neuronal mechanism in which enkephalin, or another endogenous ligand, has a controlling influence, requires a reconsideration of our views on tolerance and dependence.

There are, in principle, three possibilities of control of an inhibitory mechanism by enkephalin (Fig. 2). The inhibition could be postsynaptic, presynaptic or could be due to a modulatory effect on the nerve terminal in which both enkephalin and the compound responsible for interneuronal transmission are present. In the first two circumstances two neurones would be involved **while** in the third circumstance enkephalin would be released from the nerve terminal on which it acts by inhibiting the release of the neurotransmitter.

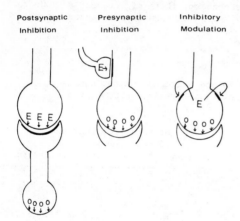

Postsynaptic Inhibition   Presynaptic Inhibition   Inhibitory Modulation

FIG. 2

Possible mechanisms for the action of enkephalin.

On present evidence, it is difficult to distinguish between the three possibilities since no decisive electrophysiological evidence is available as far as the central nervous system is concerned. In the peripheral nervous system, the action of opiates can occur in the absence of ganglion cells as, for instance, in the isolated nictitating membrane of the cat (4). In the myenteric plexus of the guinea-pig ileum, intracellular recording has shown that morphine does not alter the membrane potential of ganglion cells and does not affect intraneuronal transmission (R. A. North and G. Henderson, this volume). These observations make it unlikely that postsynaptic inhibition is the basis of the action of opiates although findings obtained in the peripheral nervous system may not necessarily hold for the central nervous system. The most likely options are therefore the two other models shown in Fig. 2, namely presynaptic inhibition or inhibitory modulation.

For an understanding of the phenomena of tolerance and **dependence** the interaction between endogenous enkephalin and exogenous opiates is of importance. Normally, enkephalin may be assumed to control certain inhibitory mechanisms determining the rate of transmitter release. If, however, opiates are administered with the intent of increasing the effects of these inhibitory mechanisms, e.g. for the purpose of analgesia, then control will pass from the endogenous enkephalin to the exogenous opiates. Since tachyphylaxis is an outstanding pharmacological characteristic of all opiates, a state of tolerance will arise in which increasing amounts of opiate will be required to maintain the inhibitory mechanisms at a level of activity sufficient to prevent signs of withdrawal. This situation may be made more severe by a possible negative feedback from the constantly stimulated opiate receptors, resulting in a decreased rate of enkephalin synthesis. Thus, the central nervous system will now be wholly dependent on the concentration of exogenously supplied opiates for the maintenance of essential inhibitory mechanisms.

When the opiates are withdrawn suddenly, these inhibitory mechanisms will become inactive, because any enkephalin which may be available will be unable to stimulate the opiate receptors until they have regained their sensitivity. It may be assumed that the loss of the inhibitory mechanisms normally controlled by enkephalin, will account for many, but not necessarily all, of the symptoms of the withdrawal syndrome. The duration of this syndrome will depend on the rate at which the opiate receptors regain their sensitivity and on the restoration of normal enkephalin synthesis if this had been suppressed by a feedback mechanism.

The acuteness of the withdrawal syndrome caused by the administration of naloxone or other antagonists to dependent animals could be readily explained by the proposed hypothesis. The block of the opiate receptors by the antagonists will also inactivate any action by enkephalin on these receptors and thus cause an even more severe inactivation of the inhibitory mechanisms than withdrawal of exogenous opiates.

On the other hand, it has to be postulated that administration of antagonists should produce signs of inactivation of the inhibitory mechanisms also in non-dependent animals although they would be expected to be less dramatic than in dependent animals. Observations which support this concept, are the increase in the nociceptive response of rats and mice to thermal stimuli (14) and the inhibition of the antinociceptive effect of electrical stimulation of the periaqueductal grey of the brain stem of rats (15). Recently, it has been shown that release of acetylcholine evoked by electrical stimulation of the myenteric plexus is enhanced by naloxone and by the (-)-isomer but not the (+)-isomer of the pure antagonist, β-5-phenyl-9-methyl-2-allyl-2'-hydroxy-6,7-benzomorphan (A. A. Waterfield and H. W. Kosterlitz, this volume). This finding is best explained by an inactivation of enkephalin which has been shown to be present in guinea-pig ileum in a concentration of about 0.8 μg-equivalents of normorphine/g tissue (J. Hughes and T. W. Smith, unpublished observations).

In conclusion, it would appear that enkephalin has physico-chemical and biochemical properties which differ in important aspects from the much more stable alkaloids of the opium poppy. The interaction of endogenous enkephalin and exogenous opiate is possibly the basis of the phenomena of tolerance and dependence observed after chronic administration of opiates.

Acknowledgements

Supported by grants from the U.S. National Institute on Drug Abuse (DA 00662) and the Medical Research Council.

References

1. W. D. M. PATON, Brit. J. Pharmacol. 12, 119-127 (1957)
2. A. L. COWIE, H. W. KOSTERLITZ and A. J. WATT, Nature, Lond. 220, 1040-1042 (1968)

3. J. HUGHES, H. W. KOSTERLITZ and F. M. LESLIE, <u>Brit. J. Pharmacol.</u> <u>53</u>, 371-381 (1975)

4. G. HENDERSON, J. HUGHES and H. W. KOSTERLITZ, <u>Brit. J. Pharmacol.</u> <u>53</u> 505-512 (1975)

5. H. W. KOSTERLITZ, F. M. LESLIE and A. A. WATERFIELD, <u>Eur. J. Pharmacol.</u> (1975) in press

6. A. HERZ and H.-J. TESCHEMACHER, <u>Adv. Drug Res.</u> <u>6</u>, 79-119 (1971)

7. J. HUGHES, <u>Brain Res.</u> <u>88</u>, 295-308 (1975)

8. L. TERENIUS and A. WAHLSTRÖM, <u>Acta pharmac. tox.</u> <u>35</u>, Suppl. 1, 55 (1974)

9. G. W. PASTERNAK and S. H. SNYDER, <u>Neurosciences Res. Prog. Bull.</u> <u>13</u>, 58 (1975)

10. N. B. EDDY and E. L. MAY, <u>Synthetic Analgesics</u>, <u>International Series of Monographs in Organic Chemistry</u>, <u>8</u>, 113-182.   Pergamon Press, London (1966)

11. J. E. VILLARREAL and M. H. SEEVERS, <u>Rep. Committee on Problems of Drug Dependence</u>, <u>34</u>, Addendum 7, 1040-1053 (1972)

12. H. H. SWAIN and M. H. SEEVERS, <u>Rep. Committee on Problems of Drug Dependence</u>, <u>36</u>, Addendum, 1168-1195 (1974)

13. H. W. KOSTERLITZ, J. A. H. LORD and A. J. WATT, <u>Agonist and Antagonist Actions of Narcotic Analgesic Drugs</u>, pp. 45-61.   Macmillan, London (1972)

14. J. J. JACOB, E. C. TREMBLAY and M.-C. COLOMBEL, <u>Psychopharmacologia</u> <u>37</u> 217-223 (1974)

15. H. AKIL, D. J. MAYER and J. C. LIEBESKIND, <u>C.r. hebd. Séanc. Acad. Sci., Paris</u> <u>274</u>, 3603-3605 (1972)

THE OPIATE NARCOTICS: NEUROCHEMICAL MECHANISMS IN ANALGESIA AND DEPENDENCE.
SUMMATION OF THE 1975 INTERNATIONAL NARCOTIC RESEARCH CLUB CONFERENCE.

Floyd E. Bloom

Division of Special Mental Health Research, National Institute of Mental
Health, St. Elizabeths Hospital, Washington, D. C. 20032

I appreciate the opportunity of participating in this highly active field
by offering my own interpretations of the sessions in terms of constructive
commentary. I was, quite frankly, amazed at the extent of progress that has
occured in this field in one year since the NRP Work Session on opiate receptor mechanisms (1) and I congratulate you on this achievement. Being heavily
invested in another area of neuropharmacology, namely, schizophrenia research,
I envy the more specific pharmacological agonists and antagonists with which
you are able to work, and the fact that you can produce experimentally the
disease syndrome in which you are interested.

My comments will be organized along lines different from the program, so
that may give us a little different slant on the situation. I propose to
discuss four sub-divisions of research items:

  (1) points on which we seem to be in agreement

  (2) points on which we clearly are not in agreement

  (3) important methological differences to be solved

  (4) and some points of interest for future research orientation.

Points of Agreement

Now among the points of consensus were certain scientific aphorisms presented here that seem to me to transcend the field of opiate research and in
a sense epitomize the progress of the meeting. For example, Kosterlitz's frequent admonition that "I absolutely insist on demonstrations of stereospecificity" is virtually an absolute requirement for this field with which everyone must agree. The other ones are a little bit more humorous. For example,
Takagi said two days ago, while referring to cyclic nucleotide components,
"I think this is a very complicated topic," and certainly everyone would agree
with that. Ian Creese and Avram Goldstein made analogous comments referring
to slightly different contexts which I have synthesized into one generalizable
aphorism, "Rigorous kinetic analysis requires rigorous attention to strict
equilibrium conditions," I think that's generally acceptable to everyone.
Avram's addendum specified that when unpurified membrane receptors or enzymes
are employed, use of the kinetic equations under these conditions may not
actually tell you anything about the true systems involved in the phenomena.

Yesterday, Lomax said with reference to the effects of opiates on
thermoregulatory systems, "measurement of the body temperature is probably the
worst way to assess the action of drugs on thermoregulatory systems." Candace
Pert said "the density of receptors (in a given brain region) need not indicate the significance of the function of those receptors." Coming from
Candace I think that takes on added significance. Finally I want to conclude
with Jose Musacchio's absolutely precious quotation, "It's not my fault."

Turning to the scientific level of agreed-upon topics, the one advance that is to me the most exciting is that there is not just one endogenous material that reacts chemically and pharmacologically like an opiate agonist but that there, in fact, may be several (see Hughes (2), Pasternak (3), Terenius (4), Teschemacher (5), and Cox (6) papers). While I agree with the attempts to compromise on nomenclature, I think it may be well to retain for the present the individual names while biological differences remain between the various factors.

Two general types of endogenous brain material have now been described. There is the small oligopeptide that John Hughes described, with a molecular weight of about 1000. He knows approximately the amino acid composition, not yet the sequence. With the possible exception of kinetic differences between the in vitro and the in vivo tests, the biological properties of the "enkephalin" isolated by Hughes and Kosterlitz seem to be similar to the "MLF" of Terenius and of Pasternak and Snyder. In terms of stereospecificity and naloxone reversibility enkephalin and the MLF's may well be similar biologically and yet distinguishable molecularly, or they might share some of the receptor site reactive groups. Therefore more research work ought to be done before we decide to give them one common name.

These "small factors" (the Hughes enkephalin factor and the MLF's) all exhibit heat and acid stability, and demonstrate very prominent sensitivity to exopeptidases. Quite importantly, Terenius could detect his MLF in the spinal fluid of patients with apparently pain provoking carcinomata or neuralgias. Now this may be a possible point of discrimination between neurotransmitters and neuromodulators (see Kosterlitz) (7), since for the most part neurotransmitter substances are very hard to demonstrate in the spinal fluid although neuromodulatory factors like prostaglandins or cyclic AMP may be demonstrable there. All three of the groups cautioned on the difficulty involved in detecting possibly produced changes in the natural endogenous factor (or factors) by the administration of exogenous opiates or in the tolerant state because the exogenous opiates bind so tightly to the receptor that the assay is affected. To make the kinds of interpretations Kosterlitz offered us this morning, this type of causal relationship between exogenous opiates and endogenous ligands must be probed fully.

Goldstein's group has characterized the second type of endogenous opioid material, which they found in porcine and bovine pituitary fractions as a Pituitary Opioid Peptide ("POP") (5,6). It also has stereochemical - pharmacological properties like a morphine agonist, and in several test systems acts longer and reverses less quickly on wash-out than the enkephalin/MLF's. The molecular weight of POP is about twice as high as enkephalin, and it is sensitive to endopeptidases rather than to exopeptidases. Simplistically, it would be better if POP were to be a precursor or some other form of the smaller endogenous factors, but it is hard for me to deduce why splitting POP in half would suddenly change its vulnerability to endopeptidases. Possibly the quarternary structures of the various peptides, when available, will explain these and other current mysteries. The POP of the Goldstein lab might even exist in several forms but there are really not sufficient data available at the moment to decide. It will be important for the people who work with POP to determine if it is present in the brain in the same form, and presumably the enkephalin-MLF groups have not yet looked for their ligands in the pituitary. If a conventional neuronal system is secreting this pituitary factor, it would presumably be the posterior pituitary, but this must be verified.

Returning to Kosterlitz's point of neurotransmitter or neuromodulator roles of the endogenous opioids (7), oxytocin and vasopressin can act as normal synaptic transmitters at their axon collaterals in the hypothalamus and yet these same substances also are secreted as endocrine hormones from the posterior pituitary. Thus a substance secreted from the brain could act both as a typical synaptic transmitter and as a hormone; epinephrine or norepinephrine can do this, depending upon where they are secreted. I think, all in all, the endogenous opioid factors represent a very exciting area for future brain research.

Since John Hughes mentioned that enkephalin occurs in the guinea pig ileum, it would be important to continue this line of approach and try to correlate the existence of enkephalin with other tissues where opiate receptors (as detected by binding or binding-displacement assays) are presumed to occur. Unless the enkephalin occurs in sympathetic ganglia, it is hard for me to envision what significance opiate receptors have on cultured neuroblastoma or glioma cells, which are derived from sympathetic ganglia, unless in those culture systems (see Hamprecht (8) and Klee (9) papers) some more silent cell types have induced or failed to repress the existence of that kind of opioid receptor.

The second major point that seemed to be generally agreed upon until this morning (when Goldstein expressed some doubts) was that development of opiate tolerance is not associated with any significant changes in the number of opiate ligand receptors or in the affinity of these receptors for opiates. Parenthetically, it should be noted that considerable research progress had to occur in order to develop the techniques by which the question of opiate receptor number and the affinity of such receptors for opioids could be measured. As noted by Snyder and Mathysse (1), this entire avenue of research arose conceptually from the 1971 observations of Goldstein and his colleagues (10), that stereospecific binding of opiates to subcellular components of mouse brain might be detected by radio-isotopic labelling experiments. Subsequent modifications of this approach (1,3,4,11-15) have indeed made possible a molecular appreciation of the opiate receptor which exceeds that of any other ligand-binding material in brain at this time.

I found the apparent lack of change in receptor number or property during tolerance to be striking; certainly, it defeated all the ideas I had about what tolerance was from reading the NRP conference report (1). Therefore it will be very important to consider experimentally Goldstein's rejoinder that present data may not absolutely eliminate the possibility that a more permanent binding of the exogenous opioid agonist to tolerant receptors only makes it appear as though the number of receptors has not increased. Until this point is settled our conceptual notions of the phenomenon of tolerance remain fluid.

It was widely agreed that the opiate receptor is on the external surface of the receptive cell; several good experiments pointing to that interpretation were just reviewed by Kosterlitz (7). I do think the use of Goldstein's photoaffinity label for this receptor (16) has other uses besides demonstrating that the receptor is on the external surface, especially such purposes as tracking and mapping of the receptor.

The only other possibly discordant feature in the external surface receptor idea were the autoradiographs which Candace Pert presented from her work with Mike Kuhar (14), indicating that locus coeruleus and substantia nigra pars compacta neurons were labeled over their cytoplasm. I understand the authors themselves are still pursuing the question as to what those grains mean. Opiate receptor activity over these cells will be crucial to define, because of the behavioral possibilities which arise from these circuits (see Agu Pert paper) (17).

The fourth thing that was generally agreed upon was that the number of receptors on a given cell type is roughly proportional to their pharmacological response, depending upon how you measure that pharmacological response. However, this confronts us with what I'll call the "Pert Paradox". Candace Pert was sitting next to me when Satoh presented the data from the Herz laboratory (18); they used microiontophoresis to characterize the opiate sensitivity of neurons in somatosensory cortex because the affinity-receptor data indicated to them that there were a lot of opiate receptors there. But Candace said "There aren't actually a lot of receptors in the somatosensory cortex." I looked up their tables last night (1); there are a lot of receptors in the frontal cortex according to Kuhar and Pert's dissection, but in the pre- and post- central gyri, the receptors are about as low in density as in the cerebellum, or possibly a unit or two higher. So the question arises, if you have a highly characterized, pharmacologically reproducible receptor that is stereospecific for the action of opiates, and reversed by naloxone, that is detectable on a very high proportion of the cells Satoh et al test, and yet by receptor binding studies there are only a "few receptors" there compared to other areas, how are we to interpret either the iontophoretic responses to opiates or the receptor binding densities?

I try to be a conservative iontophoresis "spritzer" in general, and I think in this case the answers are not in. We need a "spritzing" study of the same depth as that of Satoh et al (18), on an area that has a higher density of receptors. One such area that would be of interest to test is the amygdala, since Kuhar and Pert (1) found almost an order of magnitude higher opiate binding there than in cortex, and since amygdala contains both norepinephrine and dopamine synapses. Certainly by the present data of Satoh et al, there is a reproducible opiate receptor on cells in brain regions where finite but low numbers of receptors are known to exist, but whether one responsive cell yields physiologically significant responses with a low number of receptors or whether a large number of receptors per responsive cell is required seems to me still unclear. The present data would indicate that at worst, a very low number of receptors per cell could be adequate to evoke the response that has been demonstrated so specifically.

Points of Disagreement

There were many points of disagreement from which I selected a few that I thought could be resolvable experimentally before the 1976 INRC meeting. One close to resolution is the manner in which sulfhydryl reagents change either permanently (3) or transiently (13) the nature of the opiate receptor in either its agonist or antagonist forms, and the underlying question as to whether there is really one form of the opiate receptor, or multiple forms of the receptor, or multiple receptors. The groups are really doing quite similar experiments but performing them under different conditions, so that points of reproducibility cannot be easily visualized.

Another unclear point concerns the electrophysiological effects of morphine and other opiate agonists on neurons, a datum essential for resolving how we might expect the natural opioid factors to work (if they are secreted or naturally released). In Hamprecht's study (8), the neuroblastoma-fibroblast cells responded to norepinephrine, acetylcholine, and opiates by excitation, i.e., a depolarizing response. Yet Marshall Nirenberg reported in discussion that some neuroblastoma-glioma hybrids were excited by opiates while others were depressed; those that were excited showed increased membrane impedance during the excitation (see Klee paper) (9).

Bradley (19) reported that a mixed population of cells in the cat brain stem exhibited mixed excitatory and inhibitory responses, but that only the inhibitions (as was also reported by Herz's group, for the rat cortex) (18) were naloxone reversible and stereospecific responses.

It is hard for me to reconcile these inhibitions with the adenylate cyclase effects of opiates that have been proposed (see Collier) (20). If opiates caused their effects by inhibiting adenylate cyclase I would have anticipated that the effective functional response would have been excitation, based on what I know about the generally depressant actions of cyclic nucleotides in other test systems.

Now let me move back a step and say that the number of cells that have been properly tested with cyclic nucleotides is quite small; furthermore we know that the cells that Collier (20) and Hamprecht (8) are dealing with are a relatively infrequent sort that demonstrate a very striking activation to adenylate cyclase by prostaglandins of the E family. It may be that none of the nerve cells that have been properly tested so far with cyclic nucleotides are of this prostaglandin-sensitive class; in most test cases in the central nervous system, prostaglandins ordinarily do the opposite of cAMP. Possibly, under the conditions of most iontophoresis experiments, namely, in anesthetised animals, the cells which remain spontaneously active happen not to be the ones in which the biochemical results of Collier are observed in vitro. A combination of autoradiographic and iontophoretic approaches is needed to correlate these actions but I suppose that more than a year will be required to make that work.

Considerable separation also seems to exist between the data involving the cyclic nucleotide components and the effects of opiates, tolerance, or withdrawal on various transmitter substances. We heard often in the past sessions about a transmitter substance not being affected in its levels but being affected in its turnover, only to find that another speaker would find different changes in turnover, depending on how his tolerance state was evoked or how the withdrawal from the opiate was induced.

Those interested in labile substances must now heed very closely Costa's and Hosoya's admonitions that standard methods of sacrificing the brain and extracting transmitters or cyclic nucleotides are really inadequate to measure the levels as they were immediately before the animal was killed. Under such conditions of known lability, it makes little sense to try to measure subcellular fractions for their cyclic nucleotide content.

I was particularly impressed by Hamprecht's (8) demonstration that possibly the first change to occur in the neuroblastoma-fibroblast cell, was the activation of cGMP accumulation. If one takes the cGMP accumulation as a possible primary effect of the opiate receptor, then this event could also account for the reported impairment of cAMP accumulation when challenged with opiates and prostaglandins; one of the simplest ways that could occur is through a cGMP-activated cAMP phosphodiesterase. Having activated cAMP phosphodiesterase, it would be much harder for a given agonist to elevate the cAMP level. The cAMP system is extremely complicated and almost daily we have new ways of understanding the regulation of adenylate cyclase and probably guanylate cyclase. The most recent advance seems to be that the Brostrom concept of regulatory and catalytic sub-units of protein kinase (21) also applies to the phosphodiesterase and to the cyclases themselves. A general class of proteins, which depend upon calcium for their activity, appear to be able to activate adenylate cyclase phosphodiesterase, guanylate cyclase and protein kinases of various types. In trying to assess these systems in brain homogenates in vitro only slight variations in ionic content would be capable of causing totally opposing results.

For example, in the cerebral cortex and in sympathetic ganglia much evidence indicates that muscarinic cholinergic receptors (which in general are excitatory) oppose, both functionally and biochemically, the actions of inhibitory adrenergic receptors. Both of these functions may be accounted for by inactivation of resting conductances of ions as a mechanism by which the biophysical properties are generated. Thus the "Sodium-Free" preferred state proposed by Snyder for the agonist form of the opiate receptor (1) could reflect on either cyclic nucleotide synaptic function.

Just as iontophoretic studies of opiates could be done more profitably in a brain area where there is a higher density of opiate receptors, it may also be that in biochemical studies on transmitters, we have not yet attacked the most pertinent areas of the brain. There was a lot of emphasis on nucleus accumbens septi and striatum but they are not really the highest ones in the Pert-Kuhar or Simon rank ordering of binding affinities. Furthermore, we have a lot of reconciling to do between the in vivo data from micro-injections of opiates and opiate antagonists which induce or prevent the induction of withdrawal (22) and the in vitro physical binding assay of brain opiate receptor distributions. At present, we can only recognize certain bio-behavioral actions of the opiates in experimental animals, but it is unclear whether the whole population of opiate receptors acts equally to produce this range of behavioral effects or whether each effect arises in a particular set or subset of receptors. Perhaps anatomical maps of in vivo effects have to be overlaid on the in vitro receptor assays in order to get at areas of special physiological significance.

To summarize my impression of the available biochemical studies of opiates on transmitters and transmitter turnover, consider the following analogy. If we place on a pond several model boats, each representing one of the transmitters, and then throw into the pond at various times rocks representing the convulsions produced by morphine administration or withdrawal, all those little boats will naturally jiggle. They will jiggle to a degree depending on how close they are to where the rock hit the water, but none of them can really be said to have evoked the response of the pond. They do reflect the response of the pond, but only epiphenomenologically.

Methodological Points

It goes without saying that every drug assessment or drug competition reaction in which an opiate is to be evaluated has to be verified for the specificity of its action by determining if it is stereospecific and whether it is susceptible to opiate antagonists. While I know that everyone here appreciates that point, in the abstract, it still seemed not to be practiced universally. More recently stated are the precautions which the Snyder group offered concerning the characterization of a new opiate as an agonist or antagonist based on the effects of added or subtracted sodium. Since this test seems now to be more widely applied than it was a year ago, it would seem important to do it in the way Pasternak, Pert, Creese et al do it (15), namely, to use sodium at 5mM but no higher; concentrations higher than 5mM cause a nonspecific effect. The opposite effect, perhaps even more important functionally, is the effect of Mn, which in 1 mM concentrations increases the potency of agonists. Presumably by next year's conference a lot of people will be doing these ionic manipulations. Before you go off on your own to do them, it would be important, I think, to characterize the compounds by the procedure first described.

When Gero (23) was describing the binding of agonists and antagonists to purified serum cholinesterase he made a provocative point: since an agonist occupies the receptor and causes a conformational shift which will require some molecular energy, the distortion produced by the agonist might be expected to decrease the affinity of the receptor for the agonist more than for the antagonist, which he in fact finds. I am not sure what to do with that hypothesis but it strikes me as a testable lead.

In considering adenylate cyclase involvement with opiate receptors, several speakers have assumed that phosphodiesterase inhibitors are equivalent and monolithic in action. That is not exactly so. There are phosphodiesterase inhibitors that work more on one isozyme than another; there are phosphodiesterase inhibitors that seem to be selective for cAMP and for cGMP, as characterized by the affinity of the substrate, by subcellular location, by reaction to calcium or to other protein activators. The isozymes in different parts of the brain may vary and react differently to pharmacological agents. Theophylline is a very good phosphodiesterase inhibitor, but when you give an animal a large dose of parenteral theophylline many respiratory and cardiovascular changes occur. In the caudate nucleus, which has been a target that many people here have studied, theophylline is relatively poor as a phosphodiesterase inhibitor; the potentiation of the inhibitory response to dopamine or to cAMP requires isobutylmethylxanthine or papaverine (24).

Finally, I think a major need exists in your field to agree on standard methods of tolerance development (i.e., rapid and/or slow), and extent or level of tolerance in a given species of animal, so that when people talk about tolerance or non-tolerance they are talking about similar phenomena, obtained with similar dose levels. Arbitrary dose selections seem only to lead to confusion。

Future Points

I was very hesitant to list what I thought were points of future orientation because I have not been active in this field, and to suddenly leap in and say "That's what you ought to do" sounds like a cheap shot. However, since Kosterlitz (7) mentioned most of my ideas this morning I am just going to reemphasize a few. I think that the most burning question is really the nature of the opioid substance(s) that occurs in the brain and how its actions may relate to those of opiates applied from the outside. Trying to determine which of the actions that we see with morphine is like or unlike the functional response of the proper target cell to the natural substance is crucial but may not be totally predictable by looking at the mouse vas deferens or the guinea pig ileum. For example, if we look only at the peripheral nervous system, an excitatory effect of norepinephrine is seen on the mouse vas deferens, but no excitatory central noradrenergic transmission site is known. While the peripheral systems are very good for initially characterizing the pharmacology, they are not necessarily the end of the road in characterizing the nature of the receptor or the pharmacology of the central nervous system.

Other naturally occuring peptides also occur in intestinal smooth muscle. Substance P, which Candace Pert mentioned this morning, is probably the most relevant here since it also occurs in high concentration in the hypothalamus, the substantia gelatinosa, and dorsal root ganglion cells. Some people are moderately convinced (25) that Substance P could be an excitatory transmitter between dorsal root ganglion cells and spinal neurons. However, there is no obvious similarity in amino acid composition between excitatory Substance P and enkephalin. Nevertheless, it will be interesting to compare the aqueous conformations of these two peptides. There is another intestinal peptide called proctalin (26), which excites insect smooth muscle; it is a somewhat smaller peptide than enkephalin. Intestinal smooth muscle (if not other smooth muscle sources) may contain a large number of such active peptides in addition to enkephalin; while enkephalin is a beautiful name, it might become a more general term for a lot of peptides yet to be discovered in the central nervous system.

Lastly I want to recall the comments that Agu Pert (15) made yesterday in trying to devise experimental methods for analyzing the euphorigenic component of the actions of opiates by using the intracranial self-stimulation approach. It was striking to me that we were shown opiate receptor activity in the substantia nigra and in the locus coeruleus neurons because these are the two main ascending monoamine systems that seem to underlie most of intracranial self-stimulation. In my own selfish interest, it would be quite convenient to study some of your interesting compounds in a system that we are beginning to know how to handle with microelectrodes.

I think that the euphorigenic or reinforcing actions of opiates are a very
difficult problem to study. Perhaps your Club can enlist more people
interested in bridging this gap between cellular and behavioral observations.
It will be important, in interpreting iontophoretic responses, to compare
the responses of specific populations of neurons in awake animals to parenteral doses of opiates with effects these same cells show under anesthesia
to opiates given iontophoretically. One could assume at the beginning that
they would be similar, but not necessarily.

Now to prevent any further abuse of opiates by a bonafide member of your
observer corps, I shall stop here and hope that what I said may have been
precipitating, but not withdrawal inducing.

REFERENCES

1. S. H. SNYDER and S. MATTHYSSE, Neurosci. Res. Program Bull. 13, 1-166
    (1975).

2. J. HUGHES, T. SMITH, B. MORGAN and L. FOTHERGILL, The Opiate Narcotics:
    Neurochemical Mechanisms in Analgesia and Dependence, This book, pp. 1-
    6.

3. G. W. PASTERNAK, R. GOODMAN and S. H. SNYDER, The Opiate Narcotics:
    Neurochemical Mechanisms in Analgesia and Dependence, This book, pp. 13-
    17.

4. L. TERENIUS and A. WAHLSTROM, The Opiate Narcotics: Neurochemical
    Mechanisms in Analgesia and Dependence, This book, pp. 7-12.

5. H. TESCHEMACHER, K. E. OPHEIM, B. M. COX and A. GOLDSTEIN, The Opiate
    Narcotics: Neurochemical Mechanisms in Analgesia and Dependence, This
    book, pp. 19-23.

6. B. M. COX, K. E. OPHEIM, H. TESCHEMACHER and A. GOLDSTEIN, The Opiate
    Narcotics: Neurochemical Mechanisms in Analgesia and Dependence, This
    book, pp. 25-30.

7. H. W. KOSTERLITZ and J. HUGHES, The Opiate Narcotics: Neurochemical
    Mechanisms in Analgesia and Dependence, This book, pp. 245-250.

8. J. TRABER, R. GULLIS and B. HAMPRECHT, The Opiate Narcotics: Neuro-
    chemical Mechanisms in Analgesia and Dependence, This book, pp. 111-116.

9. W. A. KLEE, S. K. SHARMA and M. NIRENBERG, The Opiate Narcotics:
    Neurochemical Mechanisms in Analgesia and Dependence, This book, pp. 117-
    122.

10. A. GOLDSTEIN, L. I. LOWNEY and B. K. PAL, Proc. Nat. Acad. Sci. U.S.A.
    68, 1742-1747 (1971).

11. C. B. PERT, G. W. PASTERNAK and S. H. SNYDER, Science 182, 1359-1361
    (1973).

12. E. J. SIMON, J. M. HILLER and I. EDELMAN, Proc. Nat. Acad. Sci. U.S.A.
    70, 1947-1949 (1973).

13. E. J. SIMON, J. M. HILLER, I. EDELMAN, J. GROTH and K. D. STAHL, The
    Opiate Narcotics: Neurochemical Mechanisms in Analgesia and Dependence,
    This book, pp. 43-48.

14. C. B. PERT, M. J. KUHAR and S. H. SNYDER, The Opiate Narcotics: Neurochemical Mechanisms in Analgesia and Dependence, This book, pp. 97–101.

15. I. CREESE, G. W. PASTERNAK, C. B. PERT and S. H. SNYDER, The Opiate Narcotics: Neurochemical Mechanisms in Analgesia and Dependence, This book, pp. 85–90.

16. R. SCHULZ and A. GOLDSTEIN, The Opiate Narcotics: Neurochemical Mechanisms in Analgesia and Dependence, This book, pp. 91–96.

17. A. PERT and R. HULSEBUS, The Opiate Narcotics: Neurochemical Mechanisms in Analgesia and Dependence, This book, pp. 173–174.

18. M. SATOH, W. ZIEGLGANSBERGER and A. HERZ, The Opiate Narcotics: Neurochemical Mechanisms in Analgesia and Dependence, This book, pp. 229–234.

19. P. B. BRADLEY, Brit. J. Pharmacol., in press (1975).

20. H. O. J. COLLIER, D. L. FRANCIS, W. J. MCDONALD-GIBSON, A. C. ROY and S. A. SAEED, The Opiate Narcotics: Neurochemical Mechanisms in Analgesia and Dependence, This book, pp. 239–244.

21. M. A. BROSTROM, E. M. REIMANN, D. A. WALSH and E. G. KREBS, Adv. Enz. Regulation 8, 191–203 (1970).

22. E. WEI, The Opiate Narcotics: Neurochemical Mechanisms in Analgesia and Dependence, This book, pp. 171–172.

23. A. GERO and R. J. CAPETOLA, The Opiate Narcotics: Neurochemical Mechanisms in Analgesia and Dependence, This book, pp. 69–70.

24. G. R. SIGGINS, B. J. HOFFER and U. UNGERSTEDT, Life Sci. 15, 779–792 (1974).

25. S. E. LEEMAN and E. A. MROZ, Life Sci. 15, 2033–2044 (1974).

26. B. E. BROWN, Science 155, 595–597 (1967).